THE

COMPLETE

Home Health Advisor

INSTANT ACCESS TO:
LEADING CURES, RELIABLE REMEDIES, SELF-HELP STRATEGIES,
AND LIFE-SAVING FACTS

DEBORAH MITCHELL

Prentice
Hall Press

Library of Congress Cataloging-in-Publication Data

Mitchell, Deborah R.
    The complete home health advisor : instant access to leading cures, reliable remedies, self-help strategies, and life-saving facts / by Deborah Mitchell.
      p. cm.
    "A Lynn Sonberg book."
    Includes bibliographical references.
    ISBN 0-13-060564-5 — ISBN 0-7352-0288-5 (pbk.)
    1. Medicine, Popular. 2. Health. 3. Self-care, Health. I. Title.

RC81 .M584 2001
616.02'4—dc21   2001036467

Acquisitions Editor: *Edward Claflin*
Production Editor: *Mariann Hutlak*
Page Design/Layout: *Robyn Beckerman*

The information presented in this book is designed to help you make informed decisions about your health. It is not intended as a substitute for medical care or a manual for self-treatment. If you believe you have a medical problem, seek professional medical advice promptly.

Many of the drugs and products mentioned in this book are protected by registered trademarks. A reasonable effort has been made to capitalize the names of those drugs and products.

Also published as *The Home Healing Almanac.*

Printed in the United States of America

10 9 8 7 6 5 4 3 2 1

ISBN 0-7352-0288-5

ATTENTION: CORPORATIONS AND SCHOOLS

Prentice Hall Press books are available at quantity discounts with bulk purchase for educational, business, or sales promotional use. For information, please write to: Prentice Hall Special Sales, 240 Frisch Court, Paramus, New Jersey 07652. Please supply: title of book, ISBN, quantity, how the book will be used, date needed.

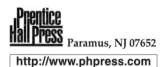 Paramus, NJ 07652

http://www.phpress.com

Contents

PART I
Help Yourself

PART II
People to See, Things to Do

PART III
Where to Go for Good Health

PART IV
Crucial Facts
about the Human Body

PART V

Health Statistics and Trivia
You Might Need to Know

PART VI
Alternative Views of Healing

PART VII
Reliable Sources

Foreword

Americans have a passion for information, especially when it concerns their health. As a physician, I certainly share that passion. My desire to find the best ways to help my patients has, over the years, driven me to learn as much as I can about various healing practices, from conventional medicine, in which I was originally trained, to alternative and complementary medicine; from the use of drugs to the use of acupuncture, herbs, and prayer.

I have found value in all forms of healing, and I have tried to pass along the elements that my patients can use at home. My patients are eager "students," because along with the desire for information, more and more people want to learn ways in which they can take charge of their health. Accumulating information is not enough; they want to:

1. prevent illness, injuries, and disease for themselves and their families;
2. take a more active role in working with health practitioners; and
3. gather the tools they need so they can do both 1 and 2 effectively.

To this end, I have found that taking a holistic view of patients and their lives and complaints is more effective than using the patch 'em up and pill 'em up approach. A Harvard University study found that the use of alternative medicine rose from 33.8 percent in 1990 to 42.1 percent in 1997, and that Americans' visits to alternative medicine practitioners increased from 36.3 percent to 46.3 percent during the same period. In fact, visits to alternative medicine providers now exceed those to primary care doctors. At the same time, our hunger for health information has caused more than 50 million of us to log on to the Internet each year in search of answers to our health care questions.

This movement toward more self-care and alternative and complementary care demonstrates a fundamental belief that each of us has the means to make dramatic lifesaving and life-enhancing changes. This is exciting news, but it isn't new news. Prevention has always been preferable to treatment, which can be painful, time-consuming, disruptive of the patient's lifestyle, and expensive.

What does any of that have to do with this book? As a physician, I am privileged to be able to help my patients become better-educated health consumers and to take steps toward more self-care. I believe *The Complete Home Health Advisor* is an excellent tool to aid in that process. This book offers a broad range of useful health information in portions you can easily digest and apply, from authoritative sources, and all in one handy volume.

In Part I, for example, the 24 chapters present hundreds of ways to "Help Yourself" and your family—from head to toe, from the inside out. You'll learn which over-the-counter medications are most popular, how to prepare a well-stocked first aid kit for your home, how to travel the world disease-free, and how to reduce your risk of disease.

In Part II, you'll learn which "People to See, Things to Do" when it comes to medical tests, procedures, and surgeries; the specialists who deal with them (and providers who don't); and the most common conventional drugs and homeopathic remedies.

Sometimes we need to know "Where to Go for Good Health," and Part III helps with that search. Whether you're in the market for an alternative practitioner, a dentist, an integrative medicine clinic, or a hospital for a special procedure, you'll find plenty of useful guidelines here. If you're looking for healing with a special touch, you'll find the "Healing Sites" presented in Chapter 33 of particular interest. And if you're evaluating the safety and health of your work or living environment, you can read about the healthiest and safest places to live in the United States, and which jobs are considered most dangerous.

Part IV, "Crucial Facts about the Human Body," is like a mini owner's manual that can help us understand our bodies and how to care for them better. The information here ranges from a body inventory to a look at common ailments that can affect us throughout our lifetimes. You will learn about some of the ways we are not kind to ourselves, including a revealing list of high-fat, high-calorie fast foods (yes, I know they taste good); harmful and safe noise levels; cancer-causing substances; and more. In Part V, "Health Statistics and Trivia You Might Need to Know," you'll learn things like just how deadly deer can be (yes, deer); how much of our tax money is spent on disease research; which plants to avoid if you have children around the house; and who some of the longest-living people in history were . . . and are.

Part VI is an eclectic look at four "Alternative Views of Healing": chakras, prayer, reflexology, and acupuncture. All four approaches allow us to explore the mysteries of healing in unique ways, and they play an interesting role in our health care system.

Part VII provides "Reliable Sources" for information, products, and services discussed throughout the book.

Here at your fingertips are thousands of ways you can improve your physical, mental, emotional, and spiritual health, well-being, and safety; protect yourself and your family; and satisfy your curiosity about various health-related topics. Just turn to any of the parts to find the topics that interest you, find the information you want, then take action or go about your life. The tone is light, even when the message is heavy, and the information is current, based on when it was gathered before publication. I hope you enjoy this book and benefit from it in good health.

Kenneth B. Singleton, M.D.

17 Youth-Preserving Tips from Top Health Authorities

We are all getting older; there's no changing that. But we can age gracefully and retain much, if not all, of the physical vigor, mental capacity, sexual energy, and spiritual fulfillment we feel right now. To do that, we need to be honest with ourselves. That means we need to stop looking for the Fountain of Youth and instead refocus on the Fountain of Health. It's not a fountain we can go up to once to get a magic potion; it's one we must drink from every day. If we want to live longer, be healthy, and look good, we need to treat our bodies with respect each moment. We have to make Life and Health our priorities.

What better way to start this book than to look at some ways to keep yourself young. Here's how.

1 *Keep your memory alive.* Age-related memory loss is not inevitable. It is caused by damage to brain cells, and there are ways to stop or even reverse such damage, says Dr. Steven J. Bock, M.D., codirector of the Center for Progressive Medicine in Rhinebeck, New York. To keep those brain cells vital, he recommends the following daily nutritional regimen:

- Vitamin A: 10,000 International Units (IU)
- Beta-carotene: 9 mg or more
- B vitamins: 50 to 100 mg
- Vitamin C: 1,000 mg

- Vitamin E: 200 to 400 IU
- Copper: 2 mg
- Manganese: 2 to 3 mg
- Chromium: 200 micrograms
- Selenium: 200 micrograms
- Zinc: 20 mg
- Essential fatty acids: 2 tablespoons flaxseed oil

2 *Recognize male menopause and do something about it.* Around the magic age of 50, men as well as women typically go through menopause. Although female menopause is well known, male menopause is less recognized—but it is just as real, say many experts. One of them, Eugene Shippen, M.D., a physician in Shillington, Pennsylvania, says that it's about this time that testosterone levels begin to decline in men. This reduction in one of the male sex hormones affects more than sex drive—it also has an impact on the heart, bones, nervous system, and brain. Symptoms of low testosterone include a less-sharp mind, reduced energy level, a few extra pounds around the midsection, sore muscles, a flagging sex drive, and less ambition. Although testosterone replacement therapy is an option, there are natural ways to stop or reverse the drop in the hormone level. Here are a few of them:

- **Exercise.** Overweight men have testosterone levels that are lower than normal. Fat manufactures more estrogen and less testosterone. When you burn fat and build muscle, estrogen levels drop and testosterone levels rise. Dr. Shippen recommends a brisk 20-minute walk at least three times a week.

- **Zinc.** Supplementation can help restore a healthy testosterone-to-estrogen ratio. Dr. Shippen recommends 50 mg twice daily until symptoms improve; then reduce to 30 to 50 mg daily.

- **Vitamin C.** Low body levels of this vitamin may be associated with low testosterone levels. Dr. Shippen suggests taking 1,000 to 3,000 mg of vitamin C daily for one to two months. If you don't experience any benefit, reduce the dosage to 1,000 mg daily.

- **High-potency multivitamin and mineral supplements.** Find one that provides the Daily Value of the vitamins it contains. The antioxidants beta-carotene and vitamin E are especially helpful in destroying the free radicals that contribute to age-related diseases.

- **Broccoli et al.** The cruciferous vegetables (for example, broccoli, brussels sprouts, cabbage, cauliflower, kale, bok choy, daikon) contain indoles, which are compounds that break down estrogen. Dr. Shippen suggests eating four servings of these vegetables per week.

- **Soy.** Forget the tofu if you want to, but you want the isoflavones found in soybeans to help you excrete excess estrogen. One cup of soy milk per day is recommended; it comes in chocolate for those who dread the thought of drinking it "straight," although several manufacturers make an excellent-tasting beverage.

3 *Keep your eyes healthy.* Cataracts are often associated with aging, but some experts believe that 90 percent of people who are in the early stages of cataract development can reverse the problem with natural remedies. Optometrist Marc Grossman, codirector of the Integral Health Centers in Rye and New Paltz, New York, says that correcting nutritional deficiencies can prevent or stop the progression of cataracts because most cataracts are caused by oxidation—destruction by free radical molecules. Taking antioxidants can halt or reverse the oxidation process.

- **Multivitamin and mineral supplements.** Dr. Grossman recommends a high-potency multivitamin and mineral supplement that contains at least 50 mg of most of the B vitamins, 15 mg of beta-carotene, 30 mg of zinc, and 200 micrograms of selenium.

- **Vitamin C.** Except for the adrenal glands, the lens of the eye contains more vitamin C than any other site in the body. A daily dosage of 1,500 mg is recommended to help prevent and heal cataracts.

- **MSM.** Methylsulfonylmethane is organic sulfur, an important component of good vision. One-half teaspoon of MSM powder per 100 pounds of body weight once daily is the recommended dosage.

- **Glutathione, ALA, and NAC.** The antioxidant glutathione is usually in low supply in people with cataracts, but the body also needs two other nutrients to make glutathione effective. Dr. Grossman recommends taking 500 mg of NAC (n-acetylcysteine) and 100 mg of ALA (alpha-lipoic acid) along with 50 mg of glutathione daily.

4 *Think good thoughts.* How can this prevent aging? According to Gary Null, Ph.D., author of *Gary Null's Ultimate Anti-Aging Program*, whenever you are experiencing aggression, fear, anger, or anxiety, "your body is in death mode." Our thoughts have a major impact on biochemistry and the immune system. Continuous negative thoughts raise the adrenal gland's production of the hormones cortisol and catecholamines, which speed up the aging of our organs. The equation is: Negative emotions = Negative hormones = Negative body impact.

The solution? Behavior modification. Begin by being aware of your stressors. Look at the reasons why you're angry or fearful. Examine your belief systems, your relationships, and your emotions. Identify your strengths and weaknesses and evaluate how they affect your life.

5 *Hang onto your hairline.*   Hair loss is one of the most upsetting parts of aging for many men and women. Although hair loss in women is a more complicated condition that usually requires professional attention, most men with this problem are experiencing genetic male-pattern baldness. For two out of three men, the solution may be to take the drug finasteride (Propecia), which is also prescribed for prostate conditions. As with all drugs, this one causes side effects, including rash, pelvic pain, dizziness, gas, headache, diarrhea, and vision changes. Consumer advocate Spencer David Kobren has conducted much research on hair products for men and, with the endorsement of physicians, suggests some natural alternatives to finasteride:

- **Black currant oil.** Taking one 500-mg capsule of this oil twice daily can improve the density and texture of hair within two months, says Kobren. This oil is rich in gamma-linolenic acid, which promotes healthy hair.

- **Nettle and pygeum.** These two herbs work together to block an enzyme called 5-alpha-reductase, which converts testosterone to DHT (dihydrotestosterone), which in turn kills hair follicles. A dosage of 50 to 100 mg nettle and 60 to 500 mg pygeum is suggested.

- **Saw palmetto.** This herb also inhibits the production of 5-alpha-reductase. Research indicates that taking 160 mg (in a product that has 85 to 95 percent fatty acids and sterols) twice daily can be effective.

- **Zinc.** This is another 5-alpha-reductase inhibitor. Taking a daily dose of 60 mg for six months can help stop hair loss.

6 *Stay heart healthy.*   Approximately 1,400 Americans die each day of a largely preventable condition—heart disease. The majority of people with heart disease have eaten, sat, and stressed their way to the problem. According to Julian Whitaker, M.D., founder and director of the Whitaker Wellness Center in Newport Beach, California, "If you have heart disease, it's possible to reverse its progress and bring your arteries to healthier condition," without the use of drugs and surgery. Dr. Whitaker finds that many people can be helped by changing their diets, taking the right supplements, learning how to manage their stress, and exercising regularly. If you already have heart disease, all of these approaches should be followed under the supervision of a qualified health care provider.

If you want to help prevent heart disease, these recommendations will get you on the road. Along with eating a healthful diet—whole, unprocessed foods such as fresh fruits and vegetables, whole grains, beans, legumes, cereals, and nuts; little or no animal protein; 3 to 6 ounces of fish several times a week; and few or no dairy products—taking the following supplements can help boost your heart health:

- **Apple cider vinegar.** There is some evidence that apple cider vinegar helps dissolve arterial plaque, says Patrick Quillin, R.D., Ph.D., director of the Rational Healing Institute in Tulsa, Oklahoma. Try adding it to your salads.

- **Coenzyme Q10.** This vitamin-like substance stimulates more energy for your cells, which in turn helps the heart pump better. This supplement is often prescribed after a heart attack, but why wait for that to happen? Cardiologist Stephen T. Sinatra, M.D., director of the New England Heart Center in Manchester, Connecticut, recommends taking 90 to 180 mg in three divided doses.

- **Magnesium.** Michael Janson, M.D., author of *The Vitamin Revolution* and *Dr. Janson's New Vitamin Revolution* recommends 500 to 1,000 mg magnesium daily in two divided doses. This mineral helps reverse heart disease.

- **Vitamin E.** Free-radical damage to the arteries can be stopped by taking vitamin E, says Dr. Janson. He recommends 400 to 800 IU daily to protect the arteries.

7 *Laugh yourself young.* Humor is a powerful stress reducer, according to the National Association for Therapeutic Humor. And it's definitely a laughing matter. Norman Cousins, author of *Anatomy of an Illness*, brought attention to the power of humor when he cured himself of a degenerative disease by surrounding himself with humor. How is that possible? When you laugh, your body "smiles" by producing more immune cells and relaxing tense muscles.

Have you ever seen people laugh so hard they fell off a chair? That's because their muscles relaxed so much they temporarily became a bag of bones.

To reduce stress, produce more immune cells, and maybe add some years to your life, make humor a part of each day. Here are a few suggestions:

- Watch some old-time cartoons. Remember Tweety Bird, Bullwinkle, and Tom and Jerry? You're never too old for a good chuckle at some of the antics of these cartoon characters. Maybe you prefer reruns of *The Honeymooners* or *I Love Lucy*. See them on cable, or rent a video. (You can tell the store clerk the cartoons are for your kids or grandkids.)

- Watch movies or comedians you find funny, and collect books on humor or funny stories. You can get these at the library; you don't need to purchase them.

- Be silly. Parents and grandparents usually find it easy to be silly with an infant or small child, often by making faces and funny sounds. You can also be silly with a pet, or just make faces at yourself in the mirror. If these ideas sound silly—well, that's the idea. Don't take yourself so seriously all the time.

- Make it a habit to look for humor. Funny things happen all the time, but we're often too busy to notice. Watch a kitten play, look for faces in the clouds, see if dogs and their owners look alike. There's laughter to be found everywhere.

8 *Say "no" to human growth hormones.*   You've probably seen the ads and books about human growth hormones and how they are virtually a Fountain of Youth. Not so, says Dean Edell, M.D., author of *Eat, Drink & Be Merry* and an Internet columnist. What human growth hormone injections do is cause sore, aching muscles that can grow tumors, says Edell. Their use should be reserved for what the Food and Drug Administration has approvedthem for: to help growth-deficient children and people with kidney disease.

9 *Get your youthful sleep.*   Lack of sufficient sleep—which most experts say is seven to eight hours a night—appears to impair the body's immune system, at least temporarily. If insufficient sleep is chronic, then you are at greater risk of developing illnesses. Christian J. Gillin, M.D., professor of psychiatry at the University of California, San Diego, has conducted sleep deprivation studies. He says that "if you get the optimal amount of quality sleep . . . you tend to live longer."

Unfortunately, about 70 million Americans have some sort of sleep problem. If you need stimulants—coffee, colas, pills—to get going in the morning or during the day; if you fight sleepiness during the day; if you fall asleep while reading or watching television; if you are so tired that you fall asleep as soon as you get into bed, you are sleep-deprived. Some people have a different problem: They are tired but so stressed out that they toss and turn and don't get quality sleep. To get more youthful sleep, here are a few tips:

- **Establish a schedule.** Go to bed and get up at the same time every day (or as close to that as possible). Don't sleep in on weekends. If you need to take a nap during the day, take a short one (30 minutes).

- **Get out of the race.** If you have trouble falling asleep because your mind is racing, use self-hypnosis or deep breathing exercises to relax.

- **Wind down.** Spend the hour before you go to bed doing something relaxing. Read a book, take a warm bath, or do light stretching.

- **Maintain your schedule.** If you work at night and must sleep during the day, keep that schedule even on your days off. Flip-flopping back and forth makes it more difficult to get quality sleep.

- **Keep it dark.** If you work a night shift, darken your bedroom as much as possible when it's time for sleep. You want to create a nighttime-like environment, says Steven Weber, Ph.D., director of the Sleep Disorder Center at the University of Wisconsin Hospital and Clinics in Madison. That's because the body responds to a day–night cycle, not to your work cycle. By creating a nighttime environment, you trick your body into thinking it is night.

10 *Care for your prostate.*   Problems with the prostate gland strike many men after age 40: a weak urinary flow, trouble with dribbling, frequent nighttime urinating, and difficulty urinating. These are the symptoms of benign prostatic hyperplasia. It can be treated with the drug finasteride (Proscar) as well as with several potent herbs, including saw palmetto, nettle, and pygeum. In some men, however, a deficiency of zinc and fatty acids may be the cause of the disease, says Julian Whitaker, M.D., director of the Tahoma Clinic in Kent, Washington.

- To help prevent benign prostatic hyperplasia, men would do well to take 30 mg zinc along with 2 mg copper daily, as well as one tablespoon flaxseed oil twice daily along with 400 IU vitamin E.

- Men who already have symptoms of benign prostatic hyperplasia should begin with 90 mg zinc daily taken in three 30-mg doses, says Dr. Whitaker. They can reduce the dosage to 60 mg daily and then to a maintenance dose of 30 mg as symptoms recede. To prevent a copper deficiency from taking too much zinc, 2 mg of copper should be taken for every 30 mg of zinc.

11 *Keep the faith.*   The power of prayer seems to extend to health and longevity. Larry Dossey, M.D., author of *Prayer Is Good Medicine*, notes that when people pray or meditate, blood pressure drops, heart rate declines, the body needs less oxygen, and over time, cholesterol levels fall. Studies show that people who attend religious services tend to handle stress better than those who don't attend, and are also far less likely to get certain diseases, such as heart disease and stroke.

You don't have to attend a church, synagogue, or mosque to get the bene-fit of prayer. Dr. Dossey says you can start with something as simple as praying before meals, taking a few moments each day to count your blessings, or con-necting with nature by taking a hike and reflecting on the splendor around you.

12 *Volunteer for youth.*   When you give back to your community by volunteering to work in a hospital, school, or an animal shelter, you do more than help others: You help yourself stay young. You'll find your spirit is revital-ized, your mind stays active, you kindle social contacts, and your energy level soars. "Volunteering gives people a feeling of mastery over their lives again," says Fred Penzel, Ph.D., a psychologist and the executive director of Western Suffolk Psychological Services in Huntington, New York. Volunteering at any age can also be a way to beat depression. When we help others, we feel better about ourselves.

13 *Detoxify your home.*   Before people can start a rejuvenation and anti-aging program, they need to detox, says Gary Null, Ph.D. He says that one of the main reasons people age prematurely is the impact of toxins in the envi-ronment on their bodies. Toxins are in our processed foods, our water supply, and our air. Hormones have been injected into the meat and dairy supply and pesti-cides are used on our fruits and vegetables. The cumulative effect of all these poisons—plus the overuse of antibiotics and other medications, toxins found in cosmetics and cleaning supplies, and exposure to radiation—is to accelerate the aging process and damage our immune systems. Because we spend many hours a day in our homes, home is one of the most important places to detoxify. Null suggests the following strategies:

- **Check airflow.** Be sure your kitchen is properly vented to prevent any accumulation of gas burnoff from pilot lights and stoves.
- **Ionize.** Use a negative ionizer in your home to eliminate airborne toxins such as dust, cigarette smoke, hydrocarbons, mold, and pet hair.
- **Exile the offenders.** Remove all toxic substances such as paint thinners, paint, gasoline, pesticides, herbicides, and fertilizers from your home, attached garage, or basement. Place them in a secured building away from your house.
- **Abandon aluminum.** Do not use aluminum-based cookware. Aluminum toxicity is believed by some to be linked with Alzheimer's disease.
- **Trash the Teflon.** Do not use Teflon or other nonstick cookware; the nonstick coating can peel and get into your food.
- **Make your house a greenhouse.** Put lots of plants (nonflowering; you don't need the pollen) in your home, as they are natural air purifiers.
- **Check your appliances.** Make sure your microwave is not leaking. A defective microwave is unsafe for up to eight feet. Also, make sure your refrigerator is not leaking freon.

14 *Put down the fork.*   This recommendation for challenging the aging process is based on more than 60 years of research in animals, which shows that they live longer and healthier lives when they eat less.

Caloric restriction is a lifelong approach to eating less food without sacrificing nutrition. According to Dr. Vincent Cristofalo, a geriatrics researcher and board member of the American Federation for Aging Research, "Caloric restriction is the only known way to significantly increase the life span of warm-blooded animals, at least mice and rats." Researchers believe they will see the same results in monkeys, who have taken part in caloric restriction studies since 1987 at the National Institute on Aging.

Although the benefits of a calorie-restricted diet won't be known until the monkeys begin to die naturally, many promising effects are already being noted. The calorie-restricted monkeys have lower levels of fat in the blood, higher levels of good cholesterol, and better control of blood glucose and insulin levels. Already they seem to be at much lower risk of developing heart disease, obesity, and diabetes, three of the biggest killers of humans.

One theory as to why caloric restriction may help increase life span is proposed by George Roth, chief of molecular physiology and genetics at the National Institute on Aging. Roth believes that taking in fewer calories reduces the flow of energy and allows the body to use the energy it has more efficiently. He compares it to a car running at a lower speed, which allows it to wear out less quickly.

15 *Avoid the sun.*   Ultraviolet light, which comes to us from the sun, accelerates aging of the skin. The best protection, says Dr. Andrew Weil, is clothing, including a wide-brimmed hat. What you don't cover up in one way, cover up in another way, which means sunscreen of at least 15 SPF on all exposed areas of the body. Dr. Weil warns not to forget the ears, bald spots on the head, and the nose.

16 *Spread on the vitamin C.*   Move over, vitamin A. Researchers in France have confirmed that applying a 5 percent vitamin C cream to the skin improves skin wrinkles significantly. Vitamin C rearranges the collagen (which is a main component of skin) and also increases its production. Although vitamin C cream is as effective as vitamin-A derived retinol creams currently being used, the vitamin C cream is associated with fewer side effects. Apply according to label directions.

17 *Move those muscles.*   Many experts have been saying it for years, and new research supports it further. In *Medicine and Science in Sports and Exercise* (vol. 32, 2000), scientists from Wageningen University in the Netherlands reported that regular exercise may help elderly people enhance the ability of the immune system to fight off infections. Although the immune system typically becomes less effective as we age, these researchers found that when compared with eating a vitamin-enriched diet or combining exercise and the diet, regular exercise alone significantly enhanced immune system function, while a vitamin-enriched diet had no benefit. In his program to reverse aging, Gary Null recommends building up to 45 minutes of aerobic exercise per day and adding in weight training three times per week.

Part I

Help Yourself

"**I** always read magazine articles about herbal remedies, for myself and my family," says Cynthia, a 29-year-old sales manager with a 5-year-old daughter.

"When I go to a bookstore, I head straight for the health section," says Cory, a 54-year-old divorced marketing analyst from Chicago. "I like to keep up on the best ways to take care of my health on my own."

"I am always cruising the Internet for the latest health information," says Martha, a 68-year-old grandmother who still works part-time as a florist. "I take an active part in staying as healthy as I can."

These people are not unusual. Health and self-help books fly off the shelves in the United States, and every week you are sure to see several health-related books among the bestsellers. Health- and nutrition-related articles in magazines are among the most widely read. And according to a Harris Interactive study, more than 98 million Americans have gone on-line to do health-related searches.

The chapters in this section offer you 24 ways to help yourself to better health and safety: at home and on the road, from your head to your toes, from better nutrition to better sex. For your home, we offer the makings of a kit of alternative home remedies, a home first aid kit, and a list of what you need to do at-home nursing care, plus dozens of guidelines on how to prevent household accidents. And because you never know when an emergency will strike, we provide instructions for how to handle the most common pediatric emergencies.

For those times when you're on the road, we discuss how to travel disease-free, show you the safest vehicles you can drive, and take a look at how safe common modes of transportation are—both in the United States and abroad. And when it comes to leisure time, you will learn about the risks of the most popular sports.

Are you one of the more than 50 million Americans who take vitamins and other supplements? Then be sure to read about the most common herbal remedies, essential oils, vitamins, minerals, and alternative supplements on the market today and how they can help improve your health. And we didn't forget about the most popular over-the-counter drugs, because we know that not everyone—or every situation—can always be treated with natural remedies.

Maintaining a healthy body–mind connection is the cornerstone of good health, so we have included chapters on "miracle" foods, exercises that make you *want* to move around and stay active, and ways to reduce your risk of disease. We offer tips for combating depression, preserving your vision, caring for your skin, and pampering your feet. We've got you covered—head to toes!

chapter one

25 Items
Every Home Remedy Kit
Should Include

You say your head has been pounding all day long? And one of your kids came home from school with a scraped knee? Just reach for your home remedy kit—if you have one. If you don't, maybe it's time to put it on your to-do list.

The recent reemergence of interest in natural medicine has turned the old-fashioned remedy kit into a must-have for every home, not so much for medical emergencies as for everyday ailments or minor traumas, such as headache, sore throat, cuts and bruises, indigestion, and insect bites. Whether you decide to purchase one of the many commercial home remedy kits available or to make one of your own, here are the ingredients that experts believe are essential. An instruction booklet or home remedy book should be kept with your kit.

Homeopathic Remedies

1 Aconite: 30c. Useful during the early stages of colds, fever, and inflammation.

2 Apis: 30c. First line of treatment for insect bites, such as bee stings and ant bites.

3 Arnica: 30c. A first-choice treatment following physical trauma, it helps reduce or prevent swelling and bruising when used soon after the injury occurs.

What You Need to Know

Infusion: An herbal infusion is like a strong tea. Generally, to make an infusion, pour 2 cups boiling water over 2 to 3 tablespoons herb and let the concoction steep for at least 10 minutes. For a home remedy kit, it is more convenient to keep herbal tea bags on hand, if they're available.

Tincture: An herbal tincture is made with the juice of a plant and mixed with alcohol.

30c: The potency of the homeopathic remedies in a home remedy kit should be 30c. The "c" refers to the centesimal (hundred) scale and indicates how much the remedy has been diluted. A 1c remedy consists of 1 part substance and 99 parts water or water and alcohol. A 30c remedy is 30 times more potent than a 1c remedy. Homeopathic remedies are available most commonly in tincture, cream, or tablet form.

4 Arsenicum: 30c. Used for abdominal pain or indigestion that may be accompanied by vomiting or diarrhea. It is best for people who are very thirsty, exhausted, and whose symptoms are worse at night.

5 Belladonna: 30c. Given for headache that starts suddenly and is throbbing or burning.

6 Cantharis: 30c. Useful for the treatment of cystitis, especially when there is burning pain before, during, and after urination.

7 Chamomilla: 30c. Effective for teething children.

8 Gelsemium: 30c. Fights the flu, especially when symptoms include shivering up and down the spine.

9 Hypericum: 30c. Effective first aid for injuries that affect nerve-rich areas, such as a fall on the tailbone or a finger slammed in a door.

10 Ignatia: 30c. A useful remedy for people who are experiencing sadness and grief and who are having trouble sleeping because of these feelings. It is especially effective when grief is unexpected, such as after a sudden death or a serious accident.

11 Ledum: 30c. First aid for black eyes and puncture wounds.

12 Mercurius vivus: 30c. An effective first aid for mouth ulcers.

13 Nux vomica: 30c. For nausea, heartburn, hangover, and burping caused by excessive intake of food, alcohol, coffee, or tobacco.

14 Rhus toxicodendron: 30c. A natural anti-inflammatory that is useful for arthritis and other aches and muscle pains. It is also effective for muscle ache and stiffness caused by flu.

15 Ruta: 30c. A remedy for injuries and strains affecting the tendons.

Herbs

16 Chamomile: The tea (infusion) or tincture can be used to treat digestive upsets and to relieve tension and stress. The infusion can be cooled and applied as a compress on wounds.

17 Cloves: This herb is effective in treating toothaches when the whole clove is placed directly on the aching spot, and for digestive problems when used as an infusion.

18 Comfrey: To promote healing, the powdered root can be sprinkled on scrapes and cuts after they have been thoroughly cleaned.

19 Echinacea: This natural antibiotic is effective against bacteria, viruses, protozoa, and fungi. Echinacea in capsules or tincture is a popular remedy for colds and flu and for hastening the healing of skin injuries.

20 Garlic: One of nature's strongest antibiotics, garlic is also used to reduce cholesterol and blood sugar levels. Deodorized garlic tablets can be used to treat bacterial infections, including tooth infections, and to hasten healing of skin wounds.

21 Peppermint: Peppermint tea is a popular remedy for stomach upset and tension headache.

22 Psyllium: An effective remedy for constipation. It is available as seeds or powdered husks.

23 Rosemary: An infusion or tincture of rosemary is effective in clearing a stuffy nose.

24 Thyme: A thyme tincture is useful as an antiseptic on minor wounds, while an infusion soothes cough, menstrual symptoms, and stomach upset.

25 Valerian: Drinking a valerian infusion before retiring helps bring on restful sleep and is good for relieving menstrual cramps.

chapter two

119

Over-the-Counter Drugs and What They're Used For

Imagine being able to buy cocaine, marijuana, and opium over-the-counter. That's what people were able to do before the creation of the Food and Drug Administration (FDA). In those days, over-the-counter (OTC) drugs, which are sold without a prescription, could contain just about anything, and often did—usually without the knowledge of the person taking the drug.

The FDA was established in 1931. The Food, Drug, and Cosmetic (FD&C) Act of 1938 gave the FDA some regulatory power, but contained no specific guidelines concerning the difference between OTC and prescription drugs. Those guidelines did not come about until 1951, when the FD&C Act was amended to define prescription drugs as substances that could be habit-forming, toxic, or unsafe unless they were used under a doctor's supervision. All other drugs, stated the Act, could be sold over-the-counter.

How Safe Are OTCs?

Some degree of risk is associated with taking any substance—whether it's a drug, a vitamin, or an herb. The FDA has defined that degree of risk as low in drugs that qualify as OTC. Naturally, anyone who takes an OTC drug must assume the responsibility to take the drug as directed on the label, and to read all accompanying printed materials. These materials include information about:

• **The ingredients.** It is best to look at the ingredients each time you buy an OTC drug, even if you think you've used exactly the same product before. Manufacturers have a habit of changing ingredients in their products or making several products whose packaging looks the same but whose ingredients are not. For example, the antacid Maalox comes in several formulations: One contains calcium carbonate and another has aluminum oxide. Checking ingredients is important, because you may be allergic to some substances.

• **Dosage.** How much of the drug to take and when to take it. Buy products that have a convenient dosing schedule.

• **Safety precautions.** Some OTC drugs should not be taken if you are going to operate heavy machinery or drive a car. Other precautions include age limits (not for children younger than 12 years, for example), not to use if pregnant or breast-feeding, not to take with certain other medications, or not to use for longer than a specific period of time.

• **Adverse reactions.** The product insert should explain which adverse reactions may occur and how often they were found to occur in studies of the product.

Guidelines for Buying OTC Drugs

- People often buy OTC drugs for conditions they have diagnosed themselves. Confirm your self-diagnosis with a medical professional.
- Compare similar product ingredient lists. Often you can get a generic brand that is equally effective but less expensive than a national brand name.
- Avoid products that claim to relieve lots of symptoms. These products tend to contain more drugs than you need, which can expose you to unnecessary risks and cost more.
- Ask a pharmacist or doctor to help you choose a product if you need help. It is always a good idea to ask about possible side effects and interactions, especially if you are taking other medications or have allergies or a medical condition.
- Do not exceed the recommended dose, and never take the drug for longer than the maximum time suggested on the label.
- Keep all drugs, including OTC drugs, out of the reach of children.

According to the FDA, there are more than 100,000 OTC drug products on the market, encompassing more than 800 active ingredients. The 119 OTC products listed here are among the most commonly used in the United States. The brand names are followed by the main generic ingredient(s) where applicable. Check individual package labels for a complete list of ingredients.

Words to Know

Acetaminophen: A drug similar to aspirin that has antifever and pain relief abilities, but not anti-inflammatory benefits like aspirin. It is recommended for people who are sensitive to aspirin.

Antiemetics: Substances that prevent vomiting and nausea.

Antihistamines: Drugs that prevent the actions of histamine, a substance that causes widening of tiny blood vessels called capillaries, resulting in a rash or hives, and increased stomach secretion, which can cause nausea and vomiting. Antihistamines can also induce sleep and relieve symptoms of the common cold.

Antiseborrheic: Drugs used to treat seborrhea, which is an alteration of the sebaceous glands. This condition can show as dandruff or as yellow-gray patches on the skin.

Coal Tar: A tar derived from coal that is used as an ingredient in ointments to treat eczema and other skin diseases.

Generic drugs: Drugs that are not protected by a trademark. They are also known as nonproprietary drugs.

NSAIDs: Nonsteroidal anti-inflammatory drugs used to reduce inflammation and the pain associated with it.

Analgesics (Pain Relievers)

The latest (2000) statistics show that the two best-selling OTC drugs in the United States are the painkillers Tylenol (generic, acetaminophen) and Advil (generic, ibuprofen).

1 Advil (NSAID, ibuprofen)   **2** Aleve (NSAID, naproxen)

3 Alka-Seltzer Effervescent Pain Reliever & Antacid (aspirin)

4 Allerest (acetaminophen)

5 Anacin (aspirin)

6 Anacin-3 (acetaminophen)

7 Anaprox (NSAID, naproxen)

8 Bayer (aspirin)

9 Bayer Select (acetaminophen)

10 Bayer Select Ibuprofen (NSAID, ibuprofen)

11 Benadryl Allergy/Sinus Headache Caplets (acetaminophen)

12 Bufferin (aspirin)

13 Comtrex (acetaminophen)

14 DayQuil Non-Drowsy Cold/Flu Formula

15 Dimetapp Sinus Caplets (NSAID, ibuprofen)

16 Dristan (aspirin)

17 Dristan AF and AF Plus (acetaminophen)

18 Excedrin-IB Caplets (NSAID, ibuprofen)

19 Midol-IB (NSAID, ibuprofen)

20 Motrin, Motrin-IB, Motrin-IB Sinus (NSAID, ibuprofen)

21 Nuprin (NSAID, ibuprofen)

22 NyQuil Hot Therapy (acetaminophen)

23 Panadol and Panadol Extra Strength (acetaminophen)

24 Robitussin Night Relief (acetaminophen)

25 Sinarest (acetaminophen)

26 Sine-Aid and Sine-Aid Maximum Strength (acetaminophen)

27 Sudafed Cold & Cough Liquid Caps (acetaminophen)

28 Synflex (NSAID, naproxen)

29 TheraFlu Maximum Strength (acetaminophen)

30 Triaminic Sore Throat Formula (acetaminophen)

31 Tylenol, Tylenol Allergy, Tylenol Caplets (acetaminophen)

Cold and Cough Remedies (Includes antihistamines, decongestants, cough suppressants.)

32 Actifed, Actifed 12-Hour (antihistamine, triprolidine)

33 Alka-Seltzer Plus Cold (antihistamine, chlorpheniramine)

34 Alka-Seltzer Plus Cold and Cough (antihistamine, chlorpheniramine; cough suppressant, dextromethorphan)

35 Allerest 12-Hour, 12-Hour Maximum Strength Caplets (antihistamine, chlorpheniramine)

36 Benadryl 25, Benadryl Cold, Cold Nighttime Liquid, Complete Allergy (antihistamine, diphenhydramine)

37 Comtrex A/S, Hot Flu Relief, Maximum Strength Liqui-Gels (antihistamine, chlorpheniramine)

38 Comtrex Cough, Comtrex Cough Formula (cough suppressant, dextromethorphan)

39 Dimetapp, Dimetapp 4-Hour, Allergy, with Codeine (antihistamine, carbinoxamine)

40 Dimetapp-DM Cough and Cold (antihistamine, carbinoxamine; cough suppressant, dextromethorphan)

41 Dristan, Dristan AF, Cold and Flu, Cold Multi-Symptom (antihistamine, chlorpheniramine)

42 Medi-Flu (cough suppressant, dextromethorphan)

43 NyQuil Liquicaps, Nighttime Colds (antihistamine, diphenhydramine)

44 NyQuil Hot Therapy, Liquicaps (cough suppressant, dextromethorphan)

45 PediaCare Allergy, Children's Cold, Children's Cough-Cold (antihistamine, chlorpheniramine)

46 Pertussin CS, ES, Cough Suppressant (cough suppressant, dextromethorphan)

47 Robitussin Night Relief, Night Relief Colds (antihistamine, pyrilamine)

48 Sinarest, Sinarest Extra Strength, Sinarest Sinus (antihistamine, chlorpheniramine)

49 Sinutab, Sinutab Extra Strength, Regular (antihistamine, chlorpheniramine)

50 Sudafed Cold & Cough Liquid Caps, Sudafed Cough (cough suppressant, dextromethorphan)

51 Tavist, Tavist-1, Tavist-D (antihistamine, clemastine fumarate)

52 Triaminic, Triaminic Allergy, Chewables, Cold, DM Nighttime for Children (antihistamine, chlorpheniramine)

53 Tylenol Allergy Sinus Gelcaps, Allergy Sinus NightTime Maximum Strength Caplets (antihistamine, diphenhydramine)

54 Vicks 44 Cold, Flu and Cough Liqui-Caps, Non-Drowsy Cold and Cough LiquiCaps (cough suppressant, dextromethorphan)

Antacids and Ulcer Treatment

Americans spend nearly $1 billion a year on antacids, making them one of the most popular OTC drugs. Antacids are used to prevent or treat gas and heartburn.

55 Di-Gel (antacid, alumina, magnesia, and simethicone)

56 Gaviscon (antacid, alumina, magnesium trisilicate, and sodium bicarbonate)

57 Gelusil (antacid, alumina, magnesia, and simethicone)

58 Maalox (antacid, alumina, and magnesia)

59 Mygel (antacid, alumina, magnesia, and simethicone)

60 Mylanta (antacid, alumina, magnesia, and simethicone)

61 Mylanta Calcium-Rich (antacid, calcium carbonate, and magnesia)

62 Pepcid AC (histamine H2 receptor antagonist, ramotidine)

63 Riopan, Riopan Extra Strength, Riopan Plus (antacid, magaldrate, and simethicone)

64 Rolaids (antacid, calcium carbonate)

65 Rolaids Calcium Rich, Rolaids Sodium Free (antacid, calcium carbonate, and magnesia)

66 Tagamet HB (histamine H2 receptor antagonist, cimetidine)

67 Tums, Tums E-X, Tums Liquid Extra Strength (antacid, calcium carbonate)

68 Zantac, Zantac 75 (histamine H2 receptor antagonist, ranitidine)

Antiacne Agents

69 Benoxyl 5 Lotion, Benoxyl 5 Wash, Benoxyl 10 Lotion (benzoyl peroxide)

70 Clearasil BP Plus 5 Cream, Maximum Strength (benzoyl peroxide)

71 Dry and Clear 5 Lotion

72 Oxy 5 Vanishing Lotion, Oxy 10 (benzoyl peroxide)

Antibiotics

Although many antibiotics are available only by prescription, there are topical OTC antibiotics that are used for cuts, scrapes, and other damage to the skin. They contain one or more of the generic drugs neomycin, bacitracin, and polymyxin. They include:

73 Bactine First Aid Antibiotic

74 Mycitracin

75 Neosporin

76 Polysporin

Antidiarrheal

77 Kaopectate Advanced Formula, Kaopectate Maximum Strength (attapulgite)

78 Pepto-Bismol (bismuth subsalicylate)

79 St. Joseph Antidiarrheal (attapulgite)

Antiemetics

80 Bonine (meclizine)

81 Dramamine, Dramamine Chewable, Dramamine Liquid (dimenhydrinate)

82 Nausene (diphenhydraminine)

83 Pedialyte (for rehydration)

Antifungals (Topical, Vaginal)

84 Desenex Antifungal (topical: cream, liquid, ointment, penetrating foam, powder, spray powder; undecylenic acid)

85 Lotrimin AF, Lotrimin (topical: cream, lotion, ointment; clotrimazole)

86 Tinactin Aerosol Liquid, Tinactin Aerosol Powder (topical: econazole)

87 Gyne-Lotrimin, Gyne-Lotrimin-3 (vaginal: clotrimazole)

88 Monistat 3, Monistat 5, Monistat 7 (vaginal: miconazole)

89 Vagistat, Vagistat-1 (vaginal: tioconazole)

Antiseborrheics

90 Denorex Extra Strength Medicated Shampoo (coal tar)

91 Head and Shoulders Antidandruff Cream Shampoo (pyrithione)

92 Selsun Blue, Selsun Blue Dry Formula (selenium sulfide)

93 Tegrin Medicated Cream Shampoo, Concentrated Gel (coal tar)

94 T-Gel (coal tar)

95 T/Gel Therapeutic Conditioner, Shampoo (coal tar)

Antismoking Agents

Nicotine replacement products are used to help people quit smoking. They should be used in conjunction with a medically supervised behavioral modification program for smoking cessation.

96 Nicoderm

97 Nicorette

98 Nicotrol

Caffeine (for Energy Boost)

99 NoDoz, NoDoz Maximum Strength Caplets

100 Pep-Back

101 Vivarin

Hair Growth Stimulant (Topical)

102 Rogaine (minoxidil)

Laxatives

103 Citrucel Orange Flavor, Citrucel Sugar-Free (methylcellulose)

104 Correctol, Correctol Caplets, Correctol Extra Gentle (docusate)

105 Dulcolax (bisacodyl)

106 Ex-Lax, Ex-Lax Pills (phenolphthalein)

107 Feen-a-Mint, Feen-a-Mint Pills (docusate)

108 Fibercon (polycarbophil)

109 Maalox Daily Fiber Therapy (psyllium)

110 Metamucil (all flavors, wafers and instant mix) (psyllium)

111 Perdiem, Perdiem Fiber (psyllium)

112 Phillips' Magnesia Tablets, Phillips' Concentrated (magnesium hydroxide)

113 Prodiem Plus (dehydrocholic acid)

114 Senokot, SenokotXTRA (senna)

Sleep Aids

115 Nytol Maximum Strength (diphenhydramine)

116 Sominex Formula 2 (diphenhydramine)

117 Sleep-Eze (diphenhydramine)

118 Unisom Nighttime Sleep Aid (doxylamine)

119 Unisom SleepGels Maximum Strength (diphenhydramine)

chapter three

58 Herbal Remedies: Effective Dosages and Forms

The popularity of herbal remedies as treatments for everything from abscesses to zits is apparent from the increasing number of people who use herbal medicine: Approximately one-third of Americans use herbal supplements and related products, and they spend more than $4 billion on them annually.

Although researchers have uncovered much fascinating information about herbs and their medicinal value, there is still a lot they do not know or understand. That is why it is common to see different experts suggest different dosages for some herbs. But we do know this: Herbal medicine can be very effective—and thus very strong—medicine.

That's good news, because you want the herbs to work; but it also means that there is the potential for adverse reactions. Even though herbal remedies are associated with many fewer problems than conventional medicines, taking more than the recommended dose of an herb can be unsafe. Therefore, consult someone who is knowledgeable about herbal remedies before you take any of them.

1 Aloe (*Aloa barbadenis*)

- Main Indications: Topical treatment for burns and wounds
- Form: Gel (the thin, clear mucilage that comes from the middle of the leaf)
- Effective Dose: Apply a little dab from a broken leaf as needed.

Herbal Remedies: What You Should Know

Here are a few things you'll see in the remedy list.

Tinctures: These products consist of an herb soaked in alcohol. The label may have a ratio, such as 1:5 or 4:1. The first number represents the amount of herb; the second, the amount of alcohol. Therefore, a 1:5 ratio means there is one part herb to five parts alcohol.

Measurements: Here are estimated conversions, from the metric system to the U.S. system, for some common amounts:

10 drops = 1 mL = 1/4 teaspoon

50 drops = 5 mL = 1 teaspoon

5 g = 1 teaspoon of dried, powdered herb

3 teaspoons = 1 tablespoon = approximately 1/2 ounce of dried, powdered herb

Standardized: A standardized herbal remedy is one that the manufacturer guarantees contains a specified potency.

Dosages: The dosages in this list are suggestions only. If you purchase a packaged herbal product that has different dosage directions, follow the package instructions.

2 Arnica (*Arnica montana*)

- Main Indications: Topical treatment of bruises and sprains, and of inflammation caused by insect bites
- Forms: Gels, creams, and ointments that contain 5 to 25 percent tincture or extract
- Effective Dose: Apply topically to the affected area according to package directions. Never use on open wounds or broken skin.

3 Ashwagandha (*Withania somnifera*)

- Main Indications: Arthritis; increases vitality and strength
- Form: Standardized tablets
- Effective Dose: Take up to three 4.5 mg tablets daily.

4 Astragalus

- Main Indications: Cold, flu, minor infections; a mainstay in traditional Chinese medicine
- Form: Capsules (usually 400 to 500 mg each)
- Effective Dose: Eight to nine capsules daily

5 Bilberry (*Vaccinium myrtillus*)

- Main Indications: Vision problems, including cataracts, glaucoma, macular degeneration, poor night vision, and retinopathy
- Forms: Standardized extracts (to 36% anthocyanosides) and standardized capsules (to 25%)
- Effective Doses: Up to four 60 mg capsules daily; or 15 to 40 drops extract in liquid up to three times daily

6 Bitter Melon (*Momordica chirantia*)

- Main Indications: Controls blood sugar and enhances the immune system
- Form: Capsules (500 mg)
- Effective Dose: One capsule 30 minutes before each meal

7 Black Cohosh (*Cimicifuga racemosa*)

- Main Indications: Menstrual and menopausal symptoms
- Forms: Capsules (20 and 40 mg) and tincture (1:5)
- Effective Doses: 40 mg daily in capsules; or 10 to 30 drops tincture in liquid daily

8 Boswella (*Boswellia serata*)

- Main Indications: Pain and swelling associated with arthritis
- Forms: Cream and capsules (500 mg)
- Effective Doses: Apply cream topically to affected areas according to package directions. Capsules: Take three daily until symptoms subside, then one daily.

9 Butcher's Broom (*Ruscus acluteatus*)

- Main Indications: Poor circulation, swelling in legs or feet
- Forms: Capsules and extract
- Effective Doses: Up to three capsules daily; or 10 to 20 drops extract in liquid daily

10 Cascara Sagrada (*Rhamnus purshiana*)

- Main Indications: Constipation
- Forms: Capsules (400 to 500 mg) and extract
- Effective Doses: Up to two capsules daily (providing 20 to 70 mg of anthraquinones, which are the active ingredients); or ½ to 1 teaspoon extract daily

11 Cat's Claw (*Uncaria tomentosa*)

- Main Indications: Inflammation; boosts the immune system
- Forms: Capsules (500 to 600 mg) and tincture
- Effective Doses: Up to three 500 to 600 mg capsules daily; or 20 to 40 drops tincture up to five times daily

12 Cayenne (*Capsicum annuum*)

- Main Indications: Enhances the immune system and reduces arthritis pain. Claims that it stimulates the digestive system have not been proven scientifically.
- Forms: Capsules (400 to 500 mg), tincture, and cream
- Effective Doses: Take up to three capsules daily, or 5 to 10 drops tincture in water daily. Topically, apply according to package directions.

13 Celery (*Apium graveolens*)

- Main Indications: Water retention, high blood pressure, inflammation, gas
- Forms: Oil and seeds
- Effective Doses: For gas, chew 1 teaspoon celery seeds (add to food to make more palatable). To use oil, mix 6 to 8 drops in water and drink twice daily.

14 Chamomile (*Matricaria recutita*)

- Main Indications: Indigestion, insomnia, nausea
- Forms: Capsules (300 to 400 mg) and tincture
- Effective Doses: Up to six capsules daily; or 10 to 40 drops tincture three times daily

15 Chaste Tree Berry (*Vitex agnus-castus*)

- Main Indications: Premenstrual syndrome (PMS), menopausal symptoms
- Forms: Capsules and tincture
- Effective Doses: One capsule up to three times daily; or 20 drops tincture one or two times daily

16 Cloves (*Caryophyllum aromaticus*)

- Main Indications: Tooth pain; vomiting
- Form: Oil
- Effective Doses: For tooth pain, rub oil on the affected area. For vomiting, mix 2 drops oil in 8 ounces water and drink.

17 Dandelion (*Taraxacum officinale*)

- Main Indications: Water retention, high blood pressure
- Forms: Capsules and extract
- Effective Doses: Up to three capsules daily; or 10 to 30 drops extract in liquid daily

18 Devil's Claw (*Harpagophytum procumbens*)

- Main Indications: Inflammation, pain relief, high cholesterol
- Forms: Capsules (400 to 500 mg) and tincture
- Effective Doses: Up to three capsules daily; or 30 drops tincture three times daily

19 Dong Quai (*Angelica sinesis*)

- Main Indications: Menstrual and menopausal symptoms

- Forms: Capsules (500 to 600 mg) and tincture (1:5)
- Effective Doses: Up to three capsules daily; or 10 to 20 drops tincture up to three times daily

20 Echinacea (*Echinacea angustifolia, E. pallida, E. purpurea*)

- Main Indications: Colds and flu (when taken at start of symptoms), urinary tract infections
- Forms: Capsules (300 to 400 mg) and tincture
- Effective Doses: Take up to three capsules daily; or 15 to 30 drops tincture in liquid three times daily. Varro E. Tyler, Ph.D., professor emeritus of pharmacognosy at Purdue University, recommends swishing the tincture (in water) in the mouth for several seconds before swallowing to help stimulate the lymphatic system in the mouth.

21 Elderberry (*Sambucus canadensis*)

- Main Indications: Fever, sore throat
- Forms: Dried herb and tincture
- Effective Doses: To make an infusion (tea), pour 6 ounces boiling water over 2 teaspoons (3 g) dried herb and steep for 5 minutes. Drink up to three cups daily. For tincture, drink 3 drops in 8 ounces water three times daily.

22 Evening Primrose (*Oenothera biennis*)

- Main Indications: PMS symptoms, arteriosclerosis, asthma, eczema, endometriosis, high blood pressure, high cholesterol, rheumatoid arthritis. Evening primrose oil is rich in gamma-linolenic acid (GLA), a fatty acid that is essential for health.
- Form: Capsules (250 and 500 mg)
- Effective Doses: Up to six 250 mg or three 500 mg capsules daily

23 Eyebright (*Euphrasia officinalis*)

- Main Indications: Irritated or inflamed eyes
- Forms: Capsule and extract
- Effective Doses: One capsule up to three times daily; or 15 to 40 drops extract in liquid every three to four hours

24 Fennel (*Foeniculum vulgare*)

- Main Indications: Stomach cramps, gas, coughs and cold, painful joints
- Forms: Dried fruit and capsules (100 mg)
- Effective Doses: To make an infusion, pour 6 ounces boiling water over 1 to 2 teaspoons (2 to 5 g) of dried fruit that has been crushed immediately before use. Steep for 10 to 15 minutes and strain. The maximum daily dose is 7 g fennel. Capsules: Take one up to three times daily.

25 Fenugreek (*Trigonella foenum-graecum*)

- Main Indications: Gastritis, high cholesterol
- Forms: Capsules (600 to 700 mg) and seed
- Effective Doses: Up to six capsules daily; or 1½ teaspoons seeds daily

26 Feverfew (*Tanacetum parthenium*)

- Main Indications: Migraine headache
- Forms: Capsules (125 mg) and tincture
- Effective Doses: One capsule daily standardized to 0.2 percent parthenolide; or 15 to 30 drops tincture daily

27 Flaxseed (*Linun usitatissimum*)

- Main Indications: Constipation, irritable bowel syndrome
- Form: Seed
- Effective Dose: ½ to 1 tablespoon whole or cracked seed in 8 ounces water taken up to three times daily

28 Garlic (*Allium sativum*)

- Main Indications: Athlete's foot, candidiasis, colds and flu, high blood pressure, high cholesterol, infections (viral, bacterial, and fungal)
- Forms: Fresh garlic cloves and deodorized capsules (500 to 600 mg); look for capsules that deliver at least 5,000 mcg allicin daily.
- Effective Doses: Some alternative health experts recommend eating at least one clove (about 4 g) daily to help maintain health, or three to five cloves daily when treating a medical condition. Capsules: Take up to three daily.

29 Ginger (*Zingiber officinale*)

- Main Indications: Indigestion, motion sickness, nausea
- Forms: Capsules (250 to 500 mg) and tincture
- Effective Doses: It is safe to take up to 2,000 mg daily, as needed. For tincture, drink 10 to 20 drops in water three times daily.

30 Ginkgo (*Ginkgo biloba*)

- Main Indications: Aging-associated symptoms (memory problems, depression, poor circulation, confusion, macular degeneration, tinnitus), migraines
- Form: Standardized capsules (Look for those that deliver at least 24% flavonoids and 6% terpenoids or terpene.)
- Effective Dose: Up to three 60 mg capsules daily

31 Ginseng (*Panax quinquefolius, P. ginseng*)

- Main Indications: Fatigue, improves concentration.
- Form: Capsules (500 to 600 mg; standardized for 4 to 7% ginsenosides, 100 mg)
- Effective Doses: Up to four capsules daily if nonstandardized, one to two if standardized

32 Goldenseal (*Hydrastis canadensis*)

- Main Indications: Infections, inflammation of the mucous membranes
- Forms: Capsules (250 to 500 mg) and tincture (1:5)
- Effective Doses: Up to three capsules daily; or 20 to 50 drops tincture daily for up to three weeks

33 Green Tea (*Camellia sinensis*)

- Main Indications: Reduces risk of cancer and heart disease
- Forms: Dried in tea bags and extract in capsules
- Effective Doses: Make tea according to package directions. Research indicates that drinking four to five cups daily may help prevent cancer and heart disease. For capsules, take two daily.

34 Gotu Kola (*Centella asiatica*)

- Main Indications: May improve memory; reduces anxiety; improves circulation
- Forms: Capsules and extract
- Effective Doses: Up to three capsules daily; or 5 to 10 drops extract in liquid three times daily

35 Grapeseed Extract

- Main Indications: Antioxidant, inflammation
- Form: Tablets
- Effective Dose: One to two 100 mg tablets daily

36 Hawthorn (*Crataegus monogyna, C. oxyacantha*)

- Main Indications: Heart conditions (angina, arrhythmia, atherosclerosis, edema, high blood pressure, high cholesterol) and heart health maintenance
- Form: Capsules (200 mg)
- Effective Dose: Consult your physician before taking hawthorn: Up to three capsules daily with meals

37 Horse Chestnut (*Aesculus hippocastanum*)

- Main Indications: Bruises, hemorrhoids, varicose veins
- Forms: Tablets and extract (both standardized to 50 mg aescin, the active ingredient)
- Effective Doses: One tablet as directed on the package; 10 to 15 drops tincture daily

38 Kava (*Piper methysticum*)

- Main Indications: Depression, genitourinary infections, insomnia, hyperactivity
- Forms: Capsules, tinctures, and extracts, all standardized at 40 to 70 mg kavalactones
- Effective Doses: Up to three capsules or tablets daily; or 10 to 20 drops extract or tincture daily in water or juice

39 Lemon Balm (*Melissa officinalis*)

- Main Indications: Stress and tension, insomnia
- Form: Dried leaf
- Effective Dose: To make an infusion (tea) from the dried leaf, pour 8 ounces hot water over 2 teaspoons (2 g) dried leaf and steep 5 to 10 minutes. Drink two to three cups daily.

40 Licorice (*Glycyrrhiza glabra*)

- Main Indications: Coughs, congestion, stomach and duodenal ulcers
- Forms: Capsules (400 to 500 mg) and tincture (Look for products that contain at least 4 percent glycyrrhizin, a primary active ingredient.)
- Effective Doses: Up to three capsules daily; or 20 to 30 drops tincture up to three times daily

41 Milk Thistle (*Silybum marianum*)

- Main Indications: Liver problems (e.g., cirrhosis, hepatitis) and health maintenance; protects against harm from pollutants
- Forms: Capsules (140 mg) and tincture, both standardized at 70 to 80 percent silymarin
- Effective Doses: Up to three capsules daily; or 10 to 25 drops tincture up to three times daily

42 Neem (*Azadirachta indica*)

- Main Indications: Skin disorders, gum disease, inflammation
- Forms: Oil and creams (for topical use) and capsules (400 to 500 mg)
- Effective Doses: Use oil and creams as indicated on the packages. Capsules: Take up to six daily.

43 Nettle (*Urtica dioica*)

- Main Indications: Symptoms of hayfever
- Forms: Capsules (100 mg) and extract
- Effective Doses: Take up to three capsules daily; some sources say to take up to eight times that amount. For extract, take 5 to 10 drops in liquid daily.

44 Passion Flower (*Passiflora incarnata*)

- Main Indications: Stress, headache
- Form: Extract
- Effective Dose: Take 15 to 60 drops extract mixed in liquid as needed daily.

45 Pau D'arco (*Tabebuia ipetiginosa*)

- Main Indications: Fights bacteria, viruses, and fungi
- Forms: Capsules (300, 500, and 600 mg) and tincture
- Effective Doses: Of capsules, limit intake to about 1,800 mg daily; of tincture, take 20 to 50 drops in liquid up to four times daily.

46 Peppermint (*Mentha piperita*)

- Main Indications: Stomach pain, gas
- Form: Tea
- Effective Dose: To make your own tea from fresh, dried peppermint, pour 6 ounces boiling water over 1 to 2 tablespoons of the herb and allow it to steep for 10 minutes. Three 6-ounce cups can be taken daily. Peppermint tea is also available commercially in tea bags.

47 Psyllium (*Plantago spp*)

- Main Indications: Constipation, high cholesterol
- Forms: Dried seeds, husks, and capsules (660 mg)
- Effective Doses: To use the dried seeds or husks, mix up to 2 teaspoons seed or 1 teaspoon husks in a large glass of water and drink immediately, 30 to 60 minutes after meals. To use the capsules, take up to six daily; drink 8 ounces of water with each dose.

48 Red Clover (*Trifolium pratense*)

- Main Indications: Menopause symptoms; helps prevent cancer
- Forms: Capsules and extract
- Effective Doses: Take up to three capsules daily, or 10 to 30 drops extract in warm liquid daily.

49 Reishi Mushroom (*Ganoderma lucidum*)

- Main Indications: May be good for arthritis pain; often taken for its possible anticancer properties
- Form: Capsules
- Effective Dose: Take one capsule up to three times daily.

50 St. John's Wort (*Hypericum perforatum*)

- Main Indications: Burns, cuts, depression, herpes, HIV/AIDS
- Forms: Capsules (300 mg) and tinctures, both standardized to 0.3 percent hypericin, and oil
- Effective Doses: Capsules: Take up to three capsules daily. Tincture: Take 10 to 30 drops in liquid several times daily. Oil: Apply on burns and cuts three to four times daily as needed.

51 Saw Palmetto (*Serenoa repens*)

- Main Indications: Prostate problems, hair loss
- Form: Standardized extract
- Effective Dose: Depends on the concentration of the product. The higher the concentration of sterols, the lower the dosage needed. Take between 150 and 1,200 mg daily.

52 Shiitake Mushroom (*Lentinus edodes*)

- Main Indications: High cholesterol; boosts the immune system
- Form: Capsules
- Effective Dose: Up to three capsules daily

53 Siberian Ginseng (*Eleutherococcus senticosus*)

- Main Indications: Immune system booster
- Forms: Capsules (400 to 500 mg) and tincture (1:5)
- Effective Doses: Up to nine capsules daily; or 20 drops tincture up to three times daily

54 Skullcap (*Scutellaria lateriflora*)

- Main Indications: Stress and anxiety, insomnia
- Forms: Capsules and extract
- Effective Doses: Take one capsule up to three times daily, or 3 to 12 drops extract in liquid daily.

55 Spirulina (*Arthrospira platenis*)

- Main Indications: Iron-deficiency anemia; helps boost the immune system
- Form: Tablets
- Effective Dose: Up to six 500 mg tablets daily

56 Turmeric (*Curcuma longaI*)

- Main Indications: Athlete's foot, digestive disorders, heart disease, liver problems, wound healing
- Forms: Capsules of the main active ingredient, curcumin, and oil
- Effective Doses: One 400 mg capsule three times daily. For athlete's foot, dilute one part oil in two parts water and apply to the affected area.

57 Uva Ursi (*Arctostaphylos uva-ursi*)

- Main Indications: Mild urinary tract infections
- Forms: Capsules (400 to 500 mg) and tincture (1:5)
- Effective Doses: Up to nine 400 to 500 mg capsules daily; or 30 to 60 drops tincture in 8 ounces water three times daily

58 Valerian (*Valeriana officinalis*)

- Main Indications: Anxiety and stress, insomnia
- Forms: Capsules and tincture (1:5)
- Effective Doses: Up to three capsules daily; or 15 to 20 drops tincture in water up to three times daily

chapter four

13 Vitamins
You Can't Live Without

There's a reason why your parents always told you to eat your fruits and vegetables: You can't live without them. Okay, maybe you don't need to eat broccoli and okra and kiwi. But fruits and vegetables are especially rich in vitamins, and you need vitamins to live.

Vitamins are organic compounds that the body uses in very small amounts to help regulate and support chemical reactions. Vitamins work along with enzymes and other substances to maintain normal metabolism and the growth, development, and function of the body's cells. With few exceptions, vitamins must be obtained from the diet or from supplementation, because the body cannot manufacture them internally.

There are 13 essential vitamins, divided into two categories: fat-soluble and water-soluble. Fat-soluble vitamins can be stored by the body in the fatty tissue and the liver for long periods of time; water-soluble vitamins must be consumed daily, because the body cannot store them and excretes them within a few days. A deficiency in any of the essential vitamins can place your health and life in danger. Here are the vitamins you need for life—and for good health.

Words to Know

RDI: Reference Dietary Intake is the Food and Nutrition Board's replacement for RDA (Recommended Daily Allowance), which many experts realized did not adequately describe the amount of a nutrient needed for good health. The RDI began to replace RDA on food labels in 1998.

IU (International Unit): An internationally accepted amount of a substance, usually used to measure fat-soluble vitamins, hormones, and vaccines.

Antioxidants: This group includes vitamins, minerals, and enzymes whose purpose is to protect the body from the formation of free radicals—atoms that damage cells.

Milligrams: mg; one-thousandth of a gram.

Micrograms: mcg; one-thousandth of a milligram, or one-millionth of a gram.

Fat-Soluble Vitamins

1 VITAMIN A

Vitamin A is an unusual vitamin for several reasons. Neither plant nor animal foods actually contain it; instead, they contain what is called either a preformed or provitamin A, which is found in animals, or beta-carotene, which is found in plants. The body converts both of these substances into vitamin A once they are in the body. Beta-carotene is the preferred form because it is a powerful antioxidant and may help to reduce the risk of serious disease, such as cancer and heart disease.

- **Benefits:** Vitamin A helps in the development and maintenance of healthy teeth, mucous membranes, skin, vision, and skeletal and soft tissue. It also helps repair damaged DNA and boosts the immune system. Some experts believe vitamin A can successfully treat glaucoma.

- **Natural Sources:** Carrots are often the first vegetable that comes to mind when people think about vitamin A. Other excellent sources include apricots, asparagus, broccoli, cantaloupe, cabbage, red peppers, squash, sweet potatoes, peas, and oranges.

2 VITAMIN D

Vitamin D is one of the vitamins the body can manufacture. If you've ever heard vitamin D referred to as the sunshine vitamin, that's because when you expose your skin (face, hands, arms, and so on) to 10 to 20 minutes of sunshine each day, the ultraviolet rays that strike your skin stimulate your system to produce a form of vitamin D. In that way, you carry a little bit of sunshine with you every day.

The RDI for vitamin D is 200 to 400 IU for children; 200 to 400 for men and women 25 to 50 years old, 400 to 600 IU for men and women 50 years and older, and 200 to 500 IU for nursing women.

- **Benefits:** Vitamin D's primary function is to help absorb calcium and phosphorous to build and maintain strong bones and teeth. It also protects against rectal and colon cancers, helps prevent colds, increases muscle strength, and helps in the treatment of conjunctivitis.
- **Natural Sources:** Fortified milk and other dairy products, yeast, fortified cereals, seafood, and cooked liver.

3 VITAMIN E

Vitamin E can be broken down into two different categories: tocopherols and tocotrienols. Both are powerful antioxidants, thus you need both forms for good health. Some foods are rich sources of tocopherols (e.g., wheat bran) while others have lots of tocotrienols (e.g., rice bran). Putting the two together, however, does not always result in a tasty combination. That's one reason why vitamin E often needs to be supplemented in the diet. Another reason is that vitamin E is found primarily in very fatty foods that are not a big part of most people's diets. The RDI is 4.5 to 15 IU for children and 12 to 15 IU for adults.

- **Benefits:** Vitamin E is a very potent antioxidant. It plays a major role in keeping the heart healthy because it prevents the arteries from clogging with cholesterol and other harmful buildup. It also helps prevent cancer of the mouth, esophagus, and throat; decreases the risk of cervical and breast cancer; improves male fertility; boosts the immune system; eases leg cramps; and reduces menopausal symptoms. It is also believed to slow the effects of Alzheimer's disease and Parkinson's disease, help prevent cataracts, speed up the healing of cuts and other wounds, and control blood sugar levels.

- **Natural Sources:** Almonds, asparagus, avocados, fortified cereals, hazelnuts, peanut butter, sunflower oil, and sunflower seeds.

4 VITAMIN K

Like vitamin D, vitamin K can be manufactured in the body. For vitamin K, that process takes places in the intestines, where about 50 percent of the vitamin K you need is produced. The rest comes from your food. The RDI is 30 to 60 mcg for children, 60 to 80 mcg for adults 25 to 50 years old, and 70 to 80 mcg for adults over age 50.

- **Benefits:** Vitamin K produces the substances needed to clot blood. Without vitamin K, you could bleed to death from a bump, bruise, or cut. Vitamin K also helps bring calcium to the bones, reduces severe menstrual flow, and prevents internal bleeding. It has been used to kill cancer cells and to treat bruises, broken capillaries, and postoperative scars.
- **Natural Sources:** Asparagus, broccoli, cabbage, egg yolk, green beans, green tea leaves, lettuce, peas, spinach, seaweed, and turnips.

Water-Soluble Vitamins

5 VITAMIN B1 (THIAMIN)

Thiamin was the first B vitamin to be discovered. The RDI is 0.3 to 1.5 mg for children, 1.1 to 1.6 mg for adults 25 to 50 years old, and 1.0 to 1.2 mg for adults over age 50.

- **Benefits:** Thiamin keeps heart muscle healthy; promotes clear memory and brain function; helps metabolize amino acids into proteins, enzymes, and hormones; and promotes growth and healthy skin.
- **Natural Sources:** Asparagus, black beans, brown rice, chicken, green peas, oatmeal, potatoes, raisins, sunflower seeds, and products labeled "enriched" (e.g., breads, pastas, and cereals).

6 VITAMIN B2 (RIBOFLAVIN)

This vitamin is a spark that turns proteins, fats, and carbohydrates into energy. The equation is simple: Too little riboflavin equals not enough energy.

- **Benefits:** In addition to its role in the metabolism of proteins, fats, and carbohydrates, riboflavin also promotes healthy eyes, skin, nails, and hair. Every cell in the body needs riboflavin to grow and reproduce, and the immune system needs this vitamin to create antibodies to fight infection.
- **Natural Sources:** Almonds, avocados, brewer's yeast, chicken, eggs, green leafy vegetables, and mushrooms.

7 VITAMIN B3 (NIACIN, NIACINAMIDE)

Niacin is made up of two compounds: nicotinic acid and niacinamide. You get approximately 50 percent of your niacin from each substance. Nicotinic acid is found in food, and niacinamide is converted from the amino acid tryptophan in the body. However, this conversion doesn't happen by itself. Other B vitamins, including thiamin, riboflavin, pyridoxine, and the almost-vitamin biotin (included in this list) are needed to make the transformation.

- **Benefits:** Niacin improves circulation by widening blood vessels, converts carbohydrates into energy, provides antioxidant protection, lowers cholesterol and blood triglyceride levels, promotes healthy digestion, helps maintain a healthy nervous system, and maintains the proper function of estrogen, progesterone, cortisone, and testosterone.
- **Natural Sources:** Broccoli, carrots, corn flour, potatoes, tomatoes, and whole wheat.

8 VITAMIN B5 (PANTOTHENIC ACID)

Scientists have a feeling that pantothenic acid is responsible for many more essential functions than are currently known. Not that the list of known benefits is anything to scoff at, but there may be more waiting to be discovered. Because deficiencies of this vitamin can only be found in people who are starving, there is no RDI. However, experts believe people need 4 to 10 mg daily for health.

- **Benefits:** The main task of this vitamin is to work with other B vitamins in metabolizing fat, carbohydrates, and protein into energy. It also helps maintain healthy red blood cells, produces hormones, and promotes growth.

- **Natural Sources:** Chicken liver, corn, eggs, lima beans, cooked mushrooms, baked potatoes, and yogurt.

9 VITAMIN B6 (PYRIDOXINE)

Vitamin B6 is another vitamin that has several components. In this case, there are three: pyridoxine, pyridoxamine, and pyridoxal. The first one is found in plant foods, and the other two are found in animal products. Because they all perform the same basic functions, scientists decided to refer to them all as pyridoxine. The RDI is 0.3 to 2 mg for children, 1.6 to 2 mg for adults 25 to 50 years old, and 2 mg for adults over age 50.

- **Benefits:** Pyridoxine is one busy vitamin; it performs more than 60 different functions, including metabolizing protein for energy and converting tryptophan into niacin. It also ensures healthy functioning of the brain, helps produce red blood cells, eliminates excess water from the body, and maintains a healthy immune system. Some people use B6 supplements to treat water retention, muscle spasms, and leg cramps.

- **Natural Sources:** Avocados, bananas, brewer's yeast, brussel sprouts, cantaloupe, some cereals, eggs, grapefruit, halibut, milk, molasses, peanuts, baked potatoes, and spinach.

10 VITAMIN B12 (COBALAMIN, CYANOCOBALAMIN)

Vitamin B12 deficiency is most often associated with anemia, a condition in which there is a reduction in the number of red blood cells, the ones that are supposed to carry oxygen to all parts of your body. Elderly people and individuals with some digestive disorders have difficulty absorbing B12 properly, and may experience vitamin B12-deficiency anemia. People who do not eat animal foods (vegetarians and vegans), which are the primary source of dietary B12, also may be susceptible to anemia. All of these groups may benefit from B12 supplements.

- **Benefits:** Vitamin B12 plays a major role in cell formation, digestion, food absorption, protein synthesis, and the metabolism of carbohydrates and fats; it also helps prevent nerve damage.

- **Natural Sources:** Cheese, eggs, kidney, liver, mackerel, milk, tofu, and fortified cereals and soy products.

11 BIOTIN

Biotin is another vitamin that is produced in the body—bacteria manufacture it in your intestinal tract—although you also get it in your food. When food reaches the intestines, biotin acts on the carbohydrates, fats, and protein to help make them usable by the body. The RDI for children is 100 to 300 mcg; for adults it is 300 mcg.

- **Benefits:** Biotin plays a vital role in maintaining healthy skin and hair, and it enhances sensitivity to insulin, which makes it important for people with diabetes.

- **Natural Sources:** The two foods richest in biotin—brewer's yeast and beef liver—are not popular with most people; but plenty of other foods contain a fair amount, including bananas, cheese, milk, oatmeal, peanut butter, rice, soybeans, and whole wheat flour.

12 FOLIC ACID

Also known as folate, this B vitamin was the focus of much interest in the 1980s and 1990s, when researchers learned that it plays a critical role in the development of normal genetic factors in babies, and thus may help prevent birth defects. In 1992, the U.S. Public Health Service recommended that all women of childbearing age consume 400 mcg of folic acid daily. The Food and Drug Administration followed suit in 1996, when it required that folic acid be added to specific flours, breads, and other grains. The FDA also allowed manufacturers to make claims on the labels of these products that adequate intake may reduce the risk of neural tube defects. The RDI for children is 50 to 150 mcg; for adults, it is 180 to 200 mcg.

- **Benefits:** In addition to its "genetic duties," folic acid helps red blood cells form, synthesizes proteins, works with vitamin B12 to metabolize amino acids and sugar, helps proper functioning of neurotransmitters, helps keep the female reproductive system healthy, and prevents arteries from clogging. Researchers have found that folic acid, along with vitamins B12 and B6, can help reduce high levels of homocysteine, a naturally occurring substance in the body that has been linked with heart problems and osteoporosis.

- **Natural Sources:** Dark green leafy vegetables (e.g., kale, spinach, endive, and collard greens) and beans (e.g., soy, peas, lentils, and garbanzo) are rich sources of folic acid. Other good sources include apricots, asparagus, barley, broccoli, cantaloupe, carrots, rice, sprouts, and wheat germ.

13 VITAMIN C (ASCORBIC ACID)

Vitamin C is a powerful antioxidant that plays a great many roles in the body, as you can see from the list of benefits. Research indicates that it has an even greater antioxidant effect on the body when it works along with another antioxidant, vitamin E.

- **Benefits:** Ascorbic acid is required for tissue growth and repair, healthy gums, adrenal gland function, wound healing, and the production of anti-stress hormones. Vitamin C also helps protect against cancer and infections, boosts the immune system, and is needed in the metabolism of folic acid.

- **Natural Sources:** Green vegetables, berries, and citrus fruits, including asparagus, avocados, beet greens, broccoli, cantaloupe, grapefruit, kale, lemons, mangos, onions, oranges, papayas, parsley, green peas, sweet peppers, pineapple, radishes, spinach, strawberries, Swiss chard, tomatoes, and watercress.

Not Quite Essential . . .
But Still Very Important

These vitamins are termed nonessential because no specific diseases have been found to be related to a diet deficient in them. Still, you wouldn't want to be without them. Some experts believe they will be added to the essential vitamin list someday.

CHOLINE

Choline is another member of the B vitamin family. Its most important function is in the field of communication: It manufactures a neurotransmitter called acetylcholine, which is the messenger that transmits information about behavior and emotions. Without acetylcholine, the messages in your brain would get mixed up . . . and so would you.

A minute amount of choline is found in many foods, but the best source of choline is lecithin (phosphatidyl choline). Good vegetables sources of lecithin include cabbage, cauliflower, chick peas, green beans, lentils, rice, soybeans, and split peas. Lecithin is also found in egg yolk, liver, and milk.

INOSITOL

Inositol is sometimes referred to as Vitamin B8. It is a fat-like substance that helps prevent hardening of the arteries and plays a role in the metabolism of cholesterol and fats. Inositol also assists in removing fat from the liver, is essential for hair growth, and is important in the formation of lecithin. It is found in beans, cantaloupe, nuts, oranges, wheat, and wheat bran.

chapter five

Mining the Top Minerals:
16 "Finds"

Four elements make up 96 percent of the human body: oxygen, hydrogen, carbon, and nitrogen. The remaining 4 percent is composed of minerals. Four percent may not sound like a lot, but without minerals, you could not live. They're the catalysts nature provides to start up most of the biochemical reactions that take place in the human body. Without them, your body would behave like a light bulb that has no tungsten filament: It simply wouldn't work.

Meet Your Minerals

Minerals are classified as either macro (bulk) or micro (trace). Macro minerals are needed in larger amounts than trace minerals, but both groups are essential for life.

When you consume minerals, the blood delivers them to cells to perform specific chemical tasks. But not all of the minerals get into cells. That's because minerals are very competitive: They compete with each other for absorption. So it's important to balance the minerals you take in. For example, the effective and proper balance of calcium and magnesium is a 2:1 ratio; put another way, you should take in twice as much calcium as magnesium.

If you choose to take mineral supplements, experts generally recommend a chelated form. *Chelated* means the mineral is attached to a protein molecule, which improves its absorption by the body. When you consume minerals in your food, the digestive tract provides the ingredients necessary for absorption.

Managing Minerals

The Food and Nutrition Board of the National Academy of Sciences determines the Reference Dietary Intake (RDI) for each nutrient people need to consume to maintain basic health. The RDI has replaced the Recommended Dietary Allowance (RDA) designation. Scientists have not been able to determine the RDI for some nutrients; for these, they use two other designations: Adequate Intake (AI) and Estimated Minimum Daily Requirement (EMDR).

6 Macro Minerals

1 *Calcium*

Functions: Calcium, the most abundant mineral in the human body, is critical for the growth and maintenance of bones and teeth. Without calcium, the heart would not beat, the blood would not clot properly, and the nervous system would not function correctly. Adequate levels of calcium help prevent rickets in children and osteoporosis in adults, and keep blood pressure normal.

Natural Sources: Dark green leafy vegetables, tofu, dairy products, fortified soy products, almonds, and salmon.

RDI: For pregnant women and young adults, 1,300 mg; for adults aged 19 to 65, 1,000 mg; for those over 65, 1,200 mg.

2 *Magnesium*

Functions: Magnesium is calcium's sidekick when it comes to bones, and a proper balance of each mineral is needed to maintain healthy bones and teeth. Magnesium and calcium also work together to regulate muscle activity. Metabolism also depends on magnesium for converting food into energy, and adequate levels of magnesium are needed to help ensure a healthy cardiovascular system.

Natural Sources: Green leafy vegetables, nuts, seeds, whole grains, and milk.

RDI: Men, 350 mg; women, 280 mg; pregnant women, 320 mg.

3 *Phosphorus*

Functions: Phosphorus is the second most abundant mineral in the body. Like calcium, it is found primarily in bones and teeth. Its other roles are to stimulate muscle contraction; promote tissue growth and repair; and help with energy production, heart and kidney function, and transmission of nerve signals.

Natural Sources: Phosphorus is found in most foods, but especially in nuts, whole grains, poultry, eggs, and soft drinks.

RDI: Adults older than 25 years, 800 mg; young adults and pregnant women, 1,200 mg.

4 *Potassium*

Functions: Potassium comes in third behind calcium and phosphorus, but it works most closely with sodium and chloride to maintain the body's distribution of fluids and pH balance. It also plays major roles in muscle contraction, regulation of blood pressure and heart beat, protein synthesis, metabolism of carbohydrates, insulin secretion, and the transmission of nerve impulses.

Natural Sources: Raw vegetables and fruits (especially citrus, bananas, and avocados), potatoes, and lean meat.

EMDR: For adults, 2,000 mg.

5 *Sodium*

Functions: Along with potassium and chloride, sodium helps maintain pH balance and fluid distribution in the body. That's one reason why sodium is found in all the bodily fluids, including tears, blood, urine, and perspiration.

Natural Sources: Most Americans get the majority of their sodium from table salt, followed by processed foods and soft drinks.

EMDR: Although the daily EMDR is 500 mg, most Americans consume at least four times that amount.

6 *Chloride*

Functions: Chloride is the natural salt of the mineral chlorine. It works along with potassium and sodium to help maintain levels and distribution of bodily fluids and to promote healthy muscle and nerve function. Alone, chloride helps the digestive process as a key ingredient in hydrochloric acid, one of the juices in the stomach that help digest food.

Natural Sources: Whole, unprocessed foods contain more than enough chloride. Unfortunately, most people consume too much salt because they eat a diet of mainly processed foods, which have added salt, and therefore chloride.

EMDR: 750 mg for adults.

MICRO MINERALS

A minute amount goes a long way: That should be your motto where trace minerals are concerned. In fact, your entire body should contain less than a teaspoon of each of the minerals in the list below. There are no RDIs for most trace minerals, because there are no known deficiencies of them; however, experts have designated safe, recommended amounts.

7 Chromium

Functions: Chromium works with insulin to regulate the body's blood sugar levels, and it plays a major role in the metabolism of fatty acids. It may also help reduce the risk of cardiovascular disease.

Natural Sources: Brewer's yeast, molasses, liver, poultry, eggs, whole grains, and cheese.

EMDR: 50 to 200 mcg for adults.

8 Copper

Functions: Copper is important for many blood functions, such as production of hemoglobin, absorption of iron so the red blood cells can carry oxygen to the tissues, and regulation of blood pressure and heartbeat. It also promotes fertility; strengthens bones, tendons, nerves, and blood vessels; and helps promote normal pigmentation of the skin and hair.

Natural Sources: Blackstrap molasses, green vegetables, black pepper, nuts, seeds, and seafood. Water that is transported through copper pipes provides copper as well.

EMDR: 0.4 to 2.5 mg for children; 1.5 to 3 mg for adults.

9 *Fluoride*

Functions: Fluoride is the natural form of fluorine and is critical for healthy bones and teeth. Beginning in the 1950s, fluoride was added to the water supplies in many U.S. cities, and this practice has been credited with reducing tooth decay by up to 70 percent.

Natural Sources: Seaweed, seafood, cheese, tea, and meat.

EMDR: Adults, 1.5 to 4 mg.

10 *Iodine*

Functions: Iodine is a component of several hormones produced by the thyroid, and it plays a major role in nutrient metabolism. It is also important in muscle and nerve function, mental development, and the maintenance of healthy nails, hair, skin, and teeth.

Natural Sources: Iodized table salt provides much of the iodine people need; other sources are seafood, kelp, and vegetables grown in iodine-rich soil.

RDI: 150 mcg for adults; 175 mcg for pregnant women.

11 *Iron*

Functions: Iron is found in hemoglobin in red blood cells, where it transports oxygen to body tissues from the lungs. It is also found in myoglobin, a protein that provides energy to muscles during exercise.

Natural Sources: Iron can come from two main sources: animal products (heme iron—poultry, red meat, seafood) and plant foods (nonheme iron—dark green vegetables, whole grains, nuts, dried fruit). Although the body is better able to absorb heme iron, it can also absorb nonheme iron when plant foods containing iron are eaten along with foods rich in vitamin C.

RDI: For adults, 10 mg; for premenopausal women, 15 mg; for pregnant women, 30 mg.

12 *Manganese*

Functions: This trace mineral is important for the proper formation and maintenance of cartilage, connective tissue, and bone. It also helps with the synthesis of genetic material and proteins, and assists with blood clotting.

Natural Sources: Bananas, bran, brown rice, beans, peas, whole grains, strawberries, and orange juice.

EMDR: 2.5 to 5 mg for adults.

13 *Molybdenum*

Functions: Makes an enzyme called xanthine oxidase, which allows the body to grow and develop properly; helps the body utilize iron; and breaks down carbohydrates, protein, and fat to be used for energy.

Natural Sources: Dark green leafy vegetables, eggs, lentils, macaroni, rice, sunflower seeds, and whole grains.

RDI: For children, 15 to 250 mcg; for adults, 75 to 250 mcg.

14 *Selenium*

Functions: This antioxidant protects tissues and cells from free-radical damage and appears to help rid the body of toxins such as mercury and arsenic. Some researchers say it fights arthritis, heart disease, and cancer.

Natural Sources: Asparagus, garlic, eggs, whole grains, and mushrooms.

RDI: For men, 70 mcg; for women, 55 mcg; for pregnant women, 65 mcg.

15 *Sulfur*

Functions: Sulfur is found in every cell in the body, and is especially plentiful in protein-rich tissues such as hair, muscle, skin, and nails. This mineral makes up 10 percent of the body's mineral content. It plays a role in metabolism, helps regulate blood sugar levels, converts toxins into nontoxic substances that can be excreted from the body, and assists in blood clotting.

Natural Sources: Sulfur is found primarily in protein foods such as beans, peas, meat, poultry, eggs, and dairy.

RDI: Even though sulfur is found throughout the body and is an essential mineral, experts have not yet determined a Reference Dietary Intake for it. Therefore, its placement in the micro mineral category is questioned by some experts and accepted by others.

16 *Zinc*

Functions: Zinc is necessary for the synthesis of the genetic materials DNA and RNA. This mineral also assists in bone development and growth, energy metabolism, wound healing, immune function, cell respiration, and the ability of the liver to rid the body of toxic substances. Zinc appears to improve short-term memory, enhance taste, and promote healthy hair and skin.

Natural Sources: Soybeans, seafood, lean meat, eggs, peanuts, and wheat bran.

RDI: For adults, 15 mg; for pregnant women, 30 mg.

chapter six

43 Alternative Supplements: The Best (and a Few Not So Great) Natural Pharmaceuticals

Nutritional supplements are a hot item. Lots of people take them. Unfortunately, few people know much about them.

As researchers look more and more deeply into the biochemistry of nutritional supplements, they're gradually learning what these substances can and cannot do for our health. In the meantime, companies that manufacture them bombard us with countless claims, some of them unsubstantiated, about the wonders of their products. Fortunately, in the vast majority of cases, there is at least a thread or two of truth to the claims. Your task as a consumer is to find those threads and follow them to better health.

In the interest of helping you do just that, here is a list of the most popular natural supplements on the market today and what they are used for. The list does not include vitamins, minerals, herbs, or homeopathic remedies; entries describing these items can be found elsewhere in this book. Here, you'll find substances such as enzymes, amino acids, oils, hormones, and food fiber.

While vitamins and minerals have Recommended Daily Intake (RDI) figures assigned to them by the Food and Nutrition Board, the natural supplements listed here do not, because scientists have not determined whether they are essential enough to human health to warrant an RDI. The typical dosage given merely reflects commonly prescribed use. **Consult a naturopath or other qualified professional before taking any of these supplements.**

Words to Know

Amino acids: Proteins that the body uses to build cells. There are 22 amino acids.

Essential amino acid: An amino acid the body can only get from food or supplements.

Nonessential amino acid: An amino acid that the body can create itself from essential amino acids.

Antioxidants: Nutrients that fight and help eliminate free radicals—harmful molecules that are believed to contribute to serious diseases such as cancer and to play a major role in aging.

1 5-HTP. The body produces 5-HTP from the amino acid tryptophan. 5-HTP is a chemical precursor (something that precedes something else) of the neurotransmitter serotonin. The supplement 5-HTP is derived from a plant called *Griffonia simplicifolia*, which grows in Africa. 5-HTP is used to treat depression and to help with weight loss.

Typical dosage: 50 to 100 mg up to three times daily.

2 Acidophilus. Acidophilus are "good" bacteria that live primarily in the intestines, where they help keep that environment free of disease-causing organisms. Acidophilus combat yeast infections, urinary tract infections, and digestive disorders, and are helpful in lowering cholesterol, reducing the odds of getting breast cancer, promoting healthy skin, and decreasing constipation and gas. Available in both liquid and capsule form.

Typical dosage: two 500 mg capsules three times daily with food.

3 Alpha-lipoic acid. In 1957, researchers isolated a substance they called alpha-lipoic acid, a coenzyme and a powerful antioxidant that supports the functions of vitamins C and E. In Germany, it is a common medical treatment for peripheral neuropathy, often a complication of diabetes. Available in 50 mg capsules.

Typical dosage: from 100 to 600 mg daily.

4 **Apple cider vinegar.** You can put it on your salad or just take it by the teaspoon, say supporters of apple cider vinegar who use it as a supplement and weight loss aid. Apple cider vinegar reportedly suppresses the appetite, stimulates metabolism, and boosts the immune system. However, there are no reliable scientific studies to support these claims.

Typical dosage: 2 teaspoonfuls in the morning with breakfast.

5 **Apple pectin.** Apple pectin is a water-soluble fiber that helps suppress the appetite and lower cholesterol levels, and may inhibit the spread of cancer. Available as a powder or in capsules.

Typical dosage: 1 teaspoon powder three times daily or 1 to 3 capsules with meals.

6 **Arginine.** Arginine is a nonessential amino acid, which means the body is capable of producing it on its own. The main reason people take arginine is to boost the immune system. Arginine does this by making lymphocytes, a type of cell that fights infections. Recent research also suggests that arginine can increase blood flow in peripheral blood vessels, thus promoting healthy circulation. Arginine may also help slow tumor growth, detoxify the liver, prevent loss of muscle after injury or surgery, and accelerate the healing of wounds. This supplement is not recommended for children, because it can affect their growth. Arginine is available in capsules.

Typical dosage: one 100 mg capsule up to three times daily. Promoting better circulation requires a higher dose, up to 3 grams a day.

7 **Bee pollen.** One of the secret recipes of nature is bee pollen, which consists of pollen plus unknown ingredients added by the bees that collect it. Bee pollen is viewed as a complete food because it contains 22 amino acids, 27 minerals, and all vitamins. Supplements are used to treat allergies, viral infections, chronic fatigue, and headache, and to improve concentration. The U.S. Department of Agriculture suggests that bee pollen is helpful in fighting cancer.

Typical dosage: ¼ to ½ teaspoon once a day; more when treating specific conditions.

8 **Beta glucans.** Beta glucans are the fiber components of oats and barley and are credited with lowering cholesterol, enhancing the immune system, and helping prevent and treat cancer. Although there is evidence that beta glucans are helpful when they are given via injection, there is little evidence to support their effectiveness when taken orally.

Typical dosage: 60 to 120 mg daily.

9 **Bioflavonoids.** These nutrients, which are sometimes referred to as flavonoids or vitamin P, include a large group of substances that Western researchers have not yet determined to be as important as vitamins. But that doesn't mean they don't perform important functions in health. Bioflavonoids play a major role in strengthening capillaries and connective tissues, preventing viral infections, and improving eyesight, and they may help prevent prostate and lung cancer. Because there are many different bioflavonoids and the dosages vary by the compound, always consult a professional before taking them.

10 **Blue-green algae.** Are you ready to open wide and swallow some pond scum? Some people call this scum "brain food," because blue-green algae reportedly is rich in protein, vitamin B12, amino acids, minerals, chlorophyll, and other essential nutrients that the brain needs to function at its best. But not everyone agrees with this claim. In fact, some experts say that blue-green algae can cause nausea, vomiting, and weakness. Blue-green algae supplements come in capsules and are not recommended for children.

Typical dosage: up to four 250 mg capsules daily between meals for adults.

11 **Boswellia.** The boswellia tree, which grows in Somalia and Saudi Arabia, produces a resin that is used for its anti-inflammatory abilities. You may know boswellia resin better as frankincense. Boswellia is used to treat arthritis and ulcerative colitis and appears to boost the immune system.

Typical dosage: 350 mg three times daily.

12 **Brewer's yeast.** It's bitter, it looks unappetizing, and it's good for you. Brewer's yeast is an excellent source of the B vitamins, which are essential for a healthy immune system, a healthy heart, and high energy levels. It also supplies chromium, which helps regulate blood sugar levels; selenium, which enhances the benefits of antioxidants; and nucleic acid, which helps fight bacterial and fungal infections. If you want to enjoy the benefits of brewer's yeast, you can either add it to foods that disguise the taste or take it in capsule form.

Typical dosage: 1 to 3 teaspoons of powder or flakes daily or one 100 mg capsule up to three times daily.

13 **Bromelain.** Pineapples are the main source of bromelain, an enzyme that helps the body absorb nutrients. Some people with arthritis take a bromelain supplement because it acts as an anti-inflammatory and is reputed to be very effective at reducing swelling and pain. An article in *Neurology* reports that bromelain helps prevent blood clots, which can cause heart attack and stroke; and it can also help reduce high blood pressure, menstrual cramps, varicose veins, and carpal tunnel syndrome. Bromelain is not recommended for children.

Typical dosage: one 100 mg capsule up to three times daily or 3 drops tincture in 8 ounces of water three times daily.

14 **Carnitine.** When two essential amino acids—methionine and lysine—come together, they create the nonessential amino acid carnitine. And it's a good thing these two amino acids hook up, because carnitine is important in keeping the heart and circulatory system working properly. Carnitine also helps reduce cholesterol levels and plays a role in energy production.

Typical dosage: 2 to 6 grams daily.

15 **Cernitin.** This little-known supplement can play an important role in reducing an enlarged prostate. Cernitin is an extract of flower pollen that must be processed in a special way to retain its effectiveness. It is reportedly as effective as prescription drugs used to treat enlarged prostate, or benign prostatic hyperplasia.

Typical dosage: two 6.3 mg tablets up to three times daily.

16 **Cetyl myristoleate.** In 1971, researchers discovered a new fatty acid and named it cetyl myristoleate, or CMO. This oily substance is found in cattle, beavers, mice, and whales. It reportedly helps relieve symptoms of osteoarthritis and rheumatoid arthritis, although there is little evidence to support this claim. Available in capsules.

Typical dosage: Take according to package directions.

17 **Chitosan.** This supplement is a fiber product derived from the skeletons of marine animals, such as oysters and other shellfish. It was originally used to soak up grease, oil, and other toxic substances from liquid before it became popular as a weight-loss aid. Its effectiveness in this latter category is hotly disputed by many experts.

Typical dosage: 1 gram 30 minutes before or with lunch or dinner, along with 8 ounces of water.

18 **Chlorophyll.** The green pigment known as chlorophyll does more than keep our world green. When it comes to human health, chlorophyll is an antibacterial and an anti-inflammatory. Chlorophyll is used to promote wound healing, promote new tissue growth, relieve gas and bloating, and prevent gallstones. Perhaps chlorophyll is best known for its ability to eliminate bad breath.

Typical dosage: 1 teaspoon powder or three 100 mg tablets after each meal.

19 **Chondroitin.** According to Jason Theodosakis, M.D., author of *The Arthritis Cure*, chondroitin supplements can greatly benefit people who have osteoarthritis. The best benefits result from combining chondroitin with another natural substance, glucosamine (see number 28). Chondroitin is a substance found naturally in the body, where it helps maintain the integrity and elasticity of connective tissue, blood vessel walls, and other tissues. It does this by attracting water to cartilage, which acts as a shock absorber in the joints and promotes mobility. It also inhibits the activity of enzymes that destroy cartilage.

Typical dosage: Chondroitin is often taken along with glucosamine at a ratio of 5:4 (glucosamine:chondroitin). The dosage depends on your weight. If you weigh less than 120 pounds, the dosage of chondroitin is 800 mg; 120 to 200 pounds, 1,200 mg; and more than 200 pounds, 1,600 mg.

20 **Cod liver oil.** Just hearing the words "cod liver oil" makes some people cringe, especially those who have been subjected to endless spoonfuls of the fish oil. Cod liver oil contains essential fatty acids, which can strengthen cell membranes, prevent clogged arteries, lower high blood pressure, relieve the stiffness and swelling of rheumatoid arthritis, and reduce cholesterol. Cod liver oil is also high in vitamins A and D.

Typical dosage: one capsule up to three times daily, or 1 to 2 tablespoons daily.

21 **Coenzyme Q10.** Discovered in 1957, coenzyme Q10 (CoQ10) is a substance found naturally in the body. Although it is found throughout the body, it is most concentrated in the heart. CoQ10 is an antioxidant and a coenzyme, which means it assists enzymes in their functions. CoQ10 is taken as a supplement by people who have heart disease, diabetes, gum disease, poor circulation, and multiple sclerosis. It is also credited with raising energy levels, helping with weight loss, and increasing endurance.

Typical dosage: 30 to 60 mg three times a day.

22   **Creatine.** Creatine monohydrate is a naturally occurring chemical that provides fuel to the body's muscles and helps them contract, especially for concentrated, short-term activity. That's what makes this supplement a favorite of bodybuilders. It is a highly controversial supplement, as many experts say that it's ineffective in helping people make significant gains in strength or in building lean muscle, and it may actually be harmful, because it interferes with the body's ability to sweat.

Typical dosage: 5 grams four times a day for up to six days, then 2 to 5 grams daily.

23   **DHA.** Docosahexaenoic acid, or DHA, is an oil derived from fish or algae that reportedly boosts mental functioning and helps prevent blood clots, which can lead to heart attack and stroke. DHA is the most abundant fat in the brain and is essential for brain and eye development and function. It may help prevent heart disease and lower cholesterol levels.

Typical dosage: 500 to 3,000 mg daily in divided doses.

24   **DHEA.** Dehydroepiandrosterone, or DHEA, is a hormone secreted by the adrenal glands. With age, the body produces less and less DHEA, which is one reason why researchers believe people older than 40 may benefit from DHEA supplements. Why? DHEA is credited with reducing susceptibility to disease, helping poor memory, treating diabetes, preventing muscle loss, relieving depression, and boosting energy.

Typical dosage: Available in capsules, liquid, and tablets, it should be taken only under the supervision of a physician.

25   **Evening primrose oil.** Many women are familiar with this supplement, as it is highly recommended for premenstrual syndrome (PMS). Evening primrose oil is pressed from the seeds of the evening primrose plant. The oil contains gamma linoleic acid, an essential fatty acid that reduces inflammation of the uterus and lowers cholesterol and blood pressure levels.

Typical dosage: for PMS, two 500 mg capsules two to three times daily. You can also apply the oil to your skin to treat eczema.

26   **Flaxseed oil.** Many experts suggest taking flaxseed oil daily, as it helps fight bacteria, fungi, and viruses; regulates hormone levels; fights cancer; and reduces heart problems. Women who are experiencing menopausal symptoms can find great relief in flaxseed oil supplements.

Typical dosage: up to three 1,000 mg capsules or 2 tablespoonfuls of oil daily.

27   **Glucomannan.** This fiber supplement is often used by people who are trying to lose weight, because it creates a feeling of fullness. Glucomannan is extracted from the konnyaku root and is a good source of beta-carotene, minerals, and thiamin. It is also credited with helping prevent buildup of plaque in blood vessels.

Typical dosage: two to three capsules (450 to 665 mg each) before meals.

28   **Glucosamine.** Glucosamine sulfate is a substance that occurs naturally in the body. It is a major ingredient in the synovial fluid, which cushions the joints, and it also helps hold tissue cells together. Glucosamine, along with chondroitin, is a popular treatment for arthritis. It promotes the body's ability to supply the materials needed to replace aging tissues and is believed to repair damaged joints in some people.

Typical dosage: Glucosamine is taken according to body weight. If you weigh less than 120 pounds, the dosage is 1,000 mg; 120 to 200 pounds, 1,500 mg; and more than 200 pounds, 2,000 mg.

29   **Guggal.** Also spelled *gugal* and *guggul*, this resin from a tree found in India is especially popular in Ayurvedic medicine. While Ayurvedic doctors have long used it to cleanse the blood vessels and joints, it is now popular in the U.S. for lowering cholesterol and triglyceride levels. Guggal also stimulates the thyroid gland and protects the heart.

Typical dosage: one 500 mg tablet three times daily.

30   **Ipriflavone.** The soybean is the origin of this bioflavonoid, which is used to help promote bone strength, especially for people at risk of osteoporosis. It reportedly helps conserve and improve bone density by stimulating osteoblast cells, which build bone. Available in tablets and capsules.

Typical dosage: up to 1,800 mg daily in divided doses.

31   **Kelp.** Kelp is a type of seaweed. Maybe you can't imagine eating seaweed, yet it is a common item on Eastern tables and is highly nutritious. Because kelp is especially rich in iodine, kelp supplements are used to treat individuals who have thyroid problems. The thyroid uses iodine to help it regulate the body's development. Kelp is also rich in the B vitamins and other nutrients. Available in capsules.

Typical dosage: 600 to 700 mg daily.

32 Lutein. Lutein is a plant nutrient (in the category "carotenoid") found in fruits and vegetables. It is an antioxidant that is important for eye health, as it helps protect the macula in the eye from free-radical damage.

Typical dosage: 6 mg per day.

33 Lysine. The essential amino acid lysine is manufactured in the body and then works with other amino acids to produce hormones, antibodies, and enzymes; promote healing of damaged tissue; encourage bone growth; and assist in the formation of collagen, which is a vital ingredient in bone, ligaments, skin, and cartilage. Lysine also helps treat the cold sores, canker sores, and genital sores associated with herpes. Supplements of lysine also appear to help people who have angina or high blood pressure.

Typical dosage: one 1,500 mg capsule up to three times daily.

34 Melatonin. Melatonin is a hormone produced by the pineal gland. At about age 40, the body's production of melatonin declines significantly, which leads researchers to believe that supplements are needed. Melatonin is used to promote sleep, boost the immune system, improve sex, and slow down aging. It is often touted as an aid for people who work nights or suffer from jet lag.

Typical dosage: 1 to 3 mg daily.

35 MSM. Methylsulfonylmethane, or MSM, is a fancy name for organic sulfur. MSM is found naturally in the body and in all living things, although in very small amounts. Supplements of MSM help relieve the pain, stiffness, and inflammation associated with arthritis, and also help treat heartburn, allergies, asthma, and digestive disorders. Because MSM improves cells' ability to allow nutrients in and to eliminate toxins, it is also used as a detoxifier.

Typical dosage: Can vary considerably; 800 to 3,000 mg daily is common.

36 NADH. Nicotinamide adenine dinucleotide, or NADH, is a coenzyme found naturally in the body. The body uses NADH for the metabolism of proteins, sugars, and fats. As a supplement, NADH can treat depression and fatigue, and there have been some successful studies of its use in Parkinson's disease.

Typical dosage: 10 mg daily.

37 **Phenylalanine.** This amino acid is used to make another amino acid, tyrosine, which then works with phenylalanine to produce brain chemicals such as dopamine and epinephrine. Phenylalanine supplements are used to relieve depression, improve mental alertness, and increase memory retention.

Typical dosage: one 100 mg capsule up to three times daily.

38 **Phosphatidylserine.** If you're having trouble remembering things, phosphatidylserine (PS) may help. You already have PS in your brain, where it helps cells to transmit messages to each other. Supplementing with PS may help aging cell membranes to continue sending messages efficiently and effectively. It is believed to improve memory capacity and help prevent memory loss, even in people with Alzheimer's disease.

Typical dosage: one 100 mg tablet up to three times daily with food.

39 **Red yeast rice.** Red yeast rice is a fermented product in which yeast is grown on white rice. Once the rice has fermented, the yeast is killed and the rice is pulverized. Numerous studies in humans have shown that red yeast rice significantly lowers cholesterol and triglyceride levels as well as or better than prescription drugs, including Lovastatin.

Typical dosage: Use only under a doctor's supervision.

40 **Royal jelly.** The milky fluid produced by worker bees for the queen bee is called royal jelly. This highly nutritious food contains nearly all the B vitamins and amino acids and is an excellent source of calcium, iron, magnesium, and other minerals. It is also believed to help stimulate the adrenal glands, increase energy, relieve the stiffness and pain of arthritis, alleviate menopause symptoms, and act as an antibiotic. Although none of these claims has been proven scientifically, anecdotal reports keep this supplement popular.

Typical dosage: one 100 mg capsule up to three times daily.

41 **SAM-e.** S-adenolyl-methionine, or SAM-e, is produced naturally in the body, where it is involved in dozens of biological reactions. SAM-e supplements are used to treat depression, osteoarthritis, and liver disease. It reportedly can speed up the body's response to other medications or herbs.

Typical dosage: Depends on the condition being treated. For osteoarthritis, for example, the beginning dosage may be 1,600 mg daily, then reduced to 800 mg when improvement is evident.

42 **Soy.** If you're looking for a source of complete protein, a way to treat osteoporosis, or an effective remedy for symptoms of menopause, turn to the beans: soybeans, that is. Soy also contains nonnutritive substances that fight cancer, including isoflavones, which are considered helpful in preventing breast and prostate cancers, and protease inhibitors, which block enzymes that cause cancer. Although there are plenty of soy-based foods on the market, some people prefer to take a soy supplement in addition to eating those foods or in place of them. Soy powders are available.

Typical dosage: 20 to 50 grams per day.

43 **Trimethylglycine.** This naturally occurring substance is used by the body to lower homocysteine levels (high levels have been linked with heart disease). Supplements of trimethylglycine (TMG) are used for this purpose, as well as for treating depression. TMG is a precursor to SAM-e (see number 41) and can be used along with SAM-e to treat liver disorders. Available in capsules and tablets.

Typical dosage: Varies widely, from 375 to 2,000 mg daily in divided doses.

chapter seven

30 Ingredients for Home First Aid Kits

If a child cut himself while playing in your home, would you be able to quickly put your hands on everything you need to attend to the wound? If someone accidentally ingested a poisonous substance she found under your bathroom sink, would you have immediate access to the emergency telephone numbers you need and the antidotes for the poison?

When an emergency strikes, you need to think and respond fast. A well-stocked, easily accessible first aid kit can help you respond quickly and effectively to common medical emergencies at home.

When assembling a home first aid kit, choose a sturdy, waterproof, lightweight container with a secure lid and handle. Plastic fishing tackle boxes and plastic toolboxes are popular choices. The kit should be stored in a dry, cool place, away from young children and pets.

All adults and older children in the house should know where the box is located and how to use its contents. Ideally, every adult and older child should take a basic first aid course, such as those offered by the American Red Cross. Other community organizations and some hospitals also provide classes for the public.

Once you have the box picked out, here's what to put in it.

1 Adhesive bandages, several sizes

2 Adhesive tape

3 Triangular bandage

4 Butterfly bandage

5 Elastic bandages

6 Sterile gauze pads

7 Sterile gauze rolls

8 Sterile cotton balls

9 Sterile eye patches

10 Disposable sterile gloves or rubber gloves

11 Tissues

12 Safety pins

13 Tweezers

14 Scissors with rounded tips

15 Instant-activating cold packs

16 Medicine spoon

17 Bulb syringe

18 Candle and matches

19 Flashlight

20 Disposable face masks

21 Paper cups

22 Aspirin, ibuprofen, and acetaminophen

23 Syrup of ipecac (Use this only with the advice of a poison control center or doctor.)

24 Activated charcoal (inactivates poisons)

25 Antibiotic cream

26 Diphenhydramine (Benadryl)

27 Calamine lotion

28 A comprehensive, easy-to-follow first aid book

29 A list of emergency telephone numbers for the doctor, police, fire department, poison control center, and ambulance service

30 An epinephrine kit if anyone in your family is allergic to insect bites and stings or to certain foods, such as shellfish or peanuts

Are You Ready for a Medical Emergency?

- Know how to get to the nearest hospital emergency department or urgent care clinic if you should need to drive yourself or a victim.

- Keep a current list of any medications you and family members are taking. Keep it in a place that is easily accessible and known to all family members so it can be found for reference by emergency medical technicians, nurses, and doctors.

- Anyone in your family who has a chronic medical condition or severe allergy to medications should wear a medical emergency ID necklace or bracelet or carry a medical emergency card.

- Learn CPR and the Heimlich maneuver.

The American Red Cross provides first aid training and instruction in CPR (cardiopulmonary resuscitation) and the Heimlich maneuver. Check the yellow pages for the chapter nearest you. Also see their Web site: www.redcross.org

The National Safety Council offers first aid and CPR classes. Check the yellow pages for your local chapter. Also see their Web site: www.nsc.org

chapter eight

46 At-Home Nursing Aids: The Essentials When You Need to Care for Someone

According to the National Family Caregivers Association, about 54 million people act as caregivers in the United States within a given year. Perhaps you are one of them. You may be a daughter or a son caring for elderly parents, a spouse taking care of your partner, or a friend taking care of a friend. Often these individuals are chronically ill or permanently disabled and need long-term care or constant supervision.

Acting as a caregiver can be a daunting experience, but it doesn't have to be if you are prepared and know where to find help when you need it. We're talking about help for both the patient and you, because you cannot be an effective caregiver if you don't take care of yourself as well.

Here we offer you four lists. One includes basic essentials for everyday care. The second comprises equipment commonly needed by people who are chronically ill or permanently disabled. The third is a collection of helpful hints to make your job as a caregiver a bit easier. Together, these three lists can help you provide a healthy, safe environment for your loved one. The fourth list is just for you: things you can do to help make sure *you* stay healthy.

Essential Items

1 Sterile gauze pads

2 Adhesive tape

3 Band-Aid strips

4 Triple antibiotic ointment

5 Cortisone cream

6 Alcohol swabs

7 Baby powder or cornstarch

8 Hydrogen peroxide

9 Isopropyl alcohol (rubbing alcohol)

10 Syrup of ipecac (used to induce vomiting)

11 Glycerin suppositories

12 Over-the-counter diarrhea medication

13 Over-the-counter antinausea medication

14 Benadryl liquid (for allergic reactions)

15 Unscented premoistened wipes

16 Cotton balls

17 Q-tips

18 Latex gloves

19 Water-based lubricant gel

20 Stool softener

21 Antacids

22 Disinfectant spray

23 Pillbox. Prescription medications should be kept in one place, and dosages put into a pillbox marked off by days and hours.

24 Plastic urinal for male patients

25 Bedpan. Plastic is more "buttock friendly." A metal one can be cold but is more sanitary.

26 Over-the-counter analgesics (acetaminophen, ibuprofen, aspirin)

27 Thermometer, oral or rectal

28 Stethoscope, available from drugstores

29 Blood pressure gauge, available from drugstores

30 Canned nutritional supplements, such as Ensure

31 Sports drinks for replacing electrolytes

32 Gait belt to help unsteady person when walking or to help transfer someone from a bed to a chair or with other transfers

Equipment Needs

33 Hospital bed, electric, with side rails

34 Air mattress (to help prevent bed sores)

35 Bed tray or hospital-type tray

36 Bedside commode, for nighttime or anytime use

37 Wheelchair

38 Cane, regular or tripod

39 Walker, with or without wheels

40 Grab bars in the bathroom—next to the toilet and in the tub; more if needed

41 Handheld shower head

42 Shower bench that sits in the tub or shower

43 Elevated toilet seat, which makes it easier to get down on and up from the toilet

44 Tilt chair that assists people in getting out of the chair

45 Metal trapeze bars hung from the ceiling or from a vertical pole next to the bed. These can help a patient move as well as exercise his or her arms.

46 Long wooden tongs that allow patients to pick up nearby objects

Helpful Hints

- If the patient needs to take a large number of pills, you may want to get a large calender on which you can track the dosages and any reactions. A spiral notebook can also be used for this purpose. You will then have a written record for the doctor.

- If the patient has limited or compromised mobility, make sure all the areas of the house through which he or she will be traveling are free of hazards, such as throw rugs, electrical cords, pet dishes, and toys. Rearrange furniture to eliminate narrow pathways. Don't wax bare floors.

- Make sure there is sufficient lighting in all rooms and hallways. If the patient will be getting up during the night to use the bathroom, put a light next to the bed.

- You can reduce the spread of germs if you remember to wash your hands often. Use liquid soap, lather for 30 seconds, and then rinse. Dry your hands with paper towels. Because lots of hand washing can be rough on your hands, use lotion after you wash to reduce dryness.

- Always keep readily available a list of all the patient's doctors and telephone numbers; a list of emergency numbers (hospital, ambulance, pharmacy, fire department); and a list of medications.

- If you're caring for someone who may wander, keep doors to the outside locked and attach bells to the top so you will hear from another room if the patient tries to get out.

- Consider taking a CPR course. They are offered by the American Red Cross and often by fire departments and local hospitals as well.

- If you sleep in a different room from the patient's and need to "keep your ears open" during the night, get a baby monitoring system, which will allow you to hear if a problem occurs.

- If a wheelchair will be moving into your house, check the width of your doorways, especially the bathrooms, before you bring the wheelchair home. In some homes, the width of the doorways does not allow for a standard wheelchair.

Caring for the Caregiver

- **Take time for yourself.** You cannot be a caregiver twenty-four hours a day, seven days a week, and expect to stay healthy. Have a family member, friend, neighbor, or other dependable individual provide you with some respite for a few hours several times a week, if possible, so you can go out to dinner, see a movie, go shopping, or just spend some quiet time doing what you like to do.

- **Talk about your feelings.** Being a caregiver can be emotionally and mentally draining. Many caregivers find it helpful to attend support group meetings where they can share their feelings with others who are going through the same experience. Look in the yellow pages or contact your doctor or local hospital for a list of support groups in your area.

- **Pay attention to your diet.** Too often, caregivers worry about their patients and forget to eat properly. Talk to your doctor or a nutritionist if you need help in planning a healthful eating and supplement program.

- **Get enough sleep.** Are there times during the day when you can take a quick nap? Don't be ashamed to ask someone to take care of your loved one so you can get some much-needed sleep.

- **Maintain your hobbies and other interests.** You will feel much more fulfilled and less stressed if you continue to do things that you enjoy.

- **Write it down in a journal.** Many people find that writing down their feelings helps them cope with difficult situations and gives them a fresh perspective on life.

- **Socialize.** If you can't get away from your caregiving responsibilities, invite people over to see you. Create social occasions: Have a potluck lunch or a dessert party where everyone brings something. When you can't have company, call a friend on the telephone.

- **Laugh.** It's been shown that laughter is a very effective medicine. Watch comedy shows, rent funny videos, read humorous books, or invite friends over who make you laugh.

chapter nine

54 High-Nutrient Disease Fighters

When Hippocrates said, "Let food be your medicine, and medicine be your food," he couldn't have foreseen the arrival of greasy, fast-food burgers or artery-clogging cheese fries. You can still follow Hippocrates' advice, however, so long as you're careful about *which* foods are your medicines.

Every time you sit down to a home-cooked meal, grab a quick snack, go out to a restaurant with friends, or prepare that special intimate dinner for two, you have the opportunity to do something healthy, disease-fighting, and life-sustaining for your body and mind.

How? By choosing natural, whole foods, or at least foods prepared with minimal processing, many of which have heart-healthy, cancer-fighting, or disease-combating abilities.

Miracle Foods

With so many "miracle" foods from which to choose, you shouldn't have much trouble including some of them at every meal. When preparing these foods, think light. Batter-dipped, deep-fried onion rings and potatoes swimming in butter and cream sauce put a nix on the miracle. Season your foods with herbs, spices, salsa, fat-free tomato sauces, flavored vinegars, fat-free yogurt, and pureed vegetables and fruits.

What Makes a Miracle Food?

What are the special qualities that make a particular food a real health enhancer? More than likely, it contains one or more of the following life-promoting ingredients:

- **Antioxidants:** These include any vitamin, mineral, or other nutrient that fights and prevents the damaging effects of atoms called free radicals. Free radicals are associated with more than 60 serious and life-threatening conditions, including cancer, heart disease, liver disease, respiratory ailments, diabetes, arthritis, ulcers, and blindness.

- **Phytochemicals:** These special nutrients are derived from plants (*phyto* means "plant") and have the potential to enhance health. Perhaps the best-known phytochemical is chlorophyll, the pigment that gives green plants their color. Although researchers have established that vitamins and minerals are necessary for human health, they have not yet learned enough about the hundreds of phytochemicals to make that determination about them. They do know, however, that phytochemicals can make an important contribution to human health. The American Dietetic Association tells consumers that phytochemicals are effective in the prevention and possibly even the treatment of diabetes, cancer, hypertension, osteoporosis, arthritis, bowel dysfunction, and heart disease.

- **Vitamins and minerals:** Both vitamins and minerals are necessary for human life (see Chapters 4 and 5). Some vitamins, such as vitamins C and E, are also antioxidants.

- **Fiber:** Fiber, also called roughage, is the part of vegetables, fruits, grains, and legumes that the body does not digest. Fiber has several critical functions, including helping move stool quickly out of the body, taking with it fats, toxins, and other poisonous materials, including carcinogens. Diets high in fiber are believed to protect against cancer of the colon, mouth, stomach, esophagus, pharynx, and endometrium. When vegetable fibers reach the large intestine, they ferment and produce a substance called butyrate, which has the ability to convert precancerous cells back to normal cells. Fiber comes in two main forms: water-soluble and insoluble. The two types of water-soluble fiber—gums and pectins—are found mostly in seeds, oats, fruits, and vegetables. They bind to substances like cholesterol and bile acids, prevent them from being absorbed, and help eliminate them in the urine. The three types of insoluble fiber—cellulose, lignin, and hemicellulose—are found primarily in whole grains, nuts, fruits, and vegetables. They help move toxins out of the intestinal tract.

1 **Apples:** Contain anticancer substances called phenols and a soluble fiber called pectin.

2 **Apricots:** Dried or fresh, both are good sources of antioxidants and fiber.

3 **Asparagus:** Contains a potent antioxidant called glutathione, which helps fight cancer, cataracts, and heart disease.

4 **Avocados:** One of the few foods that contain monounsaturated fat, the healthy fat. Also an excellent source of the antioxidants glutathione and vitamin C.

5 **Bananas:** This fruit is an excellent source of potassium, and it protects against ulcers, high cholesterol, and stroke.

6 **Barley:** A high-fiber grain that also contains anticancer substances called protease inhibitors.

7 **Beans:** Excellent sources of fiber, protein, and protease inhibitors.

8 **Blueberries:** One cup of blueberries provides 315 percent RDA of vitamin C. Blueberries also help preserve vision, fight bladder infections, and treat diarrhea.

9 **Cantaloupe:** A very rich source of vitamins A and C: one-half melon contains 186 percent RDA for vitamin C and 90 percent for vitamin A.

10 **Carrots:** Carrots contain several anticancer agents, including vitamin A, p-coumaric acid, lycopene, and chloregenic acid.

11 **Celery:** The anticancer agents in celery include phthalides and polyacetylenes.

12 **Chicory:** This member of the daisy family is sometimes called curly endive. Think about adding this green to your salads, as a mere one-half cup contains nearly 50 percent of the RDA for folic acid and about 30 percent of the RDA for vitamins A and C.

13 **Cider vinegar:** This perfect condiment not only contains the benefits of apples but also acts as a disinfectant. Take 1 teaspoon in water before breakfast or during meals in small sips, or use cider vinegar on salads and other vegetables.

14 **Cranberries:** These tiny berries have a track record for the prevention and treatment of urinary tract infections. They also contain a fair amount of fiber and vitamin C.

15 **Cruciferous vegetables:** All of the vegetables in this group contain the anticancer substances sulforaphane and indole-3-carbinol. They include arugula, broccoli, broccoli sprouts, brussels sprouts, cabbage, cauliflower, Chinese cabbage, collards, daikon, kale, kohlrabi, mustard, red radishes, turnips, and watercress.

16 **Currants:** If you can find black currants, a serving of them will give you more than 300 percent of the RDA for vitamin C, while the white and red varieties contain nearly 80 percent.

17 **Eggplant:** Low in fat and high in cancer-fighting terpenes and other phytochemicals.

18 **Figs:** Fiber and cancer-fighting agents can be found in figs.

19 **Flaxseed:** The fiber lignan in flaxseed appears to fight tumors of the breast, prostate, colon, and rectum.

20 **Garlic:** Researchers have found more than 30 cancer-fighting substances in garlic. Garlic also helps lower blood pressure and improves blood circulation.

21 **Ginger:** Ginger has been used as a medicine and a food for more than 2,000 years. Research shows that ginger helps prevent heart attacks by thinning the blood and prevents nausea and motion sickness. There is also increasing evidence that it is helpful in the treatment of arthritis, gas, heartburn, and migraine.

22 **Grapes:** Ellagic acid, a substance that inhibits cancer cell growth, is found in grapes, as is the antioxidant quercetin, which is found in red grapes.

23 **Guava:** This tropical fruit contains a high amount of fiber and 275 percent of the RDA for vitamin C.

24 **Honey:** The product of busy bees, honey is an antibacterial that also aids in digestive problems, fights diarrhea and constipation, helps heal ulcers, and contains many minerals and other nutrients.

25 **Horseradish:** Besides being a great no-fat, no-cholesterol condiment, horseradish is a potent antibacterial agent against organisms that often taint our food, including *Listeria, Escherichia coli*, and *Staphylococcus aureus*.

26 **Kiwi:** An excellent source of fiber, vitamin C, and potassium.

27 **Lemons:** In addition to being a good source of vitamin C, lemon juice is a flavorful, nutritious, no-fat seasoning to perk up your food. Drinking lemon juice in water or tea each morning is recommended as a way to help detoxify the liver, and the phytochemicals in lemons can help prevent or slow the growth of certain cancers.

28 **Lentils:** Lentils are a staple protein source for many people. They also contain fiber, cancer-fighting compounds, and a high amount of folic acid.

29 **Mangoes:** Antioxidants abound in this tropical fruit—vitamins A, C, and E are plentiful—and its high fiber content is a plus.

30 **Mushrooms:** When you think about mushrooms, think exotic. Reishi, shiitake, and maitake—three popular Japanese mushrooms—enhance the immune system and have cancer-fighting abilities.

31 **Nuts (most varieties):** Fiber, protein, magnesium, and protease inhibitors can be found in nuts, yet each variety has its own special healing properties. For example, almonds are good sources of iron, magnesium, and riboflavin, and are a good source of monounsaturated fat (the good fat), while chestnuts (one of the few low-fat nuts) are good sources of folic acid, vitamin C, and fiber. Hazelnuts and peanuts contain boron, which helps keep bones healthy, and Brazil nuts have high amounts of the mineral selenium, a potent antioxidant.

32 **Oats:** This dietary staple is high in fiber, which helps reduce cholesterol and the risk of various cancers, and helps regulate blood sugar levels. Oats are also a low-fat food and a good source of iron. Some studies indicate that oats may reduce the urge for nicotine, so reach for a bowl of oatmeal instead of a cigarette.

33 **Olive oil (cold-pressed):** An excellent source of monounsaturated fat (the good fat). Drizzle it on vegetables, pasta, potatoes, and whole-grain breads, and use it in salads.

34 **Onions:** Studies show that eating one-half of a raw onion a day can increase your good cholesterol level as much as 25 to 30 percent. Onions contain adenosine, a substance that thins the blood and thus helps reduce the risk of heart disease, and the antioxidant quercetin, which is an anticancer agent. Several other ingredients in onions can help reduce bronchial inflammation in people with asthma.

35 **Oranges:** This citrus treat helps reduce the risk of certain cancers, lowers cholesterol, and has antiviral abilities.

36 **Papaya:** One papaya contains more than three times the RDA for vitamin C and more than half the RDA for vitamin A. Papaya also contains the enzyme papain, which helps digest proteins.

37 **Parsley:** A rich source of many cancer-fighting agents, including chlorophyll, vitamin C, monoterpenes, flavonoids, and other antioxidants. Bonus: It freshens your breath.

38 **Pasta (whole-grain):** A great-tasting source of fiber and protein and a good provider of iron, whole-grain pasta is also a stress reducer and sleep aid (commonly referred to as a "comfort food").

39 **Peppers:** Peppers are either sweet or hot, with varying degrees of "punch" in both categories. Hot peppers are credited with relieving pain and reducing the risk of heart attack and stroke by busting blood clots, while the medicinal value of sweet peppers lies mainly in their cancer-fighting abilities.

40 **Pollen:** Pollen is rich in amino acids and trace elements. It regulates digestion, promotes circulation, and helps maintain heart health.

41 Potatoes: Potatoes are an excellent source of potassium, which helps maintain heart health, and a good source of protein, vitamin C, and fiber. They also contain the cancer-fighters protease inhibitors and polyphenols. Don't ruin a great thing, however, by deep frying or drowning potatoes in butter and sour cream. Herbs, spices, pureed vegetables, and salsa are great toppings.

42 Pumpkin: A mere one-half cup of pumpkin provides nearly three times the RDA of vitamin A—a potent cancer fighter—plus a good amount of iron, fiber, and vitamin C.

43 Rice (preferably brown): Brown rice is an excellent source of thiamin, which helps cells function smoothly, and natural vitamin E, which helps reduce cholesterol levels. Rice also contains protease inhibitors, which help reduce the risk of cancer, while the bran contains gamma-oryzanol, which helps lower cholesterol.

44 Sea vegetables: Sea vegetables encompass a wide variety of edible plants from the oceans. Arame, dulse, kelp, kombu, nori, wakame— these are just a few of the possibilities. Sea vegetables are both low in calories and high in iron, folic acid, calcium, potassium, fiber, magnesium, and other nutrients. Sea vegetables contain a cancer-fighting substance called fuciodan, and also help slow the development of herpes.

45 Seitan: Seitan is the protein portion of wheat, or wheat gluten, that is mixed with liquid, herbs, and spices and used as a meat substitute. It is high in protein, low in fat, and contains no cholesterol.

46 Soybeans: Soybeans are a very versatile food: They are made into soy milk, curdled into tofu, mixed with barley or wheat to make miso, or combined with grains and fermented to make tempeh. Healing properties associated with soybeans include reducing the risk of cancer, relieving symptoms of menopause, and keeping bones strong. Soybeans are an excellent source of protein, calcium, and iron.

47 Spinach: Popeye had the right idea: Spinach is a nutritious food, packed with vitamin A, folic acid, and iron. It is an excellent source of phytochemicals called carotenoids and of chlorophyll, both of which are cancer fighters. Spinach is also credited with protecting vision and helping reduce the risk of depression.

48 **Strawberries:** One cup of strawberries contains nearly 150 percent of the RDA for vitamin C, a powerful antioxidant. Strawberries also contain p-coumaric acid and chloregenic acid, two compounds that help reduce the risk of cancer by ridding the body of nitric oxides.

49 **Tangerines:** These cousins of the orange contain vitamin C, beta-carotene, pectin fiber, and folic acid, substances that variously protect against cancer, reduce the risk of heart disease, boost the immune system, and lower cholesterol levels.

50 **Tea (especially green):** Research shows that green tea reduces the risk of cancer and heart disease. Scientists believe that the tannins in tea help keep the blood thin, thus reducing the risk of blockage in the arteries. Tannins are also antiviral and antibacterial agents. Substances in tea called catechins provide cancer-fighting power.

51 **Tomatoes:** Tomatoes are one of the few foods that contain a substance called lycopene, a phytochemical credited with reducing the risk of cancer, especially prostate, pancreatic, and cervical cancers.

52 **Watermelon:** This native of Africa contains high levels of the cancer-fighting phytochemical lycopene. Watermelon is also a good source of potassium and vitamin C.

53 **Wheat:** Wheat is believed to be the most important cereal crop in the world. Its very high fiber content makes it an effective food to relieve constipation, reduce the risk of colon and breast cancers, and help prevent or treat diverticular disease (inflamed pockets in the digestive tract). Whole wheat is also a good source of the B vitamins, especially thiamin.

54 **Yeast (brewer's):** Less than an ounce of Brewer's yeast a day can reduce the risk of heart disease by raising good cholesterol and lowering bad cholesterol levels. Yeast is also an excellent source of chromium, which helps the body regulate blood sugar levels.

chapter ten

The Power of Aromatherapy:
30 Essential Essences

T ake a deep breath. What do you smell? Whatever it is—an apple pie baking in the oven, a bouquet of roses, or maybe the exhaust from the street outside your house—more than five million smell-detecting cells transmitted that aroma (or bad odor) to your brain.

Aromatherapy is a natural healing modality that is based on the sense of smell. For thousands of years, people have known about the power of scents. The ancient Romans wore roses in their hair to cure headaches, and Native Americans used prickly ash to stimulate feelings of love. Today, essential oil of lavender is used in nursing homes and hospitals to help cure insomnia.

Essential oils are extremely potent extracts from plants. Some have powerful antiseptic abilities; others can ease tension, lift mood, boost energy, stimulate feelings of love, promote healing, and encourage sleep. How do they do that?

How Aromatherapy Works

When you breathe in the scent of an essential oil, the olfactory organs in your brain are stimulated. These organs are linked to the emotional centers in the brain and different scents evoke different emotions. Essential oils can also be massaged into the skin to stimulate the nerve endings and send messages to the pituitary gland, which is the master gland of emotions.

How to Use Essential Oils

Because essential oils are very potent substances, they need to be handled with care. Keep these guidelines in mind:

- Do not inhale directly from the vial. Instead, add a few drops of the oil to a bowl of hot water or to an aroma defuser (sold in herb stores), or place a few drops on a tissue or handkerchief and inhale. Or you can add 15 to 20 drops of essential oil to 6 ounces of water in a spritzer bottle and spray the mixture into the air.
- Do not take essential oils internally or apply them to broken skin.
- Do not place undiluted essential oils on the skin. Always mix essential oils with a "carrier oil," a neutral oil such as almond, safflower, avocado, wheat germ, or jojoba. The basic dilution formula is 1/2 ounce carrier oil for every 5 drops of essential oil.

Essential Oils for You

Here are some of the most popular and effective essential oils. You can find them in health food stores and herb shops, and by mail order (see Chapter 68, Herb Sources).

Essential Oil	Response
1 Basil	Happiness, peace
2 Bay leaf	Increases psychic awareness
3 Bergamot	Promotes restful sleep
4 Black pepper	Increases alertness
5 Camphor	Increases energy
6 Cardamom	Promotes feelings of love
7 Catnip	Calming
8 Chamomile	Promotes sleep and calm
9 Cinnamon	Increases awareness and energy

Essential Oil	Response
10 Clove	Promotes healing
11 Coriander	Improves memory
12 Cypress	Promotes healing
13 Eucalyptus	Promotes healing
14 Fennel	Promotes longevity
15 Frankincense	Increases spirituality
16 Garlic	Purifies the body, promotes health
17 Ginger	Increases energy
18 Hops	Promotes sleep
19 Jasmine	Promotes love, sleep, and sex
20 Lavendar	Promotes sleep, calm
21 Lemon	Promotes healing and energy
22 Lime	Increases energy
23 Mimosa	Promotes psychic dreams
24 Nutmeg	Increases energy
25 Onion	Boosts the immune system
26 Orange	Increases energy
27 Peppermint	Enhances the mind
28 Rosemary	Promotes longevity
29 Sage	Improves memory
30 Vanilla	Promotes sex and love

chapter eleven

15 Exercise Approaches: You're Guaranteed to Love at Least One

What if you could get all the benefits of exercise in one little pill? What if all the advantages of 30 minutes of heart-pounding activity could be put into a glass of juice?

Well, forget it; it's probably never going to happen. But you can have the next best thing: exercise that is *fun* as well as healthy. Really. The secret is in how you approach the big "E—exercise." If you tell yourself, "I'm going to hate this" or "I'm going to be bored"; or if you say in the middle of a workout, "I can't wait until it's over," then you're just making your exercise sessions harder on yourself.

Hurdles to Jump

Why don't you exercise? The most common answers to that question are: 1) I don't have time; 2) it's boring; and 3) it hurts when I exercise, or I'm not physically able to exercise much.

Excuse Number 1: This hurdle is easy to overcome: Find time. Get up half an hour earlier. Take a brisk walk during your lunch break or coffee break. Write it into your schedule: "30 minutes of aerobics after work, 5:30," or "yoga class, 5:15 to 6:15." Move to make a commitment, and make a commitment to move.

Excuse Number 2: You're bored because you're not doing something you enjoy. So find an activity you like to do, or make what you're doing now more enjoyable. What's one thing that makes life more enjoyable? Variety. Exercise is not just one activity. You don't have to do the same exercises, or even the same kind of exercises, every time you work out.

Excuse Number 3: No one wants to hurt, and if exercise is painful or uncomfortable, it's easy to understand why you would want to avoid it. But there are some exercise programs and activities that are therapeutic; they can help individuals who have specific physical limitations and even help correct some of them.

In this chapter, we present 15 approaches to exercise. They offer something for just about everyone. Remember: Exercise isn't just about moving; it's also about attitude and variety. Which approach(es) to exercise do you wish to take? Don't be shy. Choose several and switch every few days. If you need exercise programs that are especially therapeutic, there are options that fit into that category as well.

Terms to Know

Aerobic: Activity that requires using oxygen and the large muscle groups in a rhythmic fashion for a given amount of time. Aerobic activity involves the heart, lungs, and cardiovascular system working together to strengthen the heart and circulate more blood and oxygen throughout the body.

Anaerobic: Activity that does not require oxygen. (Yes, you need oxygen to live, but we're talking about short bursts of energy here.) An example is weight lifting.

General Approaches to Exercise

1 Chores: Can chores like vacuuming, raking leaves, shoveling snow, gardening, and washing windows be counted as exercise? Sure they can, if you approach them with vigor and either do them continuously or go from one aerobic chore to another. That means don't vacuum for 5 minutes and then sit down to have a donut and coffee.

2 **Dancing:** Dancing is in a separate category because it is a unique aerobic activity. It can be either a social (requiring a partner) or a solo exercise, or it can involve a whole group of people (a square dance or clogging group, for example). Depending on your age and physical condition, 30 minutes of steady dancing three times a week can be an excellent aerobic workout. Types of aerobic dance include ballroom, tap, jazzercize, square, clogging, swing, and ballet.

3 **Stretching:** Often referred to as a warm-up, stretching involves moving the muscle fibers in such a way that it improves flexibility and promotes good range of motion of the muscles, ligaments, tendons, and joints. Experts recommend that everyone do 5 to 10 minutes of stretching before launching into other forms of exercise, and then do 5 to 10 minutes of cool-down stretching after each exercise session.

4 **Muscle Toning:** This exercise approach involves using weights to help tighten muscles rather than build mass. The amount of weight you use should add some resistance and allow you to do many repetitions, rather than be heavy and only let you do 8 or 10 repetitions. Ankle and wrist weights as well as hand weights are included in the muscle toning category.

5 **Team Exercise:** Some people enjoy the social interaction, camaraderie, and competition inherent in team sports. Whether it's doubles tennis, your company's softball team, a weekly neighborhood basketball game, or a bowling league, team exercise is a great way to add variety to your workout program.

6 **Meditative Exercise:** The Eastern practices of tai chi, yoga, qi gong, and other similar movement practices help develop balance, muscle tone, and inner peace all at the same time. These exercises can generally be modified to accommodate people of all ages and abilities, and they provide health benefits to everyone.

7 **Machine Assisted:** Man or woman against machine—if you enjoy the challenge of pitting yourself against a machine, or if having an exercise machine in your home fits into your lifestyle, then this exercise approach may be for you. Stair climbers, treadmills, ski machines, rowing machines, and stationary bikes are the most common aerobic machines on the market and in gyms and health clubs. Many exercise machines are available with electronic counters that keep track of calories burned, distance traveled, heart rate, and other relevant information. Too often, however, these machines become clothes horses or dust collectors. If you're thinking about buying exercise equipment for your home, try it out at a gym first.

8 **Me, Myself, and I:** Some people enjoy exercising alone: It's a time for them to ruminate on their day, compose stories, solve problems, and just relax. Long-distance runners, joggers, bikers, swimmers, and rowers are often, but not always, people who like the solitude of their chosen exercise.

9 **Muscle Building:** This type of exercise is anaerobic and involves increasing muscle mass by lifting heavy weights.

10 **Isometric:** If you don't like to move, isometric exercises are for you. Isometric exercises are those in which you apply force against a resistant object; for example, pushing against a wall. Although this activity builds up tension in the muscles (muscle contraction), you remain stationary. Isometric exercises are anaerobic and help build muscle strength, but in order to be effective you need to hold each position for 6 to 8 seconds and repeat the muscle contraction at least five times. Such exercises are helpful for people who are recovering from injuries that limit their range of motion. As exercises for building strength, they are not very effective, but when combined with muscle-building exercises, they provide more benefit. People with hypertension should not do isometric exercise, as it can increase blood pressure.

Why Exercise?

The benefits of exercise are many, and include:

- Strengthens and firms muscles.
- Strengthens the heart and lungs.
- Improves blood circulation.
- Builds endurance.
- Burns excess calories and helps you lose or maintain weight.
- Strengthens bones and limbers up joints.
- Improves digestion and relieves constipation.
- Lifts mood.
- Enhances the immune system.
- Improves sleep.

Specific Exercise Programs

11 **Alexander Technique:** The Alexander Technique is a program of simple movements that help people develop more control, coordination, and balance. The technique is taught by introducing students to nonstrenuous movements that can help them gain conscious control of body movement and improve posture. The Alexander Technique can increase flexibility and energy level.

12 **Egoscue Method:** This is a type of movement therapy based on the idea that many people experience poor balance, low energy level, stiffness, and other physical limitations because they don't move enough to keep their bodies well, or they move in ways that are harmful. One of the best examples of harmful movement is poor posture. The Egoscue Method involves evaluating people's posture and movement and then performing exercises to correct any flaws in both areas. The Egoscue Method can be effective in treating back and neck pain, arthritis, poor posture, and musculoskeletal disorders, because the process helps strengthen, stretch, and relax the body.

13 **Gyrokinetics (or Gyrotonics):** This approach was started by Juliu Horvath and has been described as a combination of yoga, dance, gynmastics, tai chi, and swimming. The basis of gyrokinetics is to exercise the muscles while simultaneously mobilizing the joints, stretching and strengthening the body, enhancing coordination, and increasing range of motion, all with minimal effort. The movements stimulate the body's internal organs and reportedly strengthen bone structure and ligaments, develop coordination and flexibility, and enhance cardiovascular health. The keys to gyrokinetics are fluid motion and breathing that make the exercises look and feel like dancing. Horvath created a device that people use to go through the 130 variations of exercise that are part of gyrokinetics. Fitness and sports centers, dance studios, and rehabilitation centers around the world are using gyrokinetics.

14 **Mensendieck System:** This movement therapy was developed by Bess Mensendieck, M.D., to help improve the body's structure and function and to help eliminate any accompanying aches and pains. The system consists of more than 200 different exercises that focus on proper, smooth movements that are part of everyday activities. The Mensendieck System is taught by trained teachers and is reportedly helpful for people who have back pain, sports-related injuries, poor posture, and Parkinson's disease.

15 **Pilates Method:** Developed in the 1920s by Joseph H. Pilates, this method involves three components: Principles, Exercises, and Equipment. Pilates is a mixture of Eastern and Western philosophies that combines breathing, balance, coordination, strength, flexibility, body mechanics, and positioning of the body. The 500 or so exercises that are part of the Pilates Method utilize various types of exercise equipment and are designed to allow for individual progress. The exercises focus on working the whole body and coordinating the upper and lower muscle groups. They emphasize stretching and strengthening the muscles. Pilates exercises can be used for both fitness and rehabilitation.

chapter twelve

10 Sexual Health Aids and How to Use Them

Has your sex life been on the back burner so long that the pilot light has fizzled out? Need a little something to rekindle or stoke the flames of passion? Flowers are nice, but they die; candy is sweet, but it puts on pounds. Aphrodisiacs, on the other hand . . .

Aphrodisiacs were named after the Greek goddess Aphrodite, whose specialties were desire, beauty, and fertility. Aphrodite was not the only icon of sexuality among ancient peoples: The Romans had Venus; the Babylonians, Ishtar; and the Phoenicians, Astarte. These goddesses inspired the creation of a great variety of love potions, which often contained a combination of herbs and other ingredients, some of which were quite exotic.

According to an old English tradition, for example, asparagus can incite lust in women and men who boil this vegetable and eat it three mornings in a row. In Malaysia, bird's nest soup, made from the nests of sea swallows that live in the caves of Borneo, is considered to be an aphrodisiac. It is not the twigs but the birds' spittle that is said to hold the key to lust and desire.

Because sexual desire—or the lack of it—is such a timeless topic, modern researchers are currently investigating some of the so-called aphrodisiacs that have been passed down through the millennia. While many of these potions have proven completely ineffective, some actually do have science on their side. In recent years, the magic of chemistry and technology has brought a few synthetically produced sex aids to the market to join the natural ones.

This list is mainly composed of natural aphrodisiacs that scientists say may actually stimulate sexual desire or improve sexual function. So dim the lights, burn some incense, and give them a try.

Words to Know

Impotence, or erectile dysfunction (ED), is an inability to achieve or maintain an erection sufficient for penetration. Approximately 30 million men are believed to have this condition.

Infusion, when speaking about herbs, is like a strong tea. To make an infusion, add a given amount of dried or fresh herb leaves or flowers, depending on the herb, to boiling water and allow the herb to steep for a designated amount of time, usually 5 to 10 minutes.

Tincture is a concentration of herb in liquid form. A tincture is usually taken by adding a given number of drops to water or another liquid.

Natural Aphrodisiacs

1 **Arginine**, an amino acid, may be effective in treating impotence, according to an article in the 1997 issue of *Journal of Urology*. One reason for its success is that arginine contributes nitrogen to the body, which the body then uses to create nitric oxide. Nitric oxide is found in high levels in the nerves that serve the tissues and arteries in the penis; thus a rich supply of nitric oxide can have a positive effect on impotence.

To Rev Up the Fire: A 1999 study reported that 31 percent of impotent men who took 5 g arginine every day for six weeks achieved an erection, compared with less than 12 percent of men who took a placebo. This dosage is the standard until further tests are performed.

2 **Damiana** (*Turnera diffusa*) has been used for centuries by Mexican women to help "get them in the mood." Damiana is a small shrub with yellow flowers that grows in Mexico, Texas, and Africa. The leaves are used to make a tea that is taken one to two hours before a lovemaking session. Researchers identified two substances in damiana—beta-sitosterol and a volatile oil—which are the source of the herb's sexually enhancing powers. Damiana also contains alkaloids that may cause a testosterone-like effect. Testosterone is a hormone that increases sexual desire in men and women.

To Rev Up the Fire: Prepare a tea using 2 heaping tablespoons of dried damiana leaves in 8 ounces of boiling water. Allow the leaves to steep for less than 5 minutes. Herbalists suggest drinking one cup of this tea per day. Another way to use damiana as a love potion is to combine 1 ounce dried damiana leaves, 2 cups vodka, 12 ounces spring water, and ½ cup honey. Allow this mixture to steep for 5 days and use 1 to 3 tablespoons per day.

3 **Ginkgo** (*Ginkgo biloba*) holds the unique distinction of being the world's oldest living species of tree. One of ginkgo's proven properties is the ability to promote blood flow, which makes it useful in improving sexual function and preventing impotence. Some of the substances in ginkgo that make it effective are called glycosides. When buying ginkgo supplements, look for a product that contains 24 percent glycosides. Ginkgo is available in capsules, tablets, and tinctures.

To Rev Up the Fire: For people younger than 50, 40 mg taken three times a day has been recommended by herbalists. For older adults, 60 mg three times a day is suggested. It takes about 2 to 3 weeks for results to become evident. As a treatment for impotence, one study showed that 50 percent of men who took 60 mg ginkgo daily regained potency after six months.

4 **Muira-puama** (*Ptychopetalum olacoides*), also known as potency wood, has been used as a sexual stimulant for centuries in the Amazon. The aphrodisiac is derived from the roots and bark of the muira-puama tree, which grows in South America. Researchers believe a resin in the tree is responsible for its sexual powers. Its negative effects are similar to those of yohimbe (see number 7), but milder. Muira-puama has been used in Europe for many years and is listed in the *British Herbal Pharmacopoeia*, where it is recommended for the treatment of impotence. A study published in the *American Journal of Natural Medicine* (November 1994) claims that muira-puama improves sexual function and desire in some individuals. The research was conducted by medical sexologist Dr. Jacques Waynberg at the Institute of Sexology in Paris. Dr. Waynberg's study included 262 men with erectile dysfunction or a lack of sexual desire. Sixty-two percent of patients with a lack of sexual desire and 52 percent of men with ED said muira-puama was beneficial. The report claims that "muira-puama may provide better results than yohimbine without side effects."

To Rev Up the Fire: The typical dosage is 4 to 12 drops of tincture twice a day. Because the ingredients in muira-puama that researchers believe are responsible for its benefits are not soluble in water and cannot be broken down in the digestive tract, tincture is thought to be the best form to take.

5 **Red clover** (*Trifolium pratense*) is considered to be a weed by many North Americans, but it's a weed you may welcome in your yard. Red clover contains phytoestrogens, which can balance hormone levels and thus enhance the sexual desire of some people who take this herb. Infusions of red clover can cause a mildly intoxicating effect, not unlike the feeling of love.

To Rev Up the Fire: To make an infusion, steep 2 teaspoons dried flowers in 4 ounces hot water for 10 minutes. Enjoy up to three doses daily. If you use the tincture, use ½ to 1½ teaspoons three times daily. Pregnant or breast-feeding women should not take red clover.

6 **Saw palmetto** (*Serenoa serrulata*) is perhaps best known as an herbal remedy for prostate problems; but partly because it does have this power, it is also an effective remedy for low sexual desire in both men and women and for impotence in men. Saw palmetto is a small palm tree that grows along the southeastern coast of the United States and in the West Indies. Native Americans recognized its ability to improve sperm production, and also used it to treat urinary tract infections.

To Rev Up the Fire: You can purchase saw palmetto in capsules (take one capsule after each meal) or tincture (drink 20 to 40 drops in water three times daily).

7 **Yohimbe** (*Pausinystalia yobimbe*) has been studied since the 1930s for its lusty properties, and today a synthetic version is available. In fact, yohimbe is available by prescription in the drug Yocon (yohimbine hydrochloride) as a treatment for impotence. Scientists have found that yohimbe increases blood flow to the penis and the clitoris and restricts the blood from leaving these areas, which adds to sexual pleasure. The substances that make yohimbe effective include several alkaloids (yohimbine, yohimbilene, and ajmaline). These alkaloids can activate many different reactions in the body, including mild visual and auditory hallucinations, weakness of the limbs, dizziness, and nausea. These are soon followed, however, by a feeling of peace and relaxation, as well as stimulation of the sex organs. These effects occur over a two- to four-hour period.

To Rev Up the Fire: Yohimbe is available by prescription, or you can prepare the herb. According to experts, add 1 ounce of dried yohimbe to 2 cups boiling water. Boil the tea for 3 minutes, then reduce the heat and simmer for 20 minutes. Strain the tea and sip slowly, about one hour before you want results. Add 1,000 mg vitamin C to the tea to help increase absorption and reduce the chance of experiencing nausea. An easier route is to take yohimbe capsules or tincture: Take one 250 or 500 mg capsule, or add 15 to 20 drops of tincture to water and take one hour before results are desired. People who have heart disease, kidney disease, glaucoma, or diabetes should not take yohimbe.

8 **Zinc** is a mineral that is critical to healthy sexual function in both women and men. Although severe zinc deficiency is rare in the United States, many people have levels that are marginally low, which is enough to negatively affect sexual function.

To Rev Up the Fire: The daily recommended intake of zinc is 15 to 30 mg. The best food sources are pumpkin seeds, sea vegetables, and sesame seeds, followed by whole-grain products, wheat germ, and soybeans. Zinc is found in most multivitamin and mineral supplements, and is also available as a lone supplement. In either case, look for the best-absorbed forms, which include zinc picolinate, zinc citrate, and zinc monomethionine. To get the full benefits of zinc, make sure you're also getting enough copper. You only need 2 to 3 mg copper per day. You may find copper in your multivitamin and mineral supplement, but it also is found in beans, peas, prunes, and whole wheat.

Prescription Aphrodisiacs

9 **Alprostadil,** or prostaglandin E, is a hormone-like substance that widens the blood vessels in the penis, making erection possible. Alprostadil (brand names Caverject, Edex, Muse) has been available since the mid 1990s and is used by men who are experiencing impotence, or ED. (As a matter of interest, alprostadil is also used to treat newborns who have congenital heart defects; it helps to open up their blood vessels.) It is highly effective—between 70 and 80 percent of men get positive results—and has been endorsed by the American Urological Association.

To Rev Up the Fire: Alprostadil is (or soon will be) available in three forms. The user-friendly form is a cream that is slated for the marketplace by the year 2002 under the brand names Alprox-TD and Topiglan, if all testing goes as planned. A November 2000 report of a 12-center trial involving 161 men showed that topical alprostadil was effective in 73 percent of men with ED when compared with a placebo (23 percent). The other two forms make some men uncomfortable: They are a form that must be injected into the penis and a tiny pellet that must be inserted into the penis.

10 **Viagra** (generic, sildenafil) hit the market with a blast in March 1998, and the sound is still being heard around the world. This product became the first drug approved for the treatment of ED, and men were gobbling up the pills at the rate of more than $1 billion in sales in 1998 alone. Studies show that Viagra can be effective in up to 88 percent of men who take the drug, although some research indicates lower results. Viagra does have some drawbacks, including a tendency to cause headache, facial flushing, indigestion, and nasal congestion. A Swedish study, presented at the 49th Annual Meeting of the American College of Cardiology in 2000, showed that Viagra was safe in men with heart disease who were not taking nitrates (nitroglycerine). However, other studies indicate that taking Viagra is a risk factor for fatal and nonfatal heart attack in men with heart disease. Men with heart disease should consult their doctors before taking Viagra, as should men who have peptic ulcers, leukemia, bleeding disorders, or sickle-cell anemia.

To Rev Up the Fire: Viagra is not just for men. Women are grabbing the tablets as well, including those who need a little sexual help after a hysterectomy. Laura Berman, M.D., of the Boston University Medical Center says that "it is reasonable for women to take Viagra after hysterectomy." Effective doses for men and women range from 10 to 100 mg. Ask your doctor for the best dosage for you. Viagra will soon have some competition. ICOS/Eli Lilly will soon market Cialis, while TAP Pharmaceuticals have Uprima on tap for the market.

chapter thirteen

Everyday Habits for Lifelong Health: *13* Ways to Slash Your Risk of Disease

Y̲ou can significantly reduce your risk of major illness *and* feel better about yourself at the same time, without even thinking about it. Sound impossible? Okay, you will probably have to think about it *a little*, just until the healthy changes in your life become old habits—comfortable, like a pair of well-worn jeans or a favorite sweater.

We tend to view good habits as hard to develop, and bad habits as easy, but the fact is that all habits, beneficial or harmful, begin basically the same way: one step at a time. If you smoke, or used to smoke, do you remember your first puff? You were starting a habit; you took the first step the first time you put a cigarette into your mouth. Then you hit the repeat button, and you were on your way to creating a habit.

Quitting smoking—the single most important health decision you can make—is not so much about giving something up as it is about establishing a new habit of *not* smoking. The most deadly and debilitating diseases in the United States today—heart disease, cancer, diabetes, stroke, osteoporosis, and arthritis—are largely the product of our lifestyle choices: habits we hold on to, even when we know they are harmful to our health.

So, if you have created harmful habits, you can create healing ones that will slash your risk of disease and provide you with health and wellness. The list of healing habits you will find here includes some that have been studied extensively and were the subject of a very large study by the American Heart Association (AHA). At the November 1999 AHA meeting in Atlanta, researchers reported on the results of a 14-year study of more than 84,000 women and the risk of heart disease. Lisa Freed, M.D., noted that taking five specific steps (the first five discussed here) can reduce the risk of heart attack, congestive heart failure, and stroke by an astounding 82 percent—more than scientists had found in past studies. And the good news is, each of these steps can also reduce the risk of many other unpleasant or life-threatening conditions.

The secret is to incorporate as many of these healthy lifestyle steps into your life as possible. No one expects perfection, but every modification you make will have a positive impact on your life and on your risk of serious disease.

Make Health a Habit: Reduce Your Risk of Disease

1 **Create a nonsmoking habit.** Most experts agree that this step is the most dramatic and beneficial one all smokers can take to reduce their risk of disease. Smoking has a detrimental effect on every system in the body, and thus is a risk factor for many ailments. Get help creating your new habit: Use a nicotine patch, undergo hypnosis, meditate, join a support group, or try herbal remedies. There are many aids to help you. You might even try giving yourself a financial incentive: Every time you want a cigarette, put aside the cost of that cigarette (about 15 cents) into a special bank or jar. By the end of the week, you will probably have enough money to buy yourself a reward.

2 **Eat a low-fat, high-fiber diet.** This may be a tall order, depending on what your dietary habits are now. The Diet & Cancer Project, a four-year collaborative effort between the American Institute for Cancer Research and the World Cancer Research Fund, brought together diet and cancer experts from around the world. They issued a 660-page report titled "Food, Nutrition, and the Prevention of Cancer: A Global Perspective." Its recommendations apply not only to cancer (30 to 40 percent of all cancers are directly associated with diet), but to general health as well. Here are a few highlights of the Project's recommendations. (All the foods should have undergone little or no processing.)

- *Eat plants.* That means fruits, vegetables, legumes, and whole grains. Eat five or more servings of fruits and vegetables daily and seven or more servings of grains, legumes, tubers, roots, and plantains.

- *Skip the meat.* If you do eat animal protein, limit consumption to less than 3 ounces per day of fish or chicken.

- *Limit consumption of fatty foods.* Cut down especially on fats from animal foods. Olive oil is the preferred source of dietary fat; or use vegetable oils in moderation.

- *Limit consumption of table salt and salty foods.* Use herbs and spices to season food.

3 **Exercise one-half hour or more per day.** No time? Get up 30 minutes earlier or take a walk during lunch or your break. Blend exercise into your day; make it fun. Exercise need not be aerobics and treadmills; it can be dancing, tennis, handball, or power walking around an enclosed mall with a friend. Although 30 minutes of continuous exercise is preferred, two 15-minute sessions per day is fine as well.

4 **Maintain a healthy weight for your height.** Overweight and obesity are epidemic in the United States, and they contribute to a long list of illnesses and disease, including diabetes, hypertension, heart disease, gallstones, stroke, arthritis, and cancer.

5 **Consume alcohol in moderation.** The American Heart Association study found that four ounces of alcohol per day was beneficial to women in preventing heart disease. This does not mean you need to take up drinking if you don't drink now.

6 **Use sunscreen.** Skin cancer is the most prevalent form of the disease in the United States, and its deadly form, melanoma, is becoming more and more common. According to the American Cancer Society, there were more than 1 million new cases of skin cancer in 2000, and nearly 10,000 deaths. Everyone should wear sunscreen with an SPF (sun protection factor) of at least 15.

7 **Reduce and manage stress.** The explosion of research into mind–body medicine has made the association between stress and physical illness clear, and the need for people to learn to manage their stress even clearer. Left unchecked, daily stress becomes chronic stress, which can translate into serious medical problems, including hypertension, heart disease, stroke, irritable bowel syndrome, migraine, and chronic fatigue. Daily management of stress can be achieved by doing 20 minutes of meditation, doing deep breathing exercises several times a day, or having a massage. If the exercise you choose is fun (and you don't feel stressed while doing it), then your exercise can be your stress reduction. You will then accomplish two goals with one solution.

8   Sleep. An estimated 50 percent of adults in the United States are sleep-deprived. One common consequence of sleep deprivation is falling asleep behind the wheel of a car. One-third of all drivers will fall asleep while driving at least once in their lifetime. The human cost of this problem: about 100,000 crashes, 71,000 injuries, and 1,500 deaths each year.

9   Practice safe sex. If you are sexually active with more than one partner or are not in a long-term, exclusively monogamous sexual relationship, you need to be vigilant to avoid contracting a sexually transmitted disease (STD). Habitual condom use, although not a 100 percent guarantee against giving or receiving an STD, is your best defense. Many STDs have reached epidemic proportions. In the United States, about 20 million people have genital herpes; between 1 and 2 million people are believed to have the AIDS virus; chlamydia strikes about 5 million Americans a year; and gonorrhea affects about 2.5 million.

10   Take nutritional supplements. Nearly everyone can benefit from a good quality multivitamin and mineral supplement. Few people eat a well-balanced, nutritionally sound diet. Even if you eat only whole, organically grown foods and drink only pure water, your body is still subjected to environmental toxins, stress, and infectious diseases from people around you, all of which can compromise your immune system and affect how your body absorbs and utilizes nutrients.

11   Socialize. Wellness is a balance of physical, emotional, mental, spiritual, and social health. Social wellness is a desire and capacity to form healthy relationships with others that allow you to build self-esteem and a feeling of belonging. It's been shown that people who are socially isolated tend to develop more illness, both physical and emotional.

12   Drink water. "Water is great medicine," says Andrew Weil, M.D., author of *Optimum Health*. The human body is about 60 percent water, and water is a major portion of every cell. Lose just 2 percent of your body's water supply and you will experience a decline in brain power and performance. Drinking 64 ounces of purified or bottled water per day is optimal.

13 **Check up on yourself.** We're pretty good about keeping our cars tuned up, but we seem to forget about our own bodies. Get in the habit of doing the screenings you can do yourself and scheduling those you cannot. For example, all females in their twenties and older should do a monthly breast self-examination, and all males beginning at age 15 should check for testicular cancer. Both men and women should routinely check their skin for any abnormalities or changes in moles or other skin markings. Routine checkups for cancer (prostate, cervical, breast, colon), high blood pressure, diabetes, glaucoma, and other conditions, should be done according to a specified schedule based on age, sex, and health history. Consult with your physician about the screenings you need.

chapter fourteen

12 Ways to Combat Depression, Stress, and Anxiety

Your boss is on your back. You're fighting with your husband. The rush hour freeway traffic leaves you tense and emotionally drained by the end of the day. You feel exhausted, yet you can't sleep. You hate your job but feel helpless to make a change. You want to lose weight but you feel too depressed to even try. You're tired and irritable and find it hard to be interested in social events. Sometimes all you want to do is hide.

Does any of this sound familiar? If so, you're not alone. Stress, anxiety, and depression are three common and somewhat similar reactions to life's ups and downs.

Stress is the body's and mind's reaction to something that disrupts a normal pattern or balance. Stress can be sudden, such as an automobile accident or the death of a loved one; or it can be everyday or common events that overwhelm you, such as driving in rush hour traffic, sharing office space with a coworker you do not like, or living from paycheck to paycheck.

Continued or chronic stress can lead to chronic fatigue, overeating, chronic pain, and other reactions, including depression.

Depression can be minor and temporary, minor and chronic, or major and chronic. About 25 percent of all women, 10 percent of all men, and 5 percent of all adolescents around the world suffer with some form of depression.

Anxiety is a normal reaction to a threat, real or imagined. That reaction includes the body's release of the hormones adrenaline and cortisone, a quickened heartbeat, shallow breathing, tensed muscles, and heightened mental alertness. When anxiety is excessive, it can appear in several forms, including phobias (fear of certain things or situations), panic attacks (an extreme, unfounded fear of something), obsessive-compulsive disorder (irrational, persistent thoughts or behavior, such as washing your hands repeatedly), posttraumatic stress disorder (prolonged anxiety after a traumatic event), and generalized anxiety (apprehensiveness that lasts for months).

Nearly everyone experiences times when the demands of life are just a bit too much: times when they don't need a doctor or prescription medication, but when a little help in refocusing their lives and priorities would lift the black cloud that hovers over them. That help can come in many forms, all of which are at your disposal. (If your stress, anxiety, or depression is prolonged or severe, see a physician for help.)

1 **Meditation** has been scientifically proven to reduce the symptoms of stress, anxiety, and depression, including high blood pressure, muscle tension, headache, nervousness, insomnia, and fatigue. You can learn meditation from tapes, books, videos, or instructors.

2 **Exercise**, especially aerobic exercise such as biking, walking, jogging, dancing, and tennis, releases natural mood elevators and painkillers called endorphins. Just 20 to 30 minutes on a stationary bike before work in the morning, a brisk walk during lunch break, or a few games of tennis after work may bring your stress back down to a manageable level. Research shows that jogging for 30 minutes three times a week can be as effective as psychotherapy in the treatment of depression.

3 **Herbs** have been used to reduce stress and treat depression for centuries. Earl Mindell, R.Ph., Ph.D., and author of *Earl Mindell's New Herb Bible*, recommends the following "herbal stress busters":

- Kava: Reduces anxiety. Take 1 to 2 capsules before bedtime.
- Hops: They're not just in beer! Mix ½ teaspoon dried hops in 4 ounces of water and drink it once daily. Also, sprinkle dry hops on your pillow to help lull you to sleep.
- Passion flower: Especially helpful for acute anxiety. Use 15 to 60 drops of extract in water daily.

- St. John's wort: This is a popular and effective herb for depression. Take according to package directions.

- Skullcap: To reduce stress, make an infusion by steeping 1 teaspoon dried herb in 8 ounces hot water. If you use the extract, take 3 to 12 drops in water daily.

- Valerian: Provides a calming effect. Take 1 to 3 capsules daily, or 10 drops of extract in water.

4 **Laughter** is the best medicine, say many experts, and scientific studies are proving them right. It certainly can't hurt. Make it a point to laugh hard every day. Get some humorous books, videos, CDs, or music; rent funny movies; or spend time with people who make you laugh.

5 **Acupressure** takes only a minute or two to apply, and you can do it just about anywhere, anytime. Here's one technique; consult a book on acupressure for many more: To help reduce feelings of anxiety and uneasiness, place your thumb in the center of your inner wrist, two finger widths from the wrist crease and between the two bones of your forearm. (This spot is known as Pericardium 6.) Press firmly with your thumb for 1 minute, release for several seconds, and then repeat again, three to five times. Repeat on the other arm.

6 **Aromatherapy** is believed to be very effective in reducing stress, depression, and anxiety. The essential oil of lavender is reportedly especially helpful for anxiety and stress, and you might try basil, rose, or chamomile for depression. Put a drop or two of any of these oils on a tissue and inhale the aroma, or place several drops into a hot bath and breathe in the aroma as you soak in the water. To help at bedtime, place a few drops on the corner of your pillow.

7 **Nutritional supplements** shown to be useful in treating depression include B-complex (take according to package directions) and folic acid (400 mcg daily). Another supplement, SAM-e (short for S-adenosyl-methionine; take according to package directions), has proven effective in treating depression in dozens of studies. It is best to consult your doctor before beginning any nutritional program to treat depression.

8 **Diet** can have a significant impact on stress, anxiety, and depression. Avoid or reduce your use of caffeine, as excessive amounts can increase anxiety. A diet that is rich in complex carbohydrates, low-fat foods, and plenty of fresh fruits and vegetables and that avoids alcohol, sugar, processed foods, and excess salt can provide the nutritional balance the body needs to handle stress.

9 **Yoga and tai chi** are two popular Eastern mind–body techniques that have proven abilities to reduce stress, depression, and anxiety. You can learn these practices through videos and books, or join a class. For best results, you should practice every day, preferably a short session both in the morning and at night.

10 **Deep breathing** is one of the easiest and most convenient ways to reduce stress and anxiety, but it needs to be done correctly to be effective. Although there are several techniques, here's a basic approach: 1) Sit comfortably with your arms resting at your side. 2) Place the tip of your tongue behind your top front teeth and leave it there throughout the exercise. 3) Gently and gradually inhale through your nose to a count of eight, completely filling your lungs and allowing your abdomen to be pushed out. 4) Hold the breath for a count of five to ten, whatever is comfortable for you. 5) Holding your lips as if you were going to blow out a candle, gradually allow the breath to leave through your mouth for a count of six. Make sure the breath has left your lungs completely. 6) Relax, breathing a few breaths normally, then repeat three more times.

11 **Progressive relaxation** techniques can leave you feeling fully refreshed after only 5 or 10 minutes. One simple technique involves lying comfortably on a flat surface and closing your eyes. Beginning at your toes, concentrate on how each body part feels, relaxing it completely until it feels light as a feather, then moving on to the next part: ankles, calves, knees, and so on. This process can also be done by tensing each body part for a few seconds, then totally releasing any tension before moving on to the next part. Do this several times a day, as needed.

12 **Guided imagery** is a way to use your inner eye to take you away from stress, anxiety, and depression. Basically, visualize yourself in a pleasant setting of your choosing and then, using all your senses, imagine yourself interacting with the setting in ways that relieve your physical and emotional turmoil. There are many books, tapes, and instructors available to help you learn these techniques.

chapter fifteen

Dozens of Ways to Stay Healthy and Disease-Free Wherever You Travel

You've packed your bags, sent your dog to the kennel, and put all your lights on timers. It's finally here: your vacation. Or maybe you're getting ready to take a long business trip. You're ready . . . or are you?

The last thing you want or need while you're away is to get sick. So, did you plan ahead? Whether you're going to the jungles of Africa, the high-rise offices of Singapore, or the ski slopes of the Rockies, you should be prepared to take care of your health. True, there are more health factors to consider if you plan to spend a month traipsing through the rain forest than if you're flying to Vermont to visit your Aunt Harriet, but we think the lists here offer a little something for most travelers.

How to Avoid Travelers' Diarrhea

Travelers' diarrhea—moderate to severe diarrhea, urgency, bloating, malaise, and nausea associated with consuming certain foods and beverages in foreign countries—is a very common ailment. Although it is rarely life-threatening (it can be dangerous in young children and the elderly), it usually lasts from 3 to 7 days and can certainly ruin your vacation. Areas of highest risk include the Middle East, Central America, and most of Africa, but travelers' diarrhea can strike when visiting Europe, Asia, Australia, the Caribbean—just about anywhere. Here's what you can do to prevent it.

- **Don't drink the water.** In areas with poor sanitation or a questionable water supply, drink only water that has been boiled for several minutes, hot beverages made with boiled water (such as coffee and tea), bottled or canned carbonated beverages, wine, and beer. Do not use ice cubes, as they are likely made with the contaminated water.

- **Brush from a bottle.** In areas with contaminated water, do not use the water when you brush your teeth. Use bottled sparkling water instead.

- **Disinfect.** You can treat questionable water with a chemical disinfectant, such as iodine (tincture of iodine or tetraglycine hydroperiodide tablets) or chlorine. Iodine provides better protection than chlorine. Chemical disinfectants can be found in sporting goods stores and pharmacies.

- **Avoid the salad bar.** Beware of raw foods in regions with poor sanitation. Foods that are most likely to cause diarrhea include uncooked vegetables and fruits, unpasteurized milk and milk products, shellfish, and raw meat. All foods should be cooked thoroughly and served hot.

- **Forego the fish.** Some fish can be toxic even when cooked. Sea bass, amber jack, grouper, red snapper, and tropical reef fish are occasionally poisonous if they have been caught among the reefs rather than in the open sea. Avoid puffer fish and barracuda at all times. The areas at highest risk for contaminated fish are the West Indies, the Indian Ocean, and the tropical Pacific Ocean.

- **Bring your meds.** If you get travelers' diarrhea, antimicrobial drugs such as doxycycline, trimethoprim-sulfamethoxazole (Bactrim, Septra), and fluoroquinolones (Cipro, Noroxin) may reduce the number of days you have to suffer.

If-You-Fly Tips

Although there are no reliable statistics, many airline passengers and flight attendants experience ill effects after flying, including headache, lightheadedness, nausea, difficulty concentrating, clammy skin, and breathing problems. Colds and other infections are not uncommon. To help prevent your flight from making you sick, try the following tips:

- **Wash up.** Once on board, wash your hands with soap and hot water before you touch your nose, eyes, or mouth.

- **Cover your nose.** To combat low humidity and avoid breathing in germs, cover your nose with a water-saturated cotton handkerchief.

- **Hydrate.** Prevent dehydration by drinking at least 8 ounces of water for each hour you are in the plane. Ask for canned or bottled water from the beverage cart, or bring your own from home.

- **Oil up.** Apply vegetable oil (olive, almond, canola) inside your nostrils. This prevents the membranes from drying out and stops germs from entering your nose.

- **Walk around.** To prevent blood clots from forming in your legs during long flights (3 hours or longer), get up and walk down the aisle once an hour, or at least stand in the aisle for a few minutes.

Traveling for Two: Pregnant Travelers

The American College of Obstetricians and Gynecologists says the safest time for pregnant women to travel is during the second trimester (weeks 18 to 24), when there is the least danger of spontaneous abortion or premature labor.

- If any of the following conditions apply to you, talk with your doctor before you travel internationally. The first two conditions apply to domestic travel as well: heart or vascular disease; severe anemia; a history of miscarriage, ectopic pregnancy, premature labor, or placental abnormalities; history of hypertension, diabetes, or toxemia with any pregnancy; vaginal bleeding during current pregnancy; unstable cervix; multiple gestation; history of infertility or difficulty getting pregnant; and first-time pregnancy in a woman older than 35 or younger than 15.

- If traveling during the third trimester, make sure medical facilities at your destination can accommodate complications of pregnancy, such as cesarean section or toxemia.

- Make sure prenatal care is available at your destination.

- Know your blood type, and check whether blood is screened for hepatitis B and HIV at your destination.

- Make sure your health insurance policy is valid if you travel abroad and that delivery will be covered if it occurs overseas. Consider getting a supplemental travel insurance policy and a prepaid medical evacuation insurance policy.

- Always carry documentation stating your expected due date. International travel is usually allowed until the 32nd week of gestation; domestic travel, until the 36th week.
- Make sure your destination has bottled water and safe food and beverages.

VACCINATIONS DURING PREGNANCY

If you travel to foreign countries while you're pregnant, you need to consider the vaccination requirements of those countries. It's also good to review CDC recommendations, such as those listed in the sidebar. And of course, always check with your doctor before receiving any vaccinations while you are pregnant.

- Give if indicated: hepatitis B, immune globulins, influenza, meningococcal, pneumococcal, polio (injection), rabies, tetanus-diphtheria, yellow fever.
- Data on safety during pregnancy not available: cholera, hepatitis B, Japanese encephalitis, plague, typhoid.
- Do not give: measles, mumps, rubella, varicella (chickenpox).

General Guidelines When Traveling to Any Undeveloped Region

- Wash your hands often with soap and water.
- Don't consume unpasteurized dairy products.
- Avoid eating undercooked meat and poultry, raw eggs, and raw shellfish.
- Eat only well-cooked foods or fruits and vegetables you have peeled yourself.
- Protect yourself against insects: Use repellents, wear long-sleeved shirts and long pants, especially dusk through dawn, and stay in screened areas when possible.
- To prevent fungal and parasitic infections, don't go barefoot. Do keep your feet clean and dry.
- Don't eat food bought from street vendors.
- Carry iodine tablets and portable water filters to purify water if bottled water is not available.
- If you take prescription medications, bring a sufficient amount with you, along with a copy of your prescription.

Who You Going to Call?

Like the weather, health conditions can change quickly. A sudden outbreak of malaria, yellow fever, or flu can happen at any time. To keep travelers up to date, the Centers for Disease Control and Prevention (CDC) maintain Outbreak Notices, which can be seen at www.cdc.gov/travel/blusheet.htm, or you can call the CDC at 1-877-FYI-TRIP. For example, an Outbreak Notice in December 2000 warned of an outbreak of polio in Haiti and the Dominican Republic. No travel restrictions were posted, but visitors were urged to be up to date on their polio vaccines if they planned to enter those countries. These same contacts at the CDC can give you the latest information on the list of countries infected with cholera, yellow fever, and plague.

Destination: Tropical South America

Bolivia, Brazil, Colombia, Ecuador, French Guiana, Guyana, Paraguay, Peru, Suriname, and Venezuela

- Malaria: A problem in some urban and many outlying areas. To find out if it is a problem in the specific area you are traveling to, contact the CDC.

- Yellow fever: A vaccination certificate may be required for certain countries.

- Insect-borne diseases: dengue, filariasis, leishmaniaasis, orchocerciasis, and Chagas disease.

- Altitude sickness: If you visit the Andes Mountains, plan your ascent carefully. You can prevent altitude sickness (headache, nausea, insomnia, weakness, unsteadiness) if you allow time for your body to adjust.

- Sunblock: Use 15 SPF or better, especially when at high altitudes.

- Vaccinations: See sidebar.

Destination: Temperate South America

Argentina, Chile, Falkland Islands, Uruguay

- Malaria: In Argentina, there is risk in northern rural areas bordering Paraguay and Bolivia. Visitors to rural northern Argentina should take chloroquine to prevent malaria. There is no risk for malaria in Chile, the Falkland Islands, and Uruguay.

- Yellow fever: No vaccination certificate is required for entry into this region.

- Insect-borne diseases: dengue, Chagas disease, and leishmaniasis.
- Altitude sickness: If you visit the Andes Mountains, ascend slowly to allow time for your body to adjust to the high altitude.
- Sunblock: Use sunscreen rated 15 SPF or higher, as the risk of sunburn is great at high altitudes.
- Vaccinations: See sidebar; also recommended is yellow fever if you travel outside urban areas in Argentina.

Standard CDC-Recommended Vaccinations When You Travel

The CDC recommends receiving the following vaccinations 4 to 6 weeks before leaving on a trip to foreign countries:

- Hepatitis A or immune globulin (IG).
- Hepatitis B: if you might be exposed to blood (e.g., if you are a health care worker), are staying more than 6 months in the area, may be receiving medical treatment, or have sexual contact with the local population. The CDC also recommends hepatitis B for all infants and 11- to 12-year-olds who did not receive the series as infants.
- Rabies: if you might be exposed to domestic or wild animals.
- Typhoid: if you are visiting developing countries in this region.
- Boosters for tetanus-diphtheria and measles and a single polio dose for adults.

Destination: The Caribbean

Antigua and Barbuda, Bahamas, Barbados, Bermuda, Cayman Islands, Cuba, Dominica, Dominican Republic, Grenada, Guadeloupe, Haiti, Jamaica, Martinique (France), Montserrat, Netherlands Antilles, Puerto Rico, St. Lucia, St. Vincent and the Grenadines, St. Kitts–Nevis, Trinidad and Tobago, Turks and Caicos, Virgin Islands

- Malaria: Risk is great year-round in Haiti and rural Dominican Republic. Travelers to those regions should take chloroquine to prevent the disease.
- Yellow fever: A vaccination certificate may be required for certain areas if you arrive in Haiti or the Dominican Republic from a sub-Saharan African or tropical South American country.

- Insect-borne diseases: dengue, filariasis, and leishmaniasis.
- Swimming: Avoid swimming in fresh water in Antigua, the Dominican Republic, Guadeloupe, Martinique, Montserrat, Puerto Rico, and St. Lucia, because the parasite schistosomiasis dwells there. Chlorinated water in swimming pools is safe.
- Vaccinations: See sidebar; also recommended is yellow fever

Destination: Mexico and Central America

Belize, Costa Rica, El Salvador, Guatemala, Honduras, Mexico, Nicaragua, Panama

- Malaria: Risk exists year-round in rural lowlands and in some urban areas. Visitors to these areas and to Panama west of the Canal Zone should take chloroquine. Visitors to areas east of the Canal Zone should take mefloquine.
- Yellow fever: A vaccination certificate may be required for entry into some countries if you are coming from tropical South America or sub-Saharan Africa.
- Insect-borne diseases: dengue, filariasis, leishmaniasis, orchocenciasis, and Chagas disease.
- Vaccinations: See sidebar; also recommended is yellow fever for visitors to Panama who will travel outside urban areas.

Destination: West Africa

Benin, Burkina Faso, Cape Verde Islands, Cote d'Ivoire, Gambia, Ghana, Guinea, Guinea-Bissau, Liberia, Mali, Mauritania, Niger, Nigeria, São Tome and Principe, Senegal, Sierra Leone, Togo

- Malaria: Most visitors to malaria risk regions should take mefloquine to prevent the disease. Risk of malaria is high in all west African countries except for most of the Cape Verde Islands.
- Yellow fever: A vaccination certificate may be required for entry into some west African countries.
- Insect-borne diseases: In this region they include dengue, filariasis, leishmaniasis, orchocerciasis, and trypanosomiasis (sleeping sickness).
- Swimming: Avoid swimming in fresh water as schistosomiasis, a parasitic infection, is found in the water. Chlorinated swimming pools are safe.
- Vaccinations: See sidebar; also recommended are meningococcal for travel to most west African countries from December through June.

Destination: Southern Africa

Botswana, Lesotho, Namibia, South Africa, St. Helena, Swaziland, Zimbabwe

- Malaria: Risk exists year-round in northern Botswana, rural areas of South Africa, all nonmountainous areas of Swaziland, and all of Zimbabwe except Harare and Bulawayo. No risk has been reported in Lesotho and St. Helena. Mefloquine is recommended.
- Yellow fever: A vaccination certificate may be required in some countries if you are coming from tropical South America or sub-Saharan Africa. There is no risk for yellow fever in Southern Africa.
- Insect-borne diseases: dengue, filariasis, leishmaniasis, orchocerciasis, and trypanosomiasis.
- Swimming: Avoid swimming in fresh water as schistosomiasis is found in the region. Chlorinated pools are safe.
- Vaccinations: See sidebar.

Destination: Central Africa

Angola, Central African Republic, Cameroon, Chad, Congo, Democratic Republic of the Congo (Zaire), Equatorial Guinea, Gabon, Sudan, Zambia

- Malaria: Because a high risk exists year-round in central Africa, the CDC recommends that all travelers take mefloquine to prevent malaria.
- Yellow fever: A vaccination certificate may be required to enter Central African countries.
- Insect-borne diseases: dengue, filariasis, leishmaniasis, and orchocerciasis. Sleeping sickness has appeared in southern Sudan.
- Swimming: Avoid swimming in fresh water in Central African countries, as the parasite schistosomiasis is found in the water. Chlorinated swimming pools are safe.
- Vaccinations: See sidebar; also recommended are meningococcal if you are going to Chad, Sudan, or Central African Republic from December through June, and yellow fever if you travel outside urban areas.

Destination: North Africa

Algeria, Canary Islands, Egypt, Libyan Arab Jamahirya, Morocco, Tunisia

- Malaria: Limited risk exists in parts of Algeria, Egypt (El Faiyum area only), Libyan Arab Jamahirya, Western Sahara, and Morocco. There is no risk for visitors in major tourist areas in North Africa, including cruises on the Nile.

- Yellow fever: A vaccination certificate may be required for entry into some countries if you are coming from tropical South America or sub-Saharan Africa. There is no risk for yellow fever in North Africa.

- Insect-borne diseases: dengue, filariasis, leishmaniasis, orchocerciasis.

- Swimming: Avoid swimming in fresh water, as schistosomiasis is found in fresh water in the region, including the Nile River. Chlorinated swimming pools are safe.

- Vaccinations: See sidebar.

Destination: East Africa

Burundi, Comoros, Djibouti, Eritrea, Ethoipia, Kenya, Madagascar, Malawi, Mauritius, Mayotte, Mozambique, Reunion, Rwanda, Seychelles, Somalia, Tanzania, Uganda

- Malaria: Possibility of infection present in all areas except for the cities of Addis Ababa, Ismara, and Nairobi, the islands of Reunion and Seychelles, and in highlands above 2,500 meters.

- Yellow fever: Certificate may be required for entry into some countries. Contact the CDC for the latest update.

- Insect-borne diseases: dengue, filariasis, leishmaniasis, orchocerciasis, trypanosomiasis, and Rift Valley fever.

- Swimming: Avoid swimming in fresh water as schistosomiasis, a parasitic infection, is found in the water, including Lake Malawi. Chlorinated swimming pools are safe.

- Vaccinations: See sidebar; also recommended are meningococcal vaccine if you visit the western half of Ethiopia from December through June, and yellow fever vaccine if you travel outside of urban areas.

Destination: Western Europe

Andorra, Austria, Azores, Belgium, Denmark, Faroe Islands, Finland, France, Germany, Gibraltar, Greece, Greenland, Iceland, Ireland, Italy, Liechtenstein, Luxembourg, Madeira, Malta, Monaco, Netherlands, Norway, Portugal, San Marino, Spain, Sweden, Switzerland, United Kingdom

- Yellow fever: No risk in Western Europe. A vaccination certificate may be required for entry into certain countries if you come from tropical South America or sub-Saharan Africa.

- Tick-borne encephalitis: This viral infection is found mainly in Central and Western Europe. People at risk are those who spend time in wooded areas during the summer and who consume dairy foods that have not been pasteurized. There is no vaccine available for this disease in the United States. Avoiding tick bites is the only preventive measure.

- Vaccinations: Hepatitis A, hepatitis B, and boosters for tetanus-diphtheria are the only recommended vaccines.

Destination: Eastern Europe

Albania, Armenia, Azerbaijan, Belarus, Bosnia and Herzegovina, Bulgaria, Croatia, Czech Republic, Estonia, Georgia, Hungary, Kazakhstan, Kyrgyzstan, Latvia, Lithuania, Moldova, Poland, Romania, Russia, Serbia and Montenegro, Slovak Republic, Slovenia, Tajikistan, Turkmenistan, Ukraine, Uzbekistan

- Malaria: Risk exists only in the southern border areas of Azerbaijan and Tajikistan.

- Yellow fever: No risk in Eastern Europe. A vaccination certificate may be required for entry into some countries if you come from tropical South America or sub-Saharan Africa.

- Other diseases: Diphtheria has been a problem in the former Soviet Union. Check with the CDC before traveling there. Tick-borne encephalitis occurs primarily in Central and Western Europe. Travelers who visit or work in wooded areas during the summer and who consume dairy foods that are not pasteurized are at risk; however, a vaccine is not available in the United States. Take precautions against tick bites.

- Vaccinations: See sidebar.

Destination: Australia and the South Pacific

Australia, Christmas Island, Cook Island, Federated States of Micronesia, Fiji, French Polynesia (Tahiti), Guam, Kiribati, Marshall Islands, Nauru, New Caledonia, New Zealand, Niue, Northern Mariana Islands, Palau, Papua New Guinea, Pitcairn, Samoa, American Samoa, Solomon Islands, Tokelau, Tonga, Tuvalu, Vanuatu, Wake Island, Wallis, and Utuna

- Vaccinations: Vaccinations recommended for travel to Australia and the South Pacific include hepatitis A, rabies, typhoid, and boosters for tetanus-diphtheria and measles, and a single polio dose for adults. Hepatitis B is now recommended for all infants and children 11 to 12 years of age who did not receive the series as infants.

Destination: Southeast Asia

Brunei Darussalam, Cambodia, Indonesia, Lao People's Democratic Republic (Laos), Malaysia, Myanmar (Burma), Philippines, Singapore, Thailand, Vietnam

- Malaria: Risk is year-round in some cities and in all rural areas except for Brunei Darussalam and Singapore. Most visitors to Southeast Asia at risk for malaria should take mefloquine.
- Yellow fever: No risk in Southeast Asia. A vaccination certificate may be required for entry into some countries if you come from tropical South America or sub-Saharan Africa.
- Insect-borne diseases: dengue, filariasis, Japanese encephalitis, and plague.
- Swimming: Avoid swimming in fresh water in Indonesia, Laos, Philippines, Cambodia, and Thailand to avoid infection with schistosomiasis. Chlorinated swimming pools are safe.
- Vaccinations: See sidebar; also recommended is Japanese encephalitis if you plan to visit rural regions for 4 weeks or longer, or if there is a known outbreak of the disease.

Destination: East Asia

China, Hong Kong, Japan, Democratic People's Republic of Korea (North), Republic of Korea (South), Macao, Mongolia, Taiwan

- Malaria: A risk only in some rural areas of China.
- Yellow fever: No risk in East Asia. A vaccination certification may be required to enter certain countries if you are coming from tropical South America or sub-Saharan Africa.
- Insect-borne diseases: dengue, filariasis, Japanese encephalitis, leishmaniasis, and plague.
- Altitude sickness: If you visit the Himalayan Mountains, ascend slowly to allow time for your body to adjust to the high altitude.
- Sunblock: Use sunscreen rated 15 SPF or higher, as the risk of sunburn is great at high altitudes.
- Swimming: In China, avoid swimming in fresh water in the southeast, east, and Yangtze River valley to avoid infection with schistosomiasis. Salt water is usually safer. Chlorinated swimming pools are safe.
- Vaccinations: See sidebar.

Destination: Indian Subcontinent

Afghanistan, Bangladesh, Bhutan, India, Maldives, Nepal, Pakistan, Sri Lanka

- Malaria: Risk exists in some urban and many rural areas, depending on the elevation. Most visitors to the Indian Subcontinent at risk for malaria should take mefloquine.

- Yellow fever: A vaccination certificate may be required for entry into some countries if you enter from tropical South America or sub-Saharan Africa. There is no risk for yellow fever in the Indian Subcontinent.

- Insect-borne diseases: dengue, filariasis, Japanese encephalitis, leishmaniasis, and plague.

- Altitude sickness: If you visit the Himalayan Mountains, ascend slowly to allow time for your body to adjust to the high altitude.

- Sunblock: Use sunscreen rated 15 SPF or higher, as the risk of sunburn is great at high altitudes.

- Vaccinations: See sidebar; also recommended is Japanese encephalitis.

Destination: Middle East

Bahrain, Cyprus, Iran, Iraq, Israel, Jordan, Kuwait, Lebanon, Oman, Qatar, Saudi Arabia, Syrian Arab Republic, Turkey, United Arab Emirates, Yemen

- Malaria: Risk is low in parts of Iran, Iraq, Oman, Saudi Arabia, Syrian Arab Republic, Turkey, United Arab Emirates, and Yemen. Visitors to risk areas of Iran, Oman, Saudi Arabia, United Arab Emirates, and Yemen should take mefloquine; travelers to risk areas of Iraq, Syria, and Turkey should take chloroquine.

- Yellow fever: A vaccination certificate may be required for entry into some countries only if you are coming from tropical South America or sub-Saharan Africa. There is no risk for yellow fever in the Middle East.

- Insect-borne diseases: dengue, filariasis, leishmaniasis, orchocerciasis, and plague.

- Vaccinations: See sidebar; also recommended by the CDC is meningococcal vaccine for all travelers to Mecca.

chapter sixteen

10 Tips
for Happy Feet
and Toes

Have you ever heard the expression, "Walk a mile in my shoes"? You might want to change it to 115,000 miles. That's the estimated number of miles the average person walks in a lifetime, according to the American Podiatric Medical Association. That's four times the circumference of the globe, and a lot of wear and tear on the feet.

So it's no surprise that 75 percent of Americans will have foot health problems at some time during their lives, or that each year about 5 percent of the U.S. population goes for treatment to the more than 13,000 podiatrists (foot doctors) who practice in the United States. That adds up to more than 14 million visits.

What types of foot problems do Americans have? Here's a quick breakdown:

- About 5 percent have foot infections, including fungal infections and warts.
- About 5 percent have ingrown toenails or other problems with toenails.
- About 5 percent have calluses or corns. Of the three main types of foot problems discussed, people are least likely to seek a podiatrist's help for corns or calluses.
- About 6 percent of people have flat feet, fallen arches, foot injuries, or bunions.

Even though the feet are not physically big parts of the body, they carry a very big load. Each foot has 26 bones, 33 joints, 107 ligaments, and 19 muscles and tendons, all of which get a considerable workout. Simply walking can place pressure on your feet that exceeds your body weight, and if you run or jog, up that pressure to three or four times your weight.

If all of this information is making you break out in a sweat, your feet may be perspiring, too. There are about 252,000 sweat glands in a pair of feet, and they excrete up to 8 ounces of moisture per day. So between the walking, the pressure, and the sweating, your feet deserve some tender, loving care. Foot specialists regularly recommend that people wear sensible, supportive footwear, avoid high heels and going barefoot, and see a podiatrist if their feet hurt. How can you avoid some of the most common foot problems? Here are 10 tips to help keep your feet healthy, happy, and ready to keep on truckin'.

1 **Change shoes.** Help prevent athlete's foot by switching shoes from day to day and wearing shoes made of natural materials, such as canvas or leather, or wearing sandals whenever possible. If you do get athlete's foot, try tea tree oil, an Australian herbal remedy that has been proven scientifically to be just as effective as the prescription drug tolnaftate. Apply tea tree oil with a cotton swab to the affected areas every day.

2 **Soak your dogs.** You can get rid of corns and calluses by relaxing your feet in warm water and Epsom salts and then using any of a variety of over-the-counter products, including pumice stones, callus removers, and electric or battery-operated handheld scrub brushes.

3 **Walk.** This is the best exercise for your feet as well as for the rest of your body because it promotes circulation and overall health.

4 **Take the edge off.** Help avoid ingrown toenails by cutting your toenails correctly: straight across, leaving the nail just a bit longer than the tips of your toes. Smooth the edges of the nail with an emery board or nail file.

5 **Take a close look.** If you are diabetic, examine your feet daily, especially between the toes. Bathe your feet daily in lukewarm water, use moisturizer, avoid tight shoes and socks, and never poke under the nail or cuticle. People with diabetes are prone to foot infections because of poor circulation in their feet.

6 **Shop for shoes later in the day.** Your feet swell during the day, so you are more likely to get a good-fitting shoe if you wait until the afternoon. Always try the shoes on both feet, as many people have one foot that is slightly larger than the other.

7 **Practice good skin sense.** Prevent sunburn by applying sunscreen on the top of your feet when wearing sandals or walking on the beach.

8 **Support yourself.** Have flat feet? Wear shoes with good arch support or, even better, get custom mold orthotics from a podiatrist. Over-the-counter arch supports made by Dr. Scholl's and Spenco are helpful for many people as well.

9 **Wash away odors.** Although giving smelly feet a fancy name—bromohydrosis—won't make your feet smell any better, a tea soak may. Place 5 tea bags in a quart of hot water and soak your feet for 30 minutes every night for about a week. Repeat as needed. (You'll know when that is.)

10 **Unpolish.** To help avoid fungal infections, do not put polish on nails of toes that are swollen, red, or discolored. Polish prevents moisture from escaping from under the nail and creates a perfect environment for infection to grow.

chapter seventeen

Setting Your Sights:

18 Tips on Vision, Lenses, and Eye Care

Most of us take our vision for granted most of the time. A 1997 study showed that more people have their cars tuned up than have their eyes examined. That's not a good statistic, especially given that more than 80 percent of what we learn comes to us through our eyes.

One reason people neglect their eyes is that vision problems are usually painless and slow to develop. You may notice a slight blurring, or your eyes may burn or feel dry occasionally. You may notice that traffic signs are not as easy to see, but if you drive familiar roads much of the time, you probably don't even notice that there's a problem.

That's why preventive eye care is essential. It's the little things that can mean the most when it comes to preventing vision problems or stopping a current problem in its tracks. If you wear glasses or contact lenses, there are tips you should follow to keep your eyes well maintained.

For a Clearer View

Like most people, you probably know enough to have routine eye examinations, every year or two, depending on your needs. But what are some of the other steps you can take to keep your eyes and your lenses in tip-top shape?

1 Never watch a television or use a computer monitor in a darkened room. The contrast between the screen and the surrounding area is detrimental to efficient vision. View both of these screens in a softly illuminated area.

2 Sit at least 20 inches away from a computer monitor and a distance from a TV set of at least five times the diagonal dimension of the television screen. That means for a 19-inch television, you should sit at least eight feet away.

3 Eat your spinach. Although a well-balanced diet is essential for overall good health, several nutrients are especially good for vision. Two powerful antioxidants are lutein and zeaxanthin, which are found in spinach, kale, and other vegetables and fruits. They are found in the yellow pigment in the retina and appear to protect against two specific eye disorders: macular degeneration and cataracts.

4 When working at a computer, blink often; this rests the eyes and re-wets them.

5 Treat stressed eyes to an herbal wash. Herbs that are best for this are bilberry, chamomile, eyebright, goldenseal, and red clover. Prepare a tea according to package directions, then strain it through a piece of cheesecloth or filter paper several times until the tea runs completely clear. Allow it to cool to room temperature. Then use an eyedropper to put two drops into each eye.

6 Eyebright is an excellent herb to take as an infusion (a strong tea) or in a supplement every day, as it rejuvenates eye tissues. Take according to package directions.

7 Do eye exercises. There are books on several techniques, including the Bates Method. Check out the Web site for the American Vision Institute (www.seeclearlysolutions.com) for eye exercises. These exercises, which can be as simple as looking up, down, and to both sides for a count of 10 and then repeating the sequence several times, improve the smoothness and efficiency of the muscles that control the eyes.

8 If your eyes are overly sensitive to light, take a vitamin B complex supplement daily. The B vitamins support the health of the eye tissues.

9 To treat pinkeye (a contagious form of conjunctivitis) naturally, you can use a very warm compress several times a day if your eyes are sticking together in the morning. A chamomile or eyebright and fennel eyewash can be helpful.

10 Are your eyelids twitching? You can relieve it by placing your forefingers on either side of your nostrils where they flare, and under your eyes. Massage these two points. The Chinese believe these two acupressure points can relieve eyelid twitching and eye disease.

11 If you have cataracts, protect your eyes by wearing sunglasses and a hat to reduce the glaring effect of the sun. Also, keep the lights low when you watch television.

12 Are your eyes dry? Dry-eye syndrome is believed to be the most common eye complaint. The eyes produce about 40 percent fewer tears with advancing age. To help preserve moisture, use humidifiers in your home, avoid smoke and fumes, and try a chamomile or goldenseal eyewash.

13 Be aware that some drugs can cause eye damage. For example, nonsteroidal anti-inflammatory drugs (NSAIDS) can cause cataracts, retinal hemorrhage, and dry-eye with long-term use. Venlafaxine (an antidepressant) can cause eye hemorrhage, as can heparin and coumadin (blood thinners) and amphotericin (an antibiotic). There are many others; check with your doctor or pharmacist before taking any drug.

14 Glaucoma is the second most common cause of blindness in the United States (diabetes is number one). This condition, in which the fluid pressure inside the eye increases harmfully, can be helped with some powerful nutritional supplements, including choline and inositol (1,000 to 2,000 mg of a combination supplement daily), glutathione (500 mg twice daily), rutin (50 mg three times daily), and vitamin B5 (100 mg three times daily).

15 Never use saliva to wet your contact lenses. Saliva is full of bacteria and can cause an eye infection. Use only wetting solution.

16 Although glass lenses offer excellent scratch resistance, they are heavy and not very impact-resistant. They may be a good choice for occasional wear around the house or for reading, but most people find lenses of polycarbonate plastic, CR-39 plastic, or high-index plastic a better choice for safety (very impact-resistant) and, because of their light weight, comfort.

17 Clean your eyeglass lenses with mild detergent and water or a special lens cleaner. Don't use paper towels to dry them, as paper towels have fibers that can scratch. Use a good cloth, preferably made of microfibre.

18 Want flattering eyeglass frames? If you have a round face, try angular or geometric frames. If your face is heart-shaped, go for an "aviator" style. A person with a square face usually looks best in oval or round frames, while a rectangular face (long and narrow) looks good in frames with a round bottom.

chapter eighteen

13 Ways

to Prevent Wrinkles and

Protect Your Skin

If you think wrinkles are an inevitable part of aging, think again. Experts say that aging is responsible for only about 10 percent of wrinkles. The real culprit? Sun exposure. The not-so-good news is that most of the damage has been done by the time people are 18 years old. The encouraging news is that there are not only ways to prevent further damage, but also techniques to repair some of it.

Why Does Skin Wrinkle?

What you can't see can hurt you, and that's true of the sun's rays. Ultraviolet (UV) light reaches the earth at different frequencies, and these frequencies attack the skin in different ways. UVA rays are associated with skin aging, skin cancer, and wrinkles, while UVB rays cause sunburn.

It doesn't have to be a sunny day for you to suffer harmful effects from the sun. Rays that pass through the clouds on a cloudy day or that reflect off snow, water, and sand can cause significant skin damage as well. The sun's rays cause the elastin and collagen fibers in the skin to deteriorate, which makes the skin less flexible. When skin becomes inflexible, the sweat and oil glands don't function well, which then causes the skin to become drier. At the same time, fat under the skin can shrink and cause the skin to sag.

If you have fair skin, you can expect to wrinkle more easily than people who have dark skin. That's because light skin has less pigment, and pigment is a natural sunscreen. Less pigment equals less protection.

A WORD ABOUT SUNSCREENS

When purchasing a sunscreen, look for one that has an SPF (sun protection factor) greater than 15 and one that protects against both UVA and UVB rays. Most sunscreens provide good protection against UVB only. Check the label for ingredients that are known to protect against UVA rays, such as benzophenone, oxybenzone, titanium oxide, and zinc oxide.

13 Tips to Protect Your Skin

1 Feed your face. Take oral supplements of 1,000 mg vitamin C three times a day and 400 IU vitamin E twice a day to protect your skin. The sun causes the release of skin-damaging free radicals, and these two antioxidants help stop them in their tracks.

2 Do a facial workout. Spend 10 to 15 minutes a day doing facial exercises. Books like *5-Minute Facelift* by Robert The and *Facercise: The Dynamic Muscle-Toning Program for Renewed Vitality and More Youthful Appearance* by Carole Maggio offer some suggestions.

3 Stroke up. When putting on facial creams, always use light, upward strokes, starting at your neck and moving upward.

4 Renew with Renova. Repair skin damage with Renova, the first antiwrinkle treatment approved by the FDA. Renova is an improvement over Retin-A, which causes skin irritation in some people. Research shows that use of Renova for six months can reduce age spots and fine lines. It is available by prescription only.

5 Stay in the shade. Protect yourself against UV rays. Wear a hat when you're outside, even when you're in the shade, and use a sunscreen of 15 SPF or higher. If you're in a room that is lit with daylight from windows, you'll still need sunscreen, because glass blocks UVB well, but blocks very little UVA.

6 Don't smoke. Smoking promotes the production of free radicals and also causes wrinkles.

7 Defy gravity. If you can, sleep on your back. This exerts minimal gravitational pull on facial skin and helps reduce sagging. If you sleep with your face pressed into a pillow, you will have a puffy face in the morning.

8 Keep the cork in the wine bottle. Avoid drinking alcohol for at least three hours before going to bed. Alcohol causes the small blood vessels to leak water into the soft tissues. This process, along with lying horizontally during the night, results in facial puffiness and stretched skin.

9 Wash sparingly. Once a day is enough. Washing your face takes away moisture, and the chlorine in tap water can cause skin damage. The hotter the water, the more damage chlorine can cause.

10 Avoid tanning beds. More than 1,500 Americans need emergency room treatment each year because of burns suffered in commercial tanning salons, according to the American Academy of Dermatology. There's longer-term damage as well: The UV rays can cause wrinkles, skin cancer, eye damage, and suppression of the immune system.

11 Make up with nutrients. Look for cosmetics that contain antioxidants such as vitamins A, C, and E; beta-carotene; and green tea extract.

12 Alphahydroxize. Promote healthy skin with alphahydroxy acids (AHAs), fruit, sugarcane, and milk extracts that remove dead skin cells and allow the moister skin below to emerge. AHAs also attract moisture to the skin, which plumps up the skin and temporarily eliminates crow's feet and other fine lines. These ingredients are available in creams and lotions.

13 Drink up. Drink at least eight glasses of water a day. Water is critical to flush toxins from the skin and promote good blood circulation.

chapter nineteen

Watching Out for Kids:

14 Pediatric Emergencies and What to Do

Every parent worries about medical emergencies involving their children. We're not talking about a little cut or scrape or bruise, although these can be a bit scary for children. We're talking about medical situations that are serious or life-threatening. But worrying doesn't help; being prepared does. Every parent should be ready to provide minimal, basic care for a child in need until professional medical help arrives.

Being prepared for medical emergencies means the following:

- Know the basics of cardiopulmonary resuscitation (CPR), the Heimlich maneuver, and first aid. Classes in both are provided by the American Red Cross, the National Safety Council, as well as many community hospitals, fire stations, and other organizations.

- Keep a list of emergency phone numbers next to all the telephones in your house. The list should include the following:

  ➢ Local emergency number (911 in many areas; local police or fire station in others)

  ➢ Police department, fire department, and ambulance (In some locations, one or more of these numbers are the same.)

  ➢ Poison control center

  ➢ Family doctor or clinic

  ➢ Work telephone numbers for parent(s)

119

➤ Nearest neighbor's phone

➤ Nearest relative's phone

➤ Pager and cellular phone numbers

- Teach your children how to call for help in case of an emergency: which number to call; how to give their name, address, and phone number; and how to describe what's wrong.

- Make sure anyone who is staying with your children, such as a babysitter, friend, or relative, knows where the emergency numbers and first aid kit are located.

Here is a list of the 14 most common medical emergencies that affect children, along with some basic first aid instructions. Remember to keep a first aid kit in your home at all times (see Chapter 7). Refer to the first aid book in your kit for complete instructions, or follow the directions given to you by a health professional. The following suggestions are meant only as a guide.

1 ALLERGIC REACTIONS

During the course of daily life, your child can have an allergic reaction to foods, medications, or insect bites or stings. These reactions can vary greatly in severity. Here we discuss moderate to severe reactions only.

Symptoms of a moderate reaction include rash, itching, swelling of the tongue, throat, or face, wheezing, coughing, and lightheadedness. Allow the child to lie down and give him an antihistamine or clemastine to help relieve swelling, rash, and itching. Contact your child's doctor immediately or take your child to the emergency department.

Symptoms of a severe reaction include all of the above plus difficulty swallowing or breathing, nausea, vomiting, abdominal cramps, pale clammy skin, rapid weak pulse, an altered consciousness or unconsciousness. These are symptoms of anaphylactic shock and can lead to cardiac arrest and death if not treated immediately.

- Call 911.

- Keep the child calm. If the child feels faint, have him lie down on a flat surface and keep him warm. Raise his feet 8 to 12 inches to help maintain blood pressure.

- If the child has an emergency kit for such incidents, follow the directions for giving the injection.
- Do CPR if necessary.
- If the child is wheezing and you have an acute treatment inhaler available, have the child use it.

2 BITES (ANIMAL AND HUMAN)

- Clean the wound immediately with mild soap and water.
- If the wounds are severe, treat them as you would any large wound (see "Bleeding").
- Call your child's doctor as soon as possible, or go to the emergency room.

3 BLEEDING

Bleeding can occur from either veins or arteries. Bleeding from the latter is more serious, as the blood is under more pressure and more can escape in a short time.

The amount of blood that you see is not always an accurate sign of how serious an injury is, as internal bleeding cannot be seen. On the other hand, in cases of scalp lacerations, there may appear to be a lot of blood when in fact not much blood is lost.

- If the wound and bleeding are severe, call 911.
- Keep the child and yourself calm.
- Try to remove any loose debris from the wound. Don't attempt to remove objects that are deeply embedded in the wound or you may cause more damage.
- If possible, wear latex gloves or keep several layers of cloth or gauze between you and the wound.
- Apply direct pressure to the wound using a sterile cloth or dressing. Keep applying pressure until the bleeding stops or medical help arrives. If the cloth soaks through, don't remove it; simply place another one on top.
- If the wound is on an arm or leg and you know the limb isn't broken, elevate the limb above the level of the child's heart.

- When the bleeding stops, apply a bandage around the compress to hold it in place. Use bandaging material or strips of cloth.
- Check for a pulse below the level of the bandage. If you don't feel a pulse, loosen the bandage slightly and check for a pulse again.
- Keep the child warm by covering her with a blanket or clothing, but keep the wound in sight.

4 BROKEN BONES

When it comes to fractures, children usually break the bones in their arms or legs. The keys here are immobilizing the injury and getting the child to a hospital.

- If an arm is broken and is bent, don't try to straighten it. Place the child's arm in a sling so the injured area is at or above the level of the heart.
- If a leg is broken, apply a splint on each side of the leg. Place a towel between the two legs and bind the splinted leg to the other leg with bandaging.
- Toes and fingers usually don't need to be splinted. Keep them protected until you reach the emergency department.
- Never try to set a fracture or dislocated bone.
- If a bone is protruding or there are other open wounds, cover them with a clean cloth.

5 BURNS

All burns are not created equal. Before you can treat a burn, you must recognize its type, then react appropriately.

First-degree burns affect the outer layer of the skin only. There is redness, pain, and perhaps some slight swelling. These burns can be treated by running cool water over the affected site and placing cool towels on the area. Do not use grease, petroleum jelly, or other oily substances. Never apply ice.

Second-degree burns can penetrate into the second layer of skin and cause redness, swelling, blistering, and tenderness. These burns often result from spilled hot liquid or a serious sunburn.

- Put the burned area in cool water or apply cool cloths for a few minutes.
- Cover the burn loosely with a sterile gauze or clean cloth and take the child to a doctor.

Third-degree burns can be deadly. They are usually caused by scalding liquids, contact with electricity, or fire. Third-degree burns penetrate through the top layers of skin and can extend into the fat or muscle below. Often they are relatively painless, as the nerve endings that would normally send pain signals to the brain have been destroyed.

- Call 911 or take the child to an emergency department immediately.
- If you are waiting for help, make sure the child is breathing. If necessary, perform rescue breathing or CPR.
- If the burns are extensive, cover the child lightly with a clean blanket.
- If the burn is not extensive, place a cold, wet cloth on the area or gently pour cool water over the affected area.
- Cover the burn with a sterile dressing. Do not attempt to remove any clothing that may be sticking to the burn.

Electrical burns can be deceptive because they affect the internal tissues more than they do the skin. All electrical burns and shocks should be checked by a doctor.

- If the child is still in contact with the electrical source, turn off the source by pulling the plug or shutting off the circuit.
- If it is not possible to stop the source, separate the child from the source with a wooden broom handle, a box, a rope, or anything that does not conduct electricity. Never use metal.
- Once the child is separated from the source, check his breathing and pulse. Do rescue breathing or CPR if needed.
- Call 911.
- Cover all burns with a dry, loose dressing and then a bandage. Do not attempt to treat the burns in any other way.

6 CHOKING

A child's choking can be frightening, but if you act quickly and appropriately, you can often help the child to breath normally again.

- Do not give the child something to drink or slap the child on the back. If the coughing reflex doesn't dislodge the object and the child can breathe, call 911 or your doctor immediately for instructions.

- If the child can't breathe or cough, have someone call 911 immediately and then perform the Heimlich maneuver by standing behind the child, putting your arms around to her front, clasping your hands together, and pushing sharply in and upward, just below her ribcage. In the case of a baby, place your fingertips at the center of the trunk, just below the rib cage, and push in and up until whatever is choking the child has become dislodged.

7 DROWNING

- Perform rescue breathing or CPR immediately. (Educational groups such as the American Red Cross offer courses that can teach you how to do these techniques properly.) Every second counts. Begin the procedure in the water if necessary.
- Call 911.
- Keep the child warm, especially if she was in cold water.

8 EYE INJURIES

Whether an object has penetrated the eye, chemicals have splashed into it, or the eye has suffered a direct blow, contact your child's doctor or an ophthalmologist immediately.

- If chemicals are involved, immediately flush the eyes with a gentle stream of cool running water for at least 15 minutes. Call a poison control center or your doctor as soon as possible. Do not allow the child to touch the eyes.
- If an object has penetrated the eye or the eye has been hit, gently cover both eyes with a gauze or clean cloth and tape it loosely to the skin. Do not apply pressure. Take the child to the emergency department.

9 FAINTING

Fainting is a loss of consciousness, usually for less than one minute. Check the child's breathing and pulse. If the child is not breathing, call 911 and begin rescue breathing. If there is no pulse, begin CPR.

10 HEAD INJURIES

- If there are serious injuries to the head, don't move the child or his head. Call 911.

- Call 911 if a child has any of these symptoms following a severe head injury:
  - ➤ Unconsciousness that lasts more than a few seconds
  - ➤ Drowsiness, difficulty speaking, vomiting, nausea
  - ➤ Convulsions
  - ➤ Blood or clear fluid draining from the nose, mouth, or ears
  - ➤ Numbness or weakness in the limbs
  - ➤ Dilated pupils or vision problems
  - ➤ Headache, irritability, or sleepiness that gets worse

- A minor head injury may cause a child to lose consciousness for a few seconds and then experience a headache, double vision, a lump on the head, and confusion for an hour or two. Have the child lie down while you call the doctor for advice.

- If the child has a lump on his head, apply an ice pack to reduce swelling. If the swelling increases, it may suggest a fracture. Go to the emergency department immediately.

- If the head injury appears to be mild and the child is not in pain, observe him for a day or two. Wake the child every three hours at night to check on his alertness. If there is any vomiting, go to the emergency department immediately.

11 HEATSTROKE

Heatstroke usually follows heat exhaustion. In itself, heat exhaustion is not an emergency condition. If left untreated, however, heat exhaustion can lead to heatstroke, which is more serious.

- Symptoms of heat exhaustion include pale and clammy skin, dizziness, nausea, fatigue, and muscle cramps. These usually occur during hot weather when a child has been too active. Allow the child to lie down, rest, and sip cool water.

- If a child advances to heatstroke, symptoms include flushed, hot, dry skin and a body temperature of 104 degrees or higher. The child may be confused and may lose consciousness. The primary goal is to lower the child's body temperature. Do the following:

➤ Call 911.

➤ Move the child to a cool location indoors or in the shade and remove his clothing.

➤ Apply moist, cool towels to his skin; if possible, place the child in a partially filled tub of cool water. If you're outside, you can spray the child with water from a garden hose (make sure it's not hot).

➤ Keep checking the child's temperature. Once it reaches 101 degrees, dry him off. If his temperature begins to rise again, repeat the cooling techniques.

12 POISONING

- If you suspect your child has ingested a poisonous substance, call the poison control center immediately, even if she isn't showing any signs. Some poisons do not take effect immediately.

- Give the center the child's name and age, what she swallowed, how much, whether she has vomited, and how long it will take for you to get to the nearest hospital.

- Take the poisonous substance or its container with you, whether it's a plant, cleaning product, vitamin or medication, or other substance.

- If the child is experiencing convulsions, is unconscious, or is having difficulty breathing, call 911.

- Never give anything to induce vomiting until you have spoken with an expert at the poison control center.

13 SHOCK

Shock—a drastic reduction in the amount of blood flowing to organs and tissues, with a drop in blood pressure—can be caused by excessive vomiting or diarrhea, bleeding, burns, infections, and severe injuries. Signs of shock include:

- Confusion, anxiety
- Pale, clammy, bluish, cool skin
- Widely dilated pupils

- Weakness in the limbs
- Extreme drowsiness
- Fainting

If a child appears to be in shock, call 911 and do the following while waiting for medical help:

- Keep making sure the child is breathing. If he stops, perform rescue breathing.
- Keep the child lying down and warm. Raise his feet above the level of the heart unless there is a back, neck, or head injury.
- If the child vomits, place him on his side to prevent him from choking on his own vomit.
- Keep the child warm but not overheated. Do not give water in case the child needs surgery.

14 SKIN CAUGHT IN ZIPPER

This can be a very painful and frustrating situation, and many people don't know what to do, which is why we've included it as an emergency. Often it is the penis skin that gets caught, when a child isn't wearing underwear and gets dressed too quickly. The skin of the penis becomes crushed between the teeth and the slide of the zipper. You don't want to yank that zipper down. Here's what to do:

- Soak the area with mineral oil to lubricate the zipper's moving parts. This should allow you to free the skin without cutting the zipper. Paint the area with povidone-iodine and irrigate with plain 1 percent lidocaine. This should allow you to manipulate the zipper and the clothing.
- If the mineral oil doesn't work, then cut the zipper away from the clothing.
- Use metal snips to cut the slide of the zipper in half. This should release the skin. Because this technique can frighten a child, divert his attention away from what you're going to do.
- Clean the crushed skin with povidone-iodine.

chapter twenty

Are You Prepared?

6 Survival Kits

Pick up the newspaper any day of the week and you're likely to read about a crisis. Somewhere an earthquake, flood, fire, tornado, hurricane, mud slide, or volcanic eruption raised havoc with the local population. An elderly couple sat stranded in their car in a blizzard for three days. Two hikers lost their way in the wilderness for a week.

Whether it's devastation caused by nature or an unfortunate turn of events, a disaster can strike at any time. You can try to save your possessions, but when it comes to priorities, life is more precious by far. Whether it's your own life, your family's, your coworkers', or your family dog's, everyone has a much better chance of surviving an emergency or catastrophe if you're prepared.

Are You Prepared?

An emergency is the worst time to realize that you're not prepared. Ask yourself: If a _____ (fill in the blank with any natural disaster that could befall your region of the country) were to hit my neighborhood tomorrow, would my family and I be safe? Do I have an escape plan? Do I have basic supplies put aside in a readily accessible place that would allow me and my family to survive for several days until help arrived? If I were to get stranded in my car (or boat) do I have the supplies I need to survive until help arrives?

If you answered no to these questions, it's time for you to take stock—and stock up—for your life. We've listed some basic items every survival kit should contain, as well as other items for specific emergency situations. You can buy ready-to-use kits from the American Red Cross, from many sporting centers or marine stores, or by searching the Internet using the key words "survival kits" or "disaster kits."

1 BASIC SURVIVAL ITEMS

Minimum required for one adult for three days.

- Six all-natural food bars°
- Six 4.2-ounce leak-proof water pouches°
- Three 12-hour lightsticks°

2 WINTER SURVIVAL KIT

These items can help if you're stranded in a car or at home without electricity in the winter and you can't get out for help. Minimum required for each adult.

- Three 20-hour warm packs
- Six all-natural food bars°
- Six 4.2-ounce leakproof water pouches°
- One emergency blanket: space-age design that retains 90 percent of body heat
- 28-piece first aid kit including iodine pads, alcohol, and guide (see Chapter 7) (You don't need one kit for each adult; adjust according to the number of people you expect to be using the kit.)
- Three waste disposal bags
- One package tissues
- Three 12-hour lightsticks
- One whistle

° These items should be Coast Guard approved with a five-year shelf life. The water is purified by reverse osmosis.

3 WILDERNESS SURVIVAL KIT

In case a 6-hour hike turns into a 72-hour wilderness challenge, everyone should have the following provisions:

- All items in the Winter Survival Kit
- Waterproof matches
- One hooded rain poncho
- One flashlight with batteries
- Water purification tablets
- One multifunction knife (Swiss army knife or similar)
- One tube tent
- Signaling device (mirror, flares)

4 DISASTER SURVIVAL KIT

This kit could be for any type of disaster. You can modify the kit depending on your specific region and needs. However, it is important always to have the items from the Winter Survival Kit for each adult and each child 3 years and older. (You don't need extra lightsticks for each child.)

- All items in Winter Survival Kit
- One dust mask
- One hooded rain poncho
- One flashlight with batteries
- One multifunction knife (Swiss army knife or similar)
- One collapsible gallon water jug
- One 5' × 7' tarp (or a tube tent)
- One radio and batteries
- One 50-foot utility cord
- One pry bar
- Personal items (toothpaste, toothbrush)
- Waterproof matches and candles
- Playing cards

5 OFFICE SURVIVAL KIT

If you are responsible for the safety of coworkers, make sure an Office Survival Kit is accessible in your workplace. It should include all the items in the Disaster Survival Kit plus a toilet bucket, a toilet seat, and toilet chemicals. Most of the Survival Kit items should fit snugly inside the toilet bucket for easy storage.

6 MARINE SURVIVAL KIT

Every boat that goes out into the ocean should have a Marine Survival Kit aboard. This kit can be quite extensive, and depending on your circumstances, you may choose not to get every item on this list. The items below are considered to be standard for oceangoing crafts, but you should have some of the items on board even if you're just sailing or motoring around the bay.

- All the items in the Basic Survival Kit
- Raft
- Life jackets
- Waterproof bag with adjustable tethers that contains as many of the following as possible:
  - Life raft repair kit
  - Manual inflation pump
  - Sea anchor
  - Sponges
  - Bailer
  - Duct tape for leaks above the water line
  - Pressure release and topper valves for the raft
  - Signaling mirrors
  - Flares: smoke, handheld, and parachute-type
  - Signal streamer (a 40-foot bright plastic ribbon that is tied to the raft and drifts on top of the water and can easily be seen from the air)
  - Binoculars
  - Multipurpose tool (Swiss army knife or similar tool)
  - Raft knife

➢ Flashlight and batteries

➢ Fire starter (in case you do hit land)

➢ Gloves

➢ Spear gun

➢ Collapsible bucket (This can be your bailer as well.)

➢ Manual desalination pump

➢ First aid kit

➢ Sunscreen

chapter twenty-one

Child's Play and Beyond: How Safe Is Your Sport?

Americans love to play, and when they do, many of them get hurt. A great number of these injuries happen to children. According to the Centers for Disease Control and Prevention (CDC), approximately 6 million high school students play team sports, and another 20 million children participate in recreational or competitive sports outside of school. In addition, countless numbers of children play unsupervised, nonteam sports, such as bike riding, running, skateboarding, and in-line skating.

Although sports can help build character, teamwork, and self-esteem in children, they can also hurt them. Each year, more than 775,000 children age 15 and younger are injured playing sports. Eighty percent of the injuries are related to football, soccer, basketball, and baseball.

Surprising Survey Results

In May 2000, the National Safe Kids Campaign released the results of a survey that showed one-third of all children who participate in organized sports experience an injury at one time or other. Perhaps most surprising about the findings is that, although an estimated 50 percent of the injuries are preventable, most parents believe there is nothing they could have done to prevent them. A full 80 percent said that the injury "was part of the game and probably would have happened anyway." Fifty-three percent of parents expressed little concern about the possibility of their children being injured while playing team sports.

Not everyone shares the views of these parents. The National Safe Kids Campaign believes that more than half of the injuries—including concussions, broken bones, torn ligaments, lacerations, and dislocated joints—can be prevented through the use of protective equipment, proper conditioning, close supervision, and adequate hydration.

The survey also showed that 34 percent of parents don't make their kids take the same safety precautions during practice sessions that they do during a game. That's unfortunate, because most sports injuries occur during practice.

Finally, 41 percent of parents reported that their childrens' coaches are not certified in cardiopulmonary resuscitation and don't have a first aid kit handy during practice or games.

General Safety Guidelines

What can you do to make sure your children are safe when they participate in sports? Here are some general guidelines.

- **Get them examined.** Before children start a training program or a competitive sport, they should get a physical examination. A doctor can help identify any special risks children may have.

- **Get them properly equipped.** Children should wear all the recommended or required safety equipment every time they participate in the sport. Depending on the sport, this can include helmets, knee pads, eyewear, and elbow pads.

- **Get them warmed up.** Children should warm up and stretch before playing

- **Get them a kit.** A first aid kit should be readily available at team practices and games.

- **Get them to rest and recover.** Children should learn not to play through pain. Injured children should be brought to a doctor for an evaluation of the injury, and should not return to play until the doctor approves.

- **Get to know your child's coaches.** Coaches should encourage safe play and enforce the rules of the game being played.

How Individual Sports Fare in Injury Rates: Numbers from the CDC

Baseball and Softball

- Of the 33 million people who participate in organized baseball and softball leagues, nearly 6 million are children 5 to 14 years old.

- Each year, more than 125,000 players under age 15 seek emergency department treatment: 95,000 for baseball-related and 30,000 for softball-related injuries.

- Among high school players, about 8 percent are hurt each year.

- The majority of injuries are minor: abrasions, fractures, sprains, and strains.

- Baseball is the main cause of sports-related eye injuries in children.

- Up to 45 percent of pitchers under age 12 have chronic elbow pain; among high school pitchers, the rate is 58 percent.

- On average, three children under age 15 die each year from baseball-related injuries.

- Sliding into the bases causes more than 70 percent of recreational softball injuries and about 33 percent of baseball injuries. Use of break-away bases can prevent 1.7 million injuries per year.

Basketball

- More than 200,000 people under age 15 are treated in emergency departments each year for basketball-related injuries.

- Injuries are usually minor, mostly sprains and strains to the knees and ankle. Eye injuries are also common.

- More injuries occur during practice at the high school and recreational levels.

- More injuries occur during games at the college level.

- Girls and women have a higher rate of injury than boys and men.

Biking

- In 1997, an estimated 567,000 people needed emergency department care as a result of bike crashes in the United States, and 813 people were killed.

- Thirty-one percent of bike-related deaths occur among children under the age of 16.
- Each year an estimated 140,000 children received emergency department care for head and eye injuries related to bike riding.
- Wearing a helmet can reduce the risk of brain injury by as much as 88 percent, yet only about 25 percent of children ages 4 to 15 wear a helmet when riding a bike.

Football

- More than 150,000 football players under the age of 15 are treated in emergency departments each year. Between 15 and 20 percent of football players ages 8 to 14 are injured during football season.
- Knee injuries total about 92,000 per year, and can lead to chronic knee pain.
- About 5 percent of football injuries are concussions. Players who get a concussion are four to six times more likely to get another one.
- Repeated concussions experienced over a long period of time can lead to serious, permanent disability.
- Sprains and strains are the most frequent injuries among players of all ages.

Gymnastics

- More than 600,000 children participate in school-sponsored and club gymnastics competitions in the United States.
- About 25,000 emergency department visits are made by gymnasts under 15 years old each year.
- Among high school gymnasts, the injury rate is 56 percent.
- The majority of gymnastics-related injures are sprains, strains, and stress fractures, most often to the ankles and knees.
- Up to 50 percent of injuries lead to chronic pain.
- Floor exercises are the most common cause of injury.

Ice Hockey

- More than 500,000 amateurs play ice hockey in the United States.
- Ice hockey is the second leading cause of winter sports injuries among children.

- Collisions with other players are associated with 46 percent of all minor injuries and 75 percent of major injuries.

- The most common types of injuries are sprains and bruises to the thigh, knee, and ankle; concussions and lacerations are also common.

- Use of full-face guards on helmets has reduced the incidence of eye injuries, and neck guards have reduced the number of spinal and soft tissue injuries.

In-Line Skating and Skateboarding

- More than 100,000 people receive emergency department treatment each year for injuries related to in-line skating, and 40,000 receive such treatment for skateboarding injuries. Most of these individuals are younger than 25.

- Most injuries are the result of losing control, skating over an obstacle, performing a trick, or skating too fast.

- Although most skating injuries are minor, 36 deaths have occurred since 1992, 31 of which involved a collision with a motor vehicle.

- Use of pads can reduce injuries by about 85 percent for wrist and elbow and 32 percent for knees.

- Nearly 66 percent of in-line skaters and skateboarders were not wearing safety equipment (helmet and pads) when they crashed.

Skiing, Sledding, and Snowboarding

- According to the U.S. Consumer Product Safety Commission (CPSC), 84,200 skiing injuries and 37,600 snowboarding injuries were treated in emergency departments in the United States in 1997; of these, 17,500 were head injuries.

- The CPSC believes that 7,700 head injuries yearly could be prevented or reduced in severity if people used skiing or snowboarding helmets, and that helmet use could also prevent about 11 skiing- and snowboarding-related deaths yearly.

- The most common skiing-related injuries are ankle and knee sprains and fractures.

- Most skiing and snowboarding injuries happen to adults; most sledding injuries occur among children 5 to 14 years old.

- More than 14,500 children ages 5 to 14 were treated for sledding-related injuries in the United States in 1997.

- Between 1993 and 1997, snowboarding injuries nearly tripled and head injuries from snowboarding increased fivefold as more and more people tried the sport.

Soccer

- More than 200,000 young people seek medical treatment each year for soccer-related injuries.

- Although the injury rate is less than 1 percent for children younger than 12 years, it is nearly 8 percent among high school players and nearly 9 percent among players 19 years and older who play on community teams.

- Older players are injured more often and have more severe injuries than young players.

- Most injuries involve sprains, strains, and bruises and usually affect the ankle or knee.

- Acute head injuries make up about 5 percent of injuries.

- The most severe injuries involve hitting a goal post: There have been 22 deaths from this cause since the early 1980s.

- Tests show that padding the goal posts can reduce the force of hitting the post by 31 to 63 percent.

chapter twenty-two

Smash, Crash, and Roll: How Dangerous Is Your Vehicle?

How safe is the car you're driving? Does a car's safety record or safety rating mean much to you when it's time to buy a car? Every year, several different groups conduct crash tests and other evaluations of a vehicle's safety and then publicize the information for consumers. One of those groups, the National Highway Traffic Safety Administration (NHTSA), conducts crash and rollover tests on cars of every size, sports utility vehicles, light trucks, and vans. We've listed some of their findings below for 2001 model year cars. The crash tests were done at a speed of 35 mph. All cars were equipped with safety belts and air bags. The rating system goes from one to five: One is the most dangerous, five is the safest. The vehicles marked "NR" are not rated for that category. To help you interpret the ratings, here's an explanation of the headings:

Front Crash: The estimated chance of a life-threatening head or chest injury for the driver resulting from a frontal crash. Vehicles are twice as likely to be involved in severe frontal crashes than in severe side crashes. (The NHTSA also rates the chances for a front seat passenger, but that information is not included here.)

Side Crash: The estimated chance of a life-threatening chest injury for the driver resulting from a side crash.

Rollover: This is an estimate of your chances of rolling over if you have what is commonly referred to as a "single vehicle crash," which is a crash caused

139

by a driver's behavior—usually speeding or inattention—and not by colliding with another vehicle. Most rollover accidents occur when a vehicle runs off the road and makes contact with a curb, a ditch, soft dirt, or another object. Although this rating does not directly predict your risk of death or injury, it's a fact that rollover accidents result in a higher fatality rate than other kinds of crashes. It's been estimated that you can reduce your chance of being killed in a rollover accident by 75 percent if you are wearing your seatbelt.

Another thing to remember is that regardless of how safe a vehicle is, it's the driver that truly makes the difference. Even the car with the highest safety rating in the world isn't safe if the driver is drunk or otherwise impaired. At the end of our list is some information about alcohol-related accidents and deaths. Take a moment to look at those figures. Perhaps some of those deaths could have been avoided if all the cars involved had been Mercury Grand Marquis or Volvos, which both rank high in safety. Then again, perhaps all of them could have been avoided if the drivers hadn't been drinking.

Vehicle	Front Crash	Side Crash	Rollover
Acura TL 4-door	★ ★ ★ ★	★ ★ ★ ★	NR
Buick Century 4-door	★ ★ ★ ★	★ ★ ★	NR
Buick Lesabre 4-door	★ ★ ★ ★	★ ★ ★ ★	NR
Buick Park Avenue 4-door	★ ★ ★ ★	★ ★ ★ ★	NR
Buick Regal 4-door	★ ★ ★ ★	★ ★ ★	NR
Cadillac Deville 4-door	★ ★ ★	★ ★ ★ ★	NR
Chevrolet Camaro 2-door	★ ★ ★ ★	★ ★ ★	NR
Chevrolet Cavalier 2-door	★ ★ ★	★	NR
Chevrolet Cavalier 4-door	★ ★ ★ ★	★	★ ★ ★ ★
Chevrolet Prizm 4-door	★ ★ ★ ★	★ ★ ★	★ ★ ★ ★
Chevrolet Impala 4-door	★ ★ ★ ★ ★	★ ★ ★ ★	★ ★ ★ ★
Chevrolet Lumina 4-door	★ ★ ★ ★	★ ★ ★ ★	NR
Chevrolet Monte Carlo 2-door	★ ★ ★ ★ ★	★ ★ ★	NR
Chrysler Concorde 4-door	★ ★ ★ ★	★ ★ ★ ★	NR
Chrysler LHS 4-door	★ ★ ★	★ ★ ★ ★	NR
Dodge Intrepid 4-door	★ ★ ★ ★	★ ★ ★ ★	NR
Dodge Neon 4-door	★ ★ ★ ★	★ ★ ★	NR
Ford Crown Victoria 4-door	★ ★ ★ ★ ★	★ ★ ★ ★	★ ★ ★ ★ ★
Ford Escort 4-door	★ ★ ★	★ ★ ★	NR

Vehicle	Front Crash	Side Crash	Rollover
Ford Focus 2-door	★ ★ ★ ★ ★	★ ★ ★ ★	★ ★ ★ ★
Honda Civic 2-door	★ ★ ★ ★ ★	★ ★ ★ ★ ★	NR
Honda Civic 4-door	★ ★ ★ ★ ★	★ ★ ★ ★ ★	★ ★ ★ ★
Lincoln LS 4-door	★ ★ ★ ★ ★	★ ★ ★ ★	★ ★ ★ ★ ★
Mazda 626 4-door	★ ★ ★ ★	★ ★ ★	NR
Mercury Grand Marquis 4-door	★ ★ ★ ★ ★	★ ★ ★ ★	★ ★ ★ ★ ★
Mercury Sable 4-door	★ ★ ★ ★ ★	★ ★ ★	★ ★ ★ ★
Mitsubishi Galant 4-door	★ ★ ★ ★	★ ★ ★ ★ ★	NR
Nissan Altima 4-door	★ ★ ★ ★	★ ★ ★	NR
Oldsmobile Alero 2-door	★ ★ ★ ★	★	NR
Oldsmobile Aurora 4-door	★ ★ ★ ★ ★	★ ★ ★	NR
Plymouth Neon 4-door	★ ★ ★ ★	★ ★ ★	NR
Pontiac Bonneville	★ ★ ★ ★	★ ★ ★ ★	NR
Pontiac Firebird 2-door	★ ★ ★ ★	★ ★ ★	NR
Pontiac Grand Am 2-door	★ ★ ★ ★	★	NR
Pontiac Sunfire 2-door	★ ★ ★	★	NR
Pontiac Sunfire 4-door	★ ★ ★ ★	★	★ ★ ★ ★
Saturn L series 4-door	★ ★ ★ ★	★ ★	NR
Saturn SL 4-door	★ ★ ★ ★ ★	★ ★ ★	NR
Subaru Legacy 4-door Wagon	★ ★ ★ ★	★ ★ ★ ★	NR
Toyota Celica 2-door	★ ★ ★ ★	★ ★ ★	NR
Toyota Corolla 4-door	★ ★ ★ ★	★ ★ ★	★ ★ ★ ★
Toyota Camry 4-door	★ ★ ★ ★	★ ★ ★	★ ★ ★ ★ ★
VW Beetle 2-door	★ ★ ★ ★	★ ★ ★ ★ ★	NR
VW Jetta 4-door	★ ★ ★ ★ ★	★ ★ ★ ★	★ ★ ★ ★
VW Passat 4-door	★ ★ ★ ★ ★	★ ★ ★ ★	NR
Volvo 580 4-door	★ ★ ★ ★ ★	★ ★ ★ ★ ★	NR

Sports Utility Vehicles

Vehicle	Front Crash	Side Crash	Rollover
Chevy Blazer 4-door 4X4	★ ★ ★	★ ★ ★ ★ ★	★ ★
Chevy Tracker 4-door 4X4	★ ★ ★ ★	NR	★ ★ ★
Ford Explorer 4-door 4X4	★ ★ ★ ★	★ ★ ★ ★ ★	★ ★
GMC Jimmy 4-door 4X4	★ ★ ★	★ ★ ★ ★ ★	★ ★
Honda CR-V 4-door 4X4	★ ★ ★ ★	★ ★ ★ ★ ★	NR

Vehicle	Front Crash	Side Crash	Rollover
Honda Passport 4-door 4X4	* * * *	* * * * *	NR
Infiniti QX4, 4-door 4X4	* * * *	* * * * *	NR
Isuzu Rodeo 4-door, 4X4	* * * *	* * * * *	NR
Jeep Cherokee 4-door 4X4	* * *	* * *	NR
Jeep Grand Cherokee 4X4	* * *	* * * *	* *
Jeep Wrangler 2-door 4X4	* * * *	NR	* * *
Mercury Mountainer 4-door 4X4	* * * *	* * * * *	* *
Nissan Pathfinder 4-door 4X4	* * * *	* * * * *	NR
Nissan Xterra 4-door 4X4	* * * *	* * * *	* *
Oldsmobile Bravada 4-door 4X4	* * *	* * * * *	* *
Subaru Forester 4-door 4X4	* * * *	NR	* * *
Suzuki Vitara 4-door 4X4	* * * *	NR	* * *
Toyota 4Runner 4X4	* * * *	* * * * *	NR

Light Trucks

Chevrolet S10 PU 4X2	* * *	* * * *	NR
Chevrolet S10 Excab 4X2	* *	* * *	* * *
Chevrolet Silverado Excab 4X2	* * *	NR	* * * *
Ford F150 PU Excab 4X2	* * * *	* * * * *	NR
Ford Ranger PU Excab 4X2	* * * *	* * * *	NR
GMC Sierra PU Excab 4X2	* * *	NR	* * * *
GMC Sonoma PU 4X2	* * *	* * * *	NR
Mazda B series Excab	* * * *	* * * *	NR

Vans

Chrysler PT Cruiser	* *	* * * *	* * * *
Honda Odyssey	* * * * *	* * * * *	* * * *
Mazda MPV	* * * *	* * * * *	* * *
Mercury Villager	* * * * *	* * * * *	* * * *
Nissan Quest	* * * * *	* * * * *	* * * *
Pontiac Montana	* * * *	* * * * *	NR
Toyota Sienna	* * * * *	* * * *	* * * *

NR = Not Rated

Sites to Visit for Crash and Safety Information

- Insurance Institute for Highway Safety: www.hwysafety.org
- National Highway Traffic Safety Administration: www.nhtsa.dot.gov
- EuroNCAP (European New Car Assessment Programme): www.theaa.co.uk
- Japanese test results: www.crashtest.com

Alcohol-Related Traffic Accidents: Avoidable Deaths and Injuries

According to the National Highway Traffic Safety Administration:

- There were 15,786 alcohol-related traffic deaths in the United States in 1999, a number that is 38 percent of the total traffic-related deaths for the year.
- The 15,786 represents one fatal crash every 33 minutes.
- About 308,000 people were injured in alcohol-related traffic accidents in 1999. That's an average of one person every 2 minutes.
- About 1.4 million drivers were arrested in 1998 for driving under the influence of alcohol or drugs.
- Who is doing all the drinking? Intoxication rates for drivers of fatal crashes were highest for motorcycles (28%), followed by light trucks (20%), passenger cars (17%), and large trucks (1%). The top age groups downing the alcohol were 21 to 24 years old (27%), 25 to 34 years old (24%), and 35 to 44 years old (21%). This is based on a blood alcohol level of greater than 0.10, which is the legal limit in most states.

chapter twenty-three

The Safest and Riskiest Ways to Travel in the United States and Beyond

If you want to place your life in the hands of the world's most dangerous drivers, there may be no better way to do so than to go for a ride a minibus or minivan in a developing country. These small vehicles are equipped with a drive train that is designed to carry about four people, yet it's not uncommon to see fifteen or sixteen people crammed into them. Combine this sardine scenario with rush hour traffic, which is when they are mainly used, and you have a recipe for disaster.

The recipe doesn't fail. In South Africa, about 60,000 minivan accidents per year leave more than 900 people dead. There are about 30,000 minivans in Lima, Peru, which killed more than 370 pedestrians per year because of speeding.

Aside from the deadly minivan, how do some other modes of transportation fare in the safety department? We thought we'd take a look at some common forms of transport—cars, motorcycles, large trucks, cruise ships, airplanes, trains, and bicycles. Whether in the United States or abroad, you're sure to find some hair-raising statistics about transportation in the lists presented here. It's almost enough to make you want to stay home.

Motorcycles—United States

- In 1999, a total of 2,472 motorcyclists were killed and about 50,000 were injured. That's an 8-percent increase in deaths from 1998 and a 2-percent increase in injuries.

- The National Highway Traffic Safety Administration estimates that wearing a helmet saved the lives of 551 motorcyclists in 1999, but that 326 more motorcyclists could have been saved if they had been wearing helmets.

- Motorcycles represented less than 2 percent of all the registered vehicles on the road in 1998.

- Per vehicle mile traveled in 1998, motorcyclists were 16 times more likely than passenger car occupants to die in a motor vehicle accident in the United States.

Airplane Safety—United States and Abroad

- According to the Massachusetts Institute of Technology (MIT), your chances of dying in an airplane crash are 1 in 4.4 million when you fly an airline of any developed nation. Your chances get much better on a U.S. airline: 1 in 11 million.

- About two-thirds of major airline crashes are attributed to flight crew error.

- Seventy-five percent of airline accidents occur in countries that make up only 12 percent of the world's air traffic.

- Experts estimate that your chances of being killed in an airplane crash are less than one in one million in North America and Western Europe, and one in 50,000 in Africa. Asia, Latin America, the Middle East, and Eastern Europe are somewhere in between.

- If you really want to live dangerously, fly a local carrier in Colombia, China, India, North Korea, any country in Central Africa, or any plane that flies in the Andes Mountains.

- If you thought pirates just operated on the water, you might change your mind if you fly in China, which has the world's worst air piracy record.

- For a change of pace, fly down under. Australian airlines haven't had a fatal crash in more than 10 years.

- The International Airline Passengers Association reports that Colombia has the worst air safety record of all countries in the Americas. The organization also names India as one of the two most dangerous countries in which to fly.

Airplane Safety—United States

Before you make your next plane reservation, you may want to take a look at the safety records for the major carriers in the United States. These statistics are for a five-year period and cover three categories, explained here:

- Accidents = Number of deaths or serious injuries or occurrences of substantial damage to the airplane, per one million takeoffs
- Incidents = Number of situations that affected or could have affected safety or operation of the aircraft, per one million takeoffs
- Near Miss = The airplane came within less than 500 feet of another aircraft, per one million takeoffs

The information was compiled from data from the Federal Aviation Administration, the National Transportation Safety Board, and the U.S. Department of Transportation. Welcome aboard!

December 1995–December 1999			
Airline	Accidents	Incidents	Near Misses
Alaska Airline	5.02	8.78	20.08
America West	6.78	2.90	15.50
American Airlines	6.97	6.97	12.94
Continental	5.70	6.58	6.58
Delta	5.85	7.73	5.43
Northwest	1.04	5.94	8.03
Southwest	1.04	7.09	5.76
TWA	2.12	7.07	7.82
United	7.27	6.01	11.53
US Airways	1.89	5.41	4.60

Trains—United States

- According to the National Safety Council, trains have a terrific safety record. Compared with other modes of transportation, there were 0.96 deaths per 100 million miles traveled in a passenger car, 0.06 deaths for the same distance by commercial airline, and 0.04 deaths on railroads, including commuter trains.

- According to the Federal Railroad Administration and the Bureau of Transportation Statistics, there were 602 deaths related to train accidents in 1997 and 577 in 1998. This includes not just passengers but also railroad workers, as well as people who found themselves on the tracks and were struck. These figures compare with 660 and 621 deaths, respectively, for the airlines during the same two years.

• According to the Federal Railroad Administration, Office of Safety Analysis, the following statistics are for 1998:

Train accidents	2,575
Train accidents per million train miles	3.77
Total reported casualties	12,775
Total Dead	1,008

Boats

• Globally, there are approximately 2,000 working ferries—boats that carry cars and people across channels, streams, rivers, and bays. Most of these boats are not safe when the seas are rough. Over a recent eight-year period, major accidents have befallen ferries in Haiti, the Philippines, Hong Kong, and Bangladesh, where more than 360 ferry accidents killed 11,350 people. The causes? Mainly overloading the boat and collisions.

• If you thought the days of Captain Hook and Bluebeard were over, think again. Piracy is a major activity in Southeast Asia. Over a recent 10-year period, there were nearly 1,500 acts of piracy, mostly targeted at merchant ships. If you're on a private boat in Southeast Asia, you shouldn't worry too much, as the loot on such boats is hardly worth the pirates' trouble. However, most pirate ships are armed with submachine guns and can look rather menacing in the water.

Cruise Ships: *Titanic* Syndrome?

• One of the biggest fears of people on a cruise ship is fire, and that fear may be well founded. Cruise ships operate under Safety of Life at Sea (SOLAS), a set of international fire safety rules. As of 1997, most ships were required to have smoke detectors and emergency lighting to designate escape routes. Although sprinklers were recommended, ships built before 1994 were given until 2005 to install them. Before you bid Bon Voyage, you may want to ask your cruise line what type of provisions they have made for fire safety.

• All cruise ships are required to have enough life jackets and lifeboats for all passengers. You also won't want to miss the lifeboat safety drill that all ships are required to conduct within 24 hours of leaving port.

• Everyone knows the chefs go "overboard" when it comes to feeding cruise passengers—there's food everywhere. If you're concerned about the safety and quality of that food, you can find out which cruise ships passed and failed their latest inspections on the Centers for Disease Control and Prevention Web site: www.cdc.org. A score of 86 is passing.

Bicycling—United States

The first automobile accident occurred in New York City in 1896, when a motor vehicle collided with a bicyclist. Ever since then, bicyclists and motor vehicles have been vying for nearly the same piece of real estate. How have the bicyclists fared?

- Since 1932, when the first records were kept, more than 46,000 bicyclists have died in traffic crashes in the United States.
- In 1999, about 51,000 bicyclists were injured and 750 were killed.
- Bicyclists account for 2 percent of all traffic fatalities.
- More than 25 percent of bicyclists killed in traffic accidents in 1999 were 5 to 15 years old.
- Most of the bicyclists killed (88%) or injured (80%) in 1999 were males.
- Alcohol was involved in more than one-third of the bicycle fatalities in 1999.

Vehicular Traffic Fatalities—United States

- In 1999, there were 41,611 traffic fatalities in the United States.
- Children ages 0 to 14 years accounted for 6 percent (2,474) of those deaths.
- There were 15,786 alcohol-related vehicular deaths in 1999. That represents one fatal crash every 33 minutes.
- About 308,000 people were injured in alcohol-related accidents—that's an average of one person every two minutes.
- Intoxication rates for drivers of fatal crashes were highest for motorcyclists: 28 percent. The lowest rate was among drivers of large trucks (1%), followed by passenger cars (17%) and light trucks (20%).

Large Trucks

Although you proabably don't drive a large rig, don't you ever wonder about the accident rates of those 18-wheelers? If one of them hits a car, who is most likely to suffer any injuries? Let's look at some statistics.

- In 1999, approximately 475,000 large trucks (gross vehicle weight greater than 10,000 pounds) were involved in crashes in the United States: 4,898 were involved in fatal crashes, and 5,362 people died. The dead accounted for 13 percent of all traffic fatalities in 1999.

- Large trucks make up 3 percent of all registered vehicles on the road and 9 percent of all vehicles involved in fatal accidents.

- Of all the fatalities that result from crashes with large trucks, 78 percent involved the occupants of other vehicles, 8 percent were nonoccupants, and 14 percent were occupants of the trucks.

School Buses

You may be putting your most precious possession on a school bus each day, but do you know what kind of accident record school buses have?

- Since 1989, there have been about 411,000 fatal crashes in the United States. School buses were involved in a mere 0.31 percent (1,291) of them.

- A total of 1,445 people have died in school bus accidents since 1989. Most of the deaths (65%) involved the occupants of other vehicles.

- An average of 29 school children die in school bus crashes each year.

chapter twenty-four

Common Household Accidents and 52 Ways to Prevent Them

*H*ome sweet home. Home is a haven. Safe at home. Most people think of their homes as safe, warm, and comfortable. At first glance, most homes would probably appear to be all those things. But looks can be very deceiving.

Every year, Americans fall victim to more than 285,000 accidental injuries or deaths in their homes or apartments. Statistics show that home accidents are the number-one cause of injury and death among children—more than all childhood diseases combined.

The elderly are also prone to accidents in the home, and most of those injuries involve a fall. While a broken bone is no fun for anyone of any age, the bones of the elderly don't have the recovery power of younger bones, and many older individuals never regain the degree of independence they had before falling and breaking a hip, leg, or pelvis. According to the National Safety Council, more than 9,000 of the 28,400 accidental deaths that occurred in U.S. homes in 1997 were the result of a fall. Every year, about 200,000 elderly people (65 years and older) are hospitalized with broken hips that they sustained in a fall.

Every room in your home may be full of love and comfort, but chances are danger is lurking there as well. Accidents happen, but they don't have to. You and your family don't have to be statistics. There are many ways you can easily make your home safe and secure for people of all ages. So we offer you the following "How to Prevent" list:

Falls

1 If you have throw rugs, use only those with no-skid backing.

2 Remove all throw rugs, even those with no-skid backing, from areas where people who use a cane or walker will be ambulating.

3 If you have stairs and small children, place a safety gate at each end of the stairs.

4 Stairways should be well-lit and free of toys, clothes, and other items that people can trip over.

5 Install window guards on all windows. Children can open windows and easily fall through screens. Some local jurisdictions require window guards.

6 Use no-slip stickers on the bottom of the tub or a no-slip bath mat.

7 Make sure there are handrails for all stairs inside and outside the home and that they are sturdy.

8 Install grab bars in the bathroom if anyone in the home needs assistance when bathing or using the toilet.

9 Wipe up spills immediately. If the spill involves grease or oil, make sure you use a grease-cutting detergent to eliminate it.

Electrocution

10 Cover unused electrical outlets with outlet covers if you have small children in the home.

11 Keep a lock on the box to the main circuit breakers if you have young children at home.

12 Do not leave electrical appliances (hair dryers, curling irons, shavers) in the bathroom where children can reach them.

13 Don't use electrical appliances next to a sink. If water is splashed or spilled onto or near an appliance, unplug it before you wipe up the water.

Fire

14 Don't overload extension cords by plugging in too many items at once. Read the ratings on the appliances and on the cord to make sure the cord is not being overextended.

15 Check electrical cords regularly for damaged or loose plugs or frayed wires.

16 Don't hang curtains near the stove, where a breeze could blow them near the burners.

17 Don't hang towels on the oven door, as they can catch fire.

18 Never leave matches or lighters within reach of young children.

19 Keep a fire extinguisher in your kitchen, and make sure it's always charged.

20 Install smoke detectors, a minimum of one per level of the house. Smoke detectors should be located adjacent to bedrooms, one in front of each if they are at separate ends of the house.

Poisoning

21 Put childproof latches on all cabinets, especially those that harbor household cleaning supplies and medications, including vitamins.

22 A medicine cabinet above the bathroom sink is still accessible to curious children who can climb up on the sink. Put a lock on this cabinet as well.

23 Do not leave containers of shampoo, powder, soap, and other health and beauty items out where they can tempt children. These items are especially attractive to children if they have fruity or sweet aromas.

24 Homes that were built before 1978 may have lead paint on the walls. Children are at risk if they eat paint chips or breathe the dust. Contact the National Lead Abatement Council (800-673-8202) for help in finding someone in your area who can check to see if you have lead-based paint in your home.

25 Children are attracted to plants and will readily put leaves and other parts into their mouths. Be aware of which plants are poisonous (see Chapter 58), and do not have them in your home.

26 Don't leave decorative lamps or candles that contain lamp oil where young children can reach them.

Poisoning (Invisible)

27 Install a carbon monoxide alarm to alert you to dangerous levels of odorless carbon monoxide gas. Carbon monoxide poisoning can occur when wood, charcoal, gas, or oil doesn't burn completely. Small amounts can make you feel tired or cause chest pains; larger amounts can cause dizziness, headache, and death. If a gas leak occurs while you're sleeping, you may not realize it unless you have an alarm.

28 Install a radon detector in your home. Exposure to radon is blamed for up to 20,000 deaths a year and is the second largest cause of lung cancer. This odorless gas rises from the soil and enters buildings, where it is not quickly dispersed or diluted.

Strangulation, Suffocation, and Choking

29 If you have infants or small children in the house, make sure your blind cords are out of reach. Attach the cords on a hook near the top of the window.

30 Use cord shorteners on cords that can be reached by young children, such as those attached to table and floor lamps and televisions. You can also make cords safer by taping them down.

31 Check all toys in the home for small pieces that can be easily detached from the toy and swallowed.

32 Keep any plastic bags locked and away from small children.

Burns

33 When cooking, keep the handles of pots and pans turned toward the wall.

34 Install an antiscald valve on your showerhead or faucets in the bathroom. This is a safety precaution to prevent infants and small children from being scalded, as well as older adults who may not be as sensitive to temperature as they once were.

35 Wait one minute before you remove the lid from a dish you take out of a microwave oven.

36 When cooking with hot oil, add the food using long-handled tongs. Avoid adding frozen food that has ice crystals on it to hot oil, as the oil will splatter and may get into your eyes or onto your skin.

37 If a pot catches fire or smokes while you are cooking, don't move the pot. Slide a lid over the top and turn off the burner.

38 Always use oven mitts or pot holders when removing cooked items from the oven and the microwave.

39 Prevent steam burns by venting a pot lid away from you.

Cuts

40 Lock up any sharp knives in the kitchen. If you have young children, do not leave a butcher block knife set on the counter.

41 If you are cutting something round, like a tomato or an onion, cut it in half first, then lay the flat side against your cutting board before you slice it.

42 Place all scissors, pins, and other sharp objects in locked drawers if you have young children at home.

Drowning

43 If you have an above-ground or in-ground pool, install a fence with a lockable gate around the pool area.

44 If you have young children, keep all indoor entryways to the pool area locked.

45 If you have toddlers, do not leave buckets or basins of water around the house or leave water in the bathtub. Young children can fall into them face first and drown.

46 Never leave a young child alone in a tub, not even for a few seconds.

47 Put safety latches on all toilets if you have toddlers in the home.

Furniture and Glass Injuries

48 Crib bar spacing should be no greater than 2 3/8 inches. Get a copy of the Consumer Product Safety Commission's standards for infant furniture to make sure all your baby's furniture meets safety standards.

49 Sharp edges on tables, counters, and appliances should be padded with foam or tape, or the item should be moved so that small children or elderly individuals will not injure themselves.

50 Mark sliding glass doors with colored tape or stickers, or decorate them with calendars or children's drawings. People of any age can mistake a glass door for a walkway.

Miscellaneous Injuries

51 Keep your garage door opener out of reach of small children.

52 Lock the door of any storage freezers you may have. If you have an empty freezer that is not being used, either lock it or get rid of it.

Part II

People to See, Things to Do

Lily considers herself a savvy consumer. This 38-year-old paralegal and mother of two reads ingredient labels. She calls the Better Business Bureau before she employs any type of contractor for her home. When it's time to buy an appliance, she checks *Consumer Reports*. And when it comes to health care, she is no different. "My health and that of my family are important to me," she says. "I want to understand the tests, the procedures, the medications—everything."

More and more people are like Lily: They want to be informed health care consumers. "Before somebody sticks a needle in my arm or a tube down my throat, I want to know what to expect and what it's going to tell me," says Stan, a 45-year-old software specialist. These are certainly reasonable expectations. But rather than ask the doctor or practitioner directly, some consumers are doing their own research on tests, operations, practitioners, drugs, and alternative remedies.

In this part of the book, we address that need. We look at a variety of "People to See, Things to Do" when it comes to your health. We begin by exploring the different ways practitioners can poke, prod, and operate on you, and some of the doctors who might do these things to you. When one of these doctors writes a prescription, do you know what you're getting? We look at the one hundred most prescribed drugs in America, what they're designed to treat, and how safe they may or may not be.

If your penchant is for alternative measures, you will find information about alternative practitioners and what you can expect from each of them. One popular alternative approach is homeopathy, so we also discuss various homeopathic remedies and what they treat. If you want something a bit more exotic, take a peek at the secrets of the shamans. These centuries-old plant remedies, handed down from generation to generation, could be the secret to relieving your symptoms.

chapter twenty-five

78 Medical Tests:
What Do They Tell You?

How often have you heard these words: "The doctor would like to run a few tests," or "We need to do some tests before we make a diagnosis"? Remember the questions that popped into your mind? "What kind of tests?" and "What are they for?"

There are hundreds of tests doctors can use to help them make a more accurate diagnosis, verify their suspicions, or assist them in deciding on a treatment plan. Many tests are for very specific conditions or offer limited information; others provide a wealth of data. What matters to you is the bottom line: What information does the test give you, and what does the information mean in your particular situation?

This list of medical tests can answer the first question; it will be up to you and your doctor to determine the answer to the second. The world of medicine is always evolving and individuals have unique needs and situations, so your experience with a particular test may differ somewhat from the explanations given here. Remember, it is your right to have a test explained to you before you take it, so don't be afraid to ask your doctor to answer any questions you may have.

1 Acquired Immunodeficiency Syndrome (AIDS) Test. There are two tests used to identify AIDS: the ELISA (enzyme linked immunoabsorbent assay) and the Western Blot Test.

Reliability: The ELISA is reliable but is not always specific for human T-cell lymphotrophic virus type-III (HTLV-III), the AIDS virus. The Blot is used to check positive results of the ELISA test. The occurrence of false positives (a report that a person is positive for HIV when he or she is actually negative) is extremely unusual when the Western Blot Test is used to confirm ELISA.

2 **Ambulatory electrocardiography monitoring**, also known as Holter monitoring or ambulatory monitoring, is a test that detects abnormal heart rhythms. It is used to evaluate chest pain, the effectiveness of anti-arrhythmic drug therapy, the status of a pacemaker or a patient's cardiac status after a myocardial infarction (heart attack), and breathing and central nervous system symptoms.
Reliability: Good, although other tests and observations are needed to make a precise diagnosis.

3 **Amsler Grid** is a checkerboard-pattern grid used to detect blind or partially blind spots in the macular area of the retina, where macular degeneration develops in some people.
Reliability: Very good.

4 **Apgar test** is a quick test performed at 1, 5, or sometimes 10 minutes after birth to determine a newborn's physical condition and how well he or she tolerated the birthing process. The factors considered are heart rate, respiration, color, muscle tone, and reflexes. A score of 8 to 10 is normal, and any score less than 7 indicates that the infant needs some assistance in adjusting to his or her new environment.
Reliability: Good.

5 **Audiology test** detects how well a person can hear. Loudness is measured in decibels (dB; see Chapter 51), with a normal range of 0 to 85. Exposure to decibels above 85 may cause hearing damage. Individuals who cannot hear pure tones below 10 dB may have some hearing loss.
Reliability: Good.

6 **Barium enema** involves a thick, chalky liquid (barium sulfate) used in an enema. After the solution reaches the bowel, x-rays are taken. A barium enema helps confirm a diagnosis of colon cancer or inflammatory disease in the lower bowel. It can also detect polyps, physical changes in the large intestine, and inflammation.
Reliability: Good.

7 **Barium swallow**, also known as esophagography, diagnoses hiatal hernia and can identify ulcers, tumors, polyps, strictures, and other problems with the upper gastrointestinal tract (esophagus, pharynx, stomach, and small intestine). It involves swallowing a thick, chalky liquid (barium sulfate), and tracking the progress of the barium on various monitoring devices.

Reliability: Good.

8 **Blood culture** is a test done to detect suspected disease-causing organisms in the bloodstream. A blood sample is taken and then placed in a special container that will encourage any organisms in the blood to grow. The health care provider can then use the results to determine which treatment approach to use.

Reliability: Good, although it is often necessary to take more than one culture because organisms may not be present in the blood when the first sample is taken, and some organisms fail to survive or grow in the containers.

9 **Blood pressure test** measures the force of the blood against the walls of the arteries as it flows through the body. High blood pressure is a risk factor for heart attack, stroke, and kidney failure. The measurement is given in two numbers, with 120/80 being normal. The systolic (upper or first number) is the pressure when the heart is contracted, and diastolic (lower or second number) is the pressure when the heart is at rest.

Reliability: Good, although it may be necessary to take it several times as some people experience "white coat syndrome," which means their blood pressure goes up when they are in a doctor's office or other medical situation.

10 **Blood type test** is routinely done on pregnant women, people who are donating blood, and those who need a transfusion. It may also be used for paternity testing and genetic testing.

Reliability: Good.

11 **Bone density testing** is a noninvasive test that helps doctors monitor degenerative bone disorders such as osteoporosis, detect or rule out bone tumors, and find infections. There are several types: 1) dual-energy x-ray absorptiometry, or DEXA, checks the wrist, vertebrae, and hip; 2) dual-photon absorptiometry, or DPA, is an earlier version of DEXA and scans the spine and hip; and 3) single-photon absorptiometry, or SPA, checks density in the heel or wrist.

Reliability: For DEXA, the margin of error is 1 percent; for DPA, 8 percent. SPA, although less comprehensive than the other two tests, is considered sufficient for people without serious risk factors. If the results of any of these tests show serious loss of bone density, further testing is needed.

12 **C-Reactive protein test** is done on a blood specimen that identifies inflammatory diseases, such as rheumatic fever and rheumatoid arthritis. It also allows health care professionals to monitor how patients are responding to therapy for these conditions.
Reliability: Good.

13 **Cerebrospinal fluid (CSF) analysis** includes measurement of CSF pressure to help identify any obstructions in fluid circulation and to assist in the diagnosis of meningitis, tumors, or bleeding around the brain and spinal cord. The specimen is gathered during a lumbar puncture procedure (see Chapter 26).
Reliability: Good.

14 **CHEM-20** is really 20 tests in one. It gives an overview of a person's blood chemistry for the concentrations or levels of 20 factors, including sugars, minerals, enzymes, proteins, and metabolites. This test can help doctors uncover a lot about any problems with specific body functions.
Reliability: For best results, an 8- to 12-hour fast should precede the blood draw.

15 **Chest radiography (x-ray)** is used to detect lung problems, such as pneumonia, tumors, breathing problems, and collapsed lung; and to identify heart disease. A chest x-ray is also part of a preadmission test (PAT, see number 50) routine.
Reliability: Good.

16 **Cholesterol (total) testing** is recommended every few years for adults, because increased levels of this fatty, sticky substance are associated with coronary artery disease, atherosclerosis, and an increased risk of death. This test is usually part of a routine chemistry panel (see number 14).
Reliability: For best results, patients should fast for 12 hours before the blood is drawn. It is common for doctors to recommend a high-density and low-density lipoprotein cholesterol screening for individuals who have a total cholesterol level greater than 200 mg/dL.

17 **Complete blood count (CBC)** is a routine screening test used to diagnose and monitor many different diseases. A CBC provides measurements on the following factors: number of red blood cells (RBCs), number of white blood cells (WBCs), total amount of hemoglobin in the blood, percentage of blood composed of cells (hematocrit), number of platelets, mean corpuscular hemoglobin (MCH), mean corpuscular hemoglobin concentration (MCHC), and mean corpuscular volume (MCV). Some of the diseases or conditions that can be identified using a CBC include anemia (low hematocrit); congenital heart disease (high number of red blood cells); bone marrow failure (low white blood cells); infection or leukemia (high white blood cells); and dehydration or diarrhea (high hematocrit).

Reliability: Good as a screen; further tests needed, depending on the findings.

18 **Computerized axial tomography (CAT)** is a noninvasive diagnostic test that creates three-dimensional images of various parts of the body. It produces images of soft tissue that are about one thousand times sharper than conventional radiology.

Reliability: Good.

19 **Coomb's test** is a blood test done to determine whether the body is making antibodies against its own red blood cells. If an individual tests positive for the presence of these "autoantibodies," it may indicate one of the following conditions, among others: autoimmune hemolytic anemia, mononucleosis, arthritis, or systemic lupus erythematosus.

Reliability: Good.

20 **Digital rectal examination (DRE)** is used to detect any abnormalities on the prostate. It is done in a doctor's office and involves the physician inserting a gloved finger into the rectum to feel for abnormalities.

Reliability: Fair; a DRE's effectiveness in reducing the number of deaths from prostate cancer has not been determined.

21 **Doppler echocardiography** uses ultrasonography to evaluate blood flow, measure the size of the heart's chambers, evaluate valve disorders and heart function, diagnose abnormal heart sounds, and detect any excess fluid in the sac around the heart (pericardial effusion). Doppler can confirm a diagnosis of peripheral artery disease and can be used to monitor people who have had arterial reconstruction and bypass surgery.

Reliability: Good, although other tests, studies, and clinical observations are needed to make a precise diagnosis.

22 **Drug screening** is a quick test to determine the presence of drugs (typically cocaine, heroin, marijuana), usually in the urine.

Reliability: Initial screening tests are very reliable. When they are done for legal (forensic) purposes, the processing of the specimens is extremely important and special procedures must be followed to prevent tampering.

23 **Echoencephalography** is a noninvasive test that determines the position and size of several brain structures and helps doctors investigate suspected disease of soft tissues of the brain and spinal cord. A transducer is guided over the area to be examined. This instrument sends an ultrasound beam through the tissue, and the reflected sound waves are converted into electrical impulses seen on a screen.

Reliability: Good.

24 **Electrocardiography (ECG)** is a noninvasive test that helps identify damage to the heart and abnormalities in the minerals (electrolytes) that control the heart's electrical activity. An ECG can also identify the location and extent of damage to the heart muscle and show how well a pacemaker is functioning; for these purposes, electrodes are attached to the chest and a readout is shown on graph paper.

Reliability: Good.

25 **Electroencephalography (EEG)** is a graphic recording of the electrical currents produced by brain activity. Electrodes are placed on the scalp and lead wires from the electrodes are attached to the recording device. An EEG helps diagnose epilepsy, brain injuries, and tumors. It also helps physicians evaluate the brain's electrical activity among people who have a head injury, meningitis, encephalitis, mental retardation, and metabolic disease.

26 **Electromyography (EMG)** is a noninvasive technique that measures minute electrical signals produced in muscle that is at rest or during voluntary contraction. The doctor uses a handheld probe to test various muscles. An EMG helps in the diagnosis of neuromuscular disease, such as muscular dystrophy, amyotrophic lateral sclerosis (ALS), and nerve disorders.

Reliability: Good.

27 **ELISA (enzyme-linked immunoabsorbant assay)** is a test done on blood samples to help detect many diseases. This test detects the presence of antigens (for example, bacteria or other disease-causing organisms) or antibodies (proteins that form in response to antigens). Physicians may order an ELISA if they suspect HIV, Lyme disease, chlamydia, mumps, or rubella, or to help diagnose blood clots, allergies, immune system diseases, and other conditions.

Reliability: Good; further tests may be needed depending on the results.

28 **Erythrocyte sedimentation rate** is a blood test that helps confirm diagnosis of diseases such as tuberculosis or connective tissue disease, and also monitors inflammatory disease and cancer. This test can indicate serious illness when all other factors seem normal.

Reliability: Good; the test is sensitive but nonspecific, and may be the first indication of a medical problem when other factors seem normal.

29 **Exercise electrocardiography**, also known as a stress test, screens for heart disease when people don't have symptoms, identifies the cause of abnormal heart rhythms that occur during exercise, helps diagnose the cause of chest pain, and determines the functional capacity of the heart after myocardial infarction or surgery. The exercise is typically done on a treadmill while the individual is being monitored by electrocardiography.

Reliability: Good; however, other tests, studies, and clinical observations are needed to establish an accurate diagnosis. Some physicians prefer the thallium stress test (see number 63).

30 **Eye examination** is a group of routine tests that evaluate a person's eyes to detect normal and abnormal structures and functions as well as the possibility of disease. The examination includes many individual tests, including visual acuity (see number 69), color vision, and peripheral vision.

Reliability: Good.

31 **Fasting plasma glucose**, also referred to as fasting blood sugar, detects abnormalities in glucose (sugar) metabolism and screens for diabetes mellitus. It is also used to monitor the drug, exercise, and diet programs of individuals who have diabetes. Patients must fast for 12 hours before the blood sample is drawn.

Reliability: Good; an abnormal reading is followed up with a glucose tolerance test.

32 **Fecal occult blood test** detects gastrointestinal bleeding and is especially important for early diagnosis of bowel cancer, gastritis, and polyps in the colon.

Reliability: Good when done properly—three samples collected over several days, because blood may not appear in every sample. Eighty percent of people with bowel cancer have positive results on this test. If results are positive, further testing is necessary.

33 **Free prostate-specific antigen (PSA) test** measures the amount of free (versus bound) PSA in the blood. While the standard PSA test measures the total amount of PSA (see number 53), this test focuses on the free PSA. Some researchers believe that men with prostate cancer have more bound PSA than free PSA. The free PSA test is recommended as a follow-up test for men who have a high standard PSA level.

Reliability: Good. If the percentage of free PSA is greater than 23 percent of the total PSA, the risk of prostate cancer is minimal. If the percentage is less than 10 percent, the risk is high or more likely. Any percentage between 10 and 23 suggests uncertainty.

34 **Glomerular filtration rate (GFR),** or creatinine clearance test, determines the amount of fluid that the kidneys filter per minute. The muscles produce creatinine, nearly all of which is filtered through the kidneys. The creatinine levels obtained from a GFR test are compared with the levels in the blood to get an indication of how the kidneys are functioning. A 24-hour urine sample (total urine collected over a 24-hour period) and a single blood sample are needed for this test.

Reliability: Good.

35 **Hair analysis** is used to detect chronic poisoning by heavy metals (e.g., lead, mercury) or to evaluate the level of zinc in the diet. Hair samples are also used to detect chronic drug abuse.

Reliability: Differences in results are associated with various factors, such as race (the hair of Caucasians absorbs the least amount of heavy metals, while that of Asians absorbs the most), hair color, and environmental factors. Doctors do not agree on the reliability of hair analysis.

36 **Hematocrit** is a measure of the volume of red blood cells. This figure helps in the diagnosis of anemia, polycythemia, and abnormal hydration. A hematocrit is usually done as part of a complete blood count (CBC; see number 17), but may be done alone in some situations.

Reliability: Good.

37 **Human-leukocyte antigen (HLA) test** is a blood test that is used to ensure a match between a tissue or organ donor and the recipient. It can also be used to aid in genetic counseling and in paternity tests.

Reliability: Good; however, a recent blood transfusion will interfere with accuracy.

38 **Intravenous pylogram** is a test that uses x-rays to evaluate the structure and function of the urinary tract. It is often given to people who have blood in their urine, a urinary infection, injury to the kidneys, suspicion of cancer, and other conditions. X-rays of the urinary tract are taken both before and after a dye is injected into the patient's arm. The dye highlights abnormalities such as tumors, blockages, kidney stones, and other problems.

Reliability: Good.

39 **Liver scan** (also called liver-spleen scan, liver scintigraphy) is an imaging test used to examine the liver and spleen. A radioactive substance is injected into the veins, after which a special x-ray camera is used to take images. The test is used to detect tumors and other abnormalities of the liver and spleen and to monitor diseased livers (for example, cirrhosis, hepatitis).

Reliability: Good.

40 **Lung perfusion test** is often used to diagnose a blood clot in the lungs. People who have shortness of breath, chest pain, or a blood clot in the legs are candidates for this test. A radioactive substance, which gives off gamma rays once it is in the body, is injected into a vein and a special camera detects the gamma rays as it takes pictures of the chest. An abnormal test result indicates a blood clot or other blockage in the blood flow in the lungs.

Reliability: Good.

41 **Magnetic resonance imaging (MRI)** uses magnetic fields and radio waves linked to a computer that allows doctors to evaluate various parts of the body and to confirm diagnoses of suspected diseases. A dye is often injected into a vein to allow physicians to get a better image of the internal structures. MRI has the ability to see through bone and does not involve radiation.

Reliability: Good. It is especially effective in determining the location and size of tumors.

42 Mammography screens for breast cancer and evaluates breast symptoms, including lumps, nipple discharge, and breast pain. A mammogram is an x-ray of the breast.

Reliability: Good to fair. An estimated 10 to 15 percent of cancers are missed using mammography. Even when a lump is discovered, a mammogram cannot identify whether it is malignant or benign; it also is not effective in detecting abnormalities in dense breast tissue, which is common in women younger than 50.

43 Mini-Mental Status Examination is a psychological test used to evaluate the mental functioning of individuals who are suspected of experiencing mental decline or dementia. This five-minute test looks at a person's ability to recall facts, calculate numbers, and write.

Reliability: Good as a preliminary screen and to determine whether more comprehensive testing is needed.

44 Obstetric screening profile is a standard group of tests performed on blood samples of pregnant women to assess their baseline health status. It is given to women who have no known conditions that could make pregnancy or delivery difficult. The tests include complete blood count, differential white cell count, hepatitis B detection, test for immunity to rubella, a test for syphilis, an antibody screen, and blood typing.

Reliability: Good. Any abnormality requires further testing or other measures.

45 Ophthalmoscopy is the routine examination of the back of the eye using an ophthalmoscope. This test allows a magnified evaluation of the retina, nerves, and blood vessels to help detect and evaluate eye disorders.

Reliability: Good.

46 Pap (Papanicolaou) smear, or Pap test, is the collection of a sampling of cells from the cervix. It is one of the most commonly performed tests in medicine. A pap smear is used to detect malignant cells in the cervix and vagina as well as any viral, fungal, or parasitic infections. It is also used to evaluate the response of the cervix to chemotherapy and radiation therapy.

Reliability: Good.

47 **Platelet aggregation studies** include a group of tests done on blood samples to determine if the blood is clotting properly. This panel of tests is used to detect bleeding disorders.
Reliability: Good.

48 **Polysomnography**, also known as a sleep apnea study or cardiopulmonary sleep study, is a method for measuring different physiological problems that can occur during sleep. Patients must spend one or more nights at a test site and are hooked up to various monitoring devices. The series of tests include electrocardiography, electroencephalography, electromyography, nasal air flow, air flow through the mouth, and other measurements.
Reliability: Good.

49 **Positron Emission Tomography (PET)** is a noninvasive imaging technique used to evaluate blood flow and use of oxygen and glucose (sugar) by the brain and heart. It also helps diagnose brain disorders, including dementia, epilepsy, brain tumors, and movement disorders such as Parkinson's disease.
Reliability: Good.

50 **Preadmission tests (PAT)** are a group of tests required before a patient is admitted to a hospital for an elective procedure. A typical PAT includes a complete blood count, urinalysis, a battery of blood chemistries, an electrocardiogram, chest x-ray, and prothrombin time (the time it takes your blood to clot).
Reliability: Limited for ambulatory surgical procedures, because any abnormalities may be ignored unless they are serious.

51 **Pregnancy test (urine and blood)** detects the amount of human chorionic gonadotropin (HCG) in the urine or blood. HCG is produced by the placenta, and it is detectable in the urine and blood within 10 days after fertilization. Pregnancy tests can be done using home testing kits (see the list of over-the-counter tests) or by a clinical laboratory.
Reliability: Good.

52 **Pregnancy ultrasound** can be performed either to confirm a pregnancy or several times during pregnancy to monitor the progress of the fetus and health of the mother. A handheld instrument called a transducer is either placed into the vagina (during the first trimester only) or placed on the abdomen.

Sound waves transmitted from the transducer reflect off the body's internal structures and make two- or three-dimensional pictures that appear on a computer screen. A pregnancy ultrasound can perform many functions, including identifying the number of fetuses in the womb, detecting some birth defects (for example, cleft palate, spinal bifida), monitoring the amniotic fluid, and determining the birth date.

Reliability: Good.

53 **Prostate-specific antigen (PSA) test** is a blood test in which the presence of high levels of prostate-specific antigen may indicate prostate cancer.

Reliability: Because PSA levels may be high in men who have noncancerous prostate conditions, researchers are attempting to improve the reliability of the PSA test. However, the PSA test is the most reliable test for prostate cancer to date.

54 **Prothrombin time (PT)** is a blood test used to identify how long it takes for the blood to clot and to evaluate the activity of various coagulation factors. This test is often used to monitor the effectiveness of therapy with anticoagulants, especially Warfarin.

Reliability: Good.

55 **Radio-allergosorbent test (RAST)** identifies the cause of allergic reactions and symptoms, including rash, hay fever, and asthma.

Reliability: RAST is more specific, less painful, and less dangerous (will not cause life-threatening reaction) than skin tests to detect the cause of allergies.

56 **Rh typing** is a blood typing test performed on new mothers to see if they will need a RhoGam (Rh-immunoglobulin) injection. It is also used to assess the compatibility of a donor's blood before a transfusion is done.

Reliability: Good.

57 **Rheumatoid factor (RF)** is a blood test that helps confirm a diagnosis of rheumatoid arthritis.

Reliability: Good, although specificity is only fair because up to 25 percent of people with rheumatoid arthritis do not have a positive RF test.

58 **Rubella test** is a blood test used to determine if an individual is immune to rubella, also known as German measles, a viral infection that usually

occurs in childhood. If a pregnant woman becomes infected with the disease, major birth defects may result. Women who are planning to become pregnant and who do not know if they are immune to the disease may want to get this test.
Reliability: Good.

59 **Skin biopsy** determines whether a skin abnormality is benign or malignant. A local anesthetic is applied and a sample of the abnormality or the entire lesion is removed for analysis. A skin biopsy is also used to confirm the diagnosis of some fungal and bacterial skin infections.
Reliability: Good.

60 **Sperm antibody testing** is done for couples who are having difficulty conceiving. There is evidence that sperm antibodies in men and women can cause infertility. Sperm antibodies are chemicals found in the semen, blood, cervical mucus, and other body fluids that prevent sperm from fertilizing an egg. The sperm antibody test examines a sperm sample and identifies whether such antibodies are present.
Reliability: Good.

61 **Spirometry** measures how quickly the lungs fill and empty. It is one of the most important of the pulmonary function tests. Patients breathe into a plastic tube that is attached to a spirometer, which measures the volume of air. The results give an indication of whether the airways are narrowed; it can also help monitor the effectiveness of treatments for lung problems.
Reliability: Good.

62 **Sputum culture** is taken to help confirm diagnosis of respiratory disorders, including pneumonia, bronchitis, and tuberculosis. The sample is usually obtained through deep coughing. If this is not possible, suction or bronchoscopy may be required.
Reliability: Good.

63 **Thallium stress test and imaging** is used to evaluate blood flow through the heart muscle. During this test, the radionuclide thallium 201 is injected into the arm. The physician uses a scanner to follow the progress of the substance to detect abnormalities in flow and to determine a person's risk of heart attack or angina. This imaging technique locates narrowed arteries and evaluates the effectiveness of grafted blood vessels and angioplasty. The thallium stress test is a popular alternative for people who cannot perform the exercise test.

Reliability: Good, although other tests, studies, and clinical observations are needed to establish a precise diagnosis.

64 **Throat culture** isolates and identifies bacteria, particularly streptococcus, that infect the tonsils, throat, and pharynx, and is a screening tool for people without symptoms who may have *Neisseria meningitis*, a life-threatening bacterial infection of the central nervous system. A sterile applicator is used to swab the back of the throat and collect the specimen.

Reliability: Good.

65 **Thyroid panel**, or thyroid function test, is a group of laboratory tests done to measure the levels of various hormones in the blood to determine the status of the thyroid. The panel usually includes total thyroxine (T4), total T3 resin uptake, and thyroid-stimulating hormone tests. The panel can also help identify the cause of abnormal hormone levels.

Reliability: Good.

66 **Tuberculin skin test**, or Mantoux test, screens for tuberculosis. A short needle is used to inject the tuberculosis antigen into the top skin layer.

Reliability: Fair. The test does not provide a definitive diagnosis, nor does it distinguish between an active and a dormant infection. Other tests are necessary to get a more accurate diagnosis. Although true negatives mean that individuals don't have tuberculosis, false negatives are sometimes seen in people who have immune system deficiencies, AIDS or viral infection, or who are taking steroid therapy.

67 **Ultrasound** sends high-frequency sound waves into the body, which then send back different signals based on the density of the tissue they hit. The images are then seen on a computer screen. It is very safe and can be used on pregnant women.

Reliability: Good.

68 **Urinalysis** is a simple, inexpensive screening tool to detect urinary tract and kidney infections or metabolic disease. A urine sample is tested using a microscope or by dipping reagent strips into the sample. Chemical changes to the strips indicate different conditions.

Reliability: Good.

69 **Visual acuity** is an eye test done to evaluate distant and near vision and to identify the extent to which one is nearsighted or farsighted. It is part of a routine eye examination.
Reliability: Good.

70 **White blood count** can suggest the presence of an infection or inflammation and allows physicians to monitor response to chemotherapy or radiation therapy.
Reliability: Good; unfavorable results indicate the need for additional tests, such as a white blood cell differential.

71 **White blood cell differential test** measures the levels of the different kinds of white blood cells in the bloodstream and whether they are normal or abnormal. The test is usually ordered to check for anemia, leukemia, and infections such as mononucleosis, HIV, and tuberculosis.
Reliability: Good.

Over-the-Counter Tests

You can take your health into your own hands and perhaps even save a little money when you use home tests or over-the-counter testing monitors. Home pregnancy tests first hit the market in 1977, and today they are very popular as a way to find out whether little feet will soon be pattering their way through one's home. On a more serious note, the presence of HIV/AIDS can be tested for in the privacy of your own home as well. Be aware, however, that as of this writing, only one HIV/AIDS home test kit has approval from the Food and Drug Administration (FDA). Here's a rundown of these and other test kits you can purchase over the counter.

72 **Blood glucose monitors** allow individuals who have diabetes to monitor their own blood glucose levels. The basic procedure is to: 1) use a lancet to prick a fingertip; 2) place the blood on a test strip; 3) insert the strip into the monitor; and 4) wait 5 to 40 seconds, depending on the monitor, for the reading. All blood glucose monitors on the market are relatively accurate, but they tend to lose accuracy over time. Check the accuracy of your monitor monthly by following the manufacturer's directions. There are several brands, including

Accu-Chek bG, AccuChec Complete, BioScann 2000, FastTake, Glucometer DEX, and In Charge. A new model, Free Style, uses a smaller sample of blood than older monitors and can use the blood from areas of the body other than the fingertips. The FDA approved Free Style in January 2000.

73 **Blood pressure monitors** are now electronic and digitized, which makes it easy to track your blood pressure or that of a loved one at home. Although you can purchase the old-fashioned sphygmomanometer and inflatable cuff, the new electronic or digital blood pressure monitors are much easier to use. The new models still have a cuff, which is placed on the upper arm or wrist. The cuff is connected to an electronic monitor and automatically inflates and deflates when you press a button. Then you wait for a reading. The monitor also displays your pulse rate. There's no need to listen with a stethoscope. Reliable electronic or digital blood pressure monitors generally cost $40 to $100. Finger cuff monitors are not as accurate as arm cuff monitors, because they are extremely sensitive to body temperature and position. Brands include A&D Medica, IntelliSense, Lumiscope, Omron, and Samsung.

74 **Fecal occult blood test** can be done at home to help detect colorectal cancer. The most common test is the stool guaiac test. (Guaiac is a resin used to detect occult blood in stool.) To do the test, a small amount of stool is applied to a chemically treated card and a chemical solution is added. If the card turns blue, there is blood in the stool. The presence of blood does not necessarily indicate cancer. About half of the time, there is no abnormality that can explain a positive result.

75 **HIV home test kits** allow people to check for HIV infection in the privacy of their own homes. The test requires collection of three blood samples that are sent to a laboratory in a prepaid express envelope that comes with the kit. As of early 2001, the only FDA-approved HIV home test kit on the market was Home AccessExpress HIV-1 Test System. According to the *Archives of Internal Medicine*, this kit has an accuracy level of 99.9 percent in clinical trials. The FDA will answer consumers' questions about other HIV test kits at the Office of Special Health Issues. Phone: 301-827-4460.

76 **Home pregnancy test kits** test for the hormone human chorionic gonadotropin (HCG) in a urine sample. Instructions for using these kits vary according to brand. All are easy to use and nearly 100 percent accurate. Popular brands include Answer Plus, Clear Blue Easy, Conceive Accutip, 1 Step E.P.T., Fact Plus, and First Response 1 Step.

77 **Ovulation prediction tests** allow women to identify when they are ovulating so they will know if it's an optimal time to try to get pregnant. All of the test kits on the market require a urine sample. A positive result on the test indicates a surge in luteinizing hormone levels, the signal that ovulation will probably occur within 24 to 36 hours. Brands on the market include Answer, Clear Plan Easy, First Response, OvuSign, and Sure Step. Accuracy for OTC ovulation prediction tests is 99 percent.

78 **Urinalysis home kits** allow you to test for the presence of urinary tract infections. There are two basic types of test: a dipstick test and a culture kit. The dipstick test kits contain specially treated plastic strips that are either held in your urine stream or dipped into a urine sample. The strips can detect nitrate, a substance produced by most bacteria that cause urinary tract infections; white blood cells, which also indicate infection; or both. The culture test contains tubes or slides and a culture medium that promotes the growth of bacteria. You place a small sample of urine in the tube or on the slide, and if bacteria are present, they will grow in the culture. Home testing for urinary tract infections should be done under the supervision of your physician so no abnormal results caused by problems other than a urinary tract infection will be overlooked.

chapter twenty-six

31 Medical Procedures: What to Expect . . . and What You'll Pay

What's the difference between a medical test, a medical procedure, and a surgical procedure? The difference between a test and surgery seems pretty clear, but let's look at all three terms, according to definitions based on *Taber's Cyclopedic Medical Dictionary*:

- **Test:** An examination or a method used to identify or determine the presence or nature of a disease, symptom, or substance.
- **Procedure:** A particular way of accomplishing a desired result, in this case, using medical approaches or tools.
- **Surgery:** Manual and operative procedures used to correct deformities and defects, repair injuries, and diagnose and cure diseases; an operation.

Using these definitions, "procedure" seems to be in the middle: it's a little more than a test, but not quite an operation. Yet a procedure can be used to "test" or "identify" the presence of a disease, because that is the "desired result." Getting confused?

Let's put semantics aside. The fact is, not everyone categorizes medical tests, procedures, and operations in the same way. The important thing is to get the information you want. When you are about to undergo a medical procedure, one thing you want to know is, "What are they going to do to me?" Each of the entries here gives you a brief idea of what to expect when you roll up your sleeve, lie down on the table, or swallow that funny-tasting pink stuff. These are only general explanations; your actual experience may differ. Therefore, always request from your health care professional a full explanation of any procedure before it is done.

If you don't see the specific procedure you're interested in among the 31 in this list, look in Chapter 25 or Chapter 31. Or you can investigate some of the Web sites suggested in Chapter 70.

Procedures

1 **Amniocentesis** is the removal of fluid from the amniotic sac during pregnancy to diagnose abnormalities in an unborn child. This test can detect genetic characteristics and abnormalities before birth, and is also used to monitor and manage a difficult pregnancy. Amniocentesis is capable of identifying about 10 percent of the more than 400 possible birth defects. It is not able to identify abnormalities such as cleft palate, cleft lip, congenital heart disease, and certain types of mental retardation.

Here's what to expect:

- You will lie on your back and the doctor or technician will use ultrasound to find the exact location of the fetus.
- The chosen site is sterilized. A long, thin needle is inserted through the abdomen into the uterus and fluid is withdrawn for analysis.
- Cost: $700–$900, which includes analysis of the chromosomes.

2 **Angiography** is a procedure that allows a physician to see defects in the veins and arteries and to evaluate blood flow through the heart, lungs, and brain. It is usually performed in a hospital setting.

Here's what to expect:

- You may receive a sedative and local anesthesia.
- The insertion site for the catheter is cleaned and prepared (shaved if necessary).
- A hollow, flexible tube (catheter) is inserted into an artery or vein near the organ being studied.
- A radio-opaque dye is injected into the catheter. This allows the physician to see the vessels being studied on an x-ray.
- Cost: $4,000–$6,000

3 **Arteriography** is a general term for a procedure that allows physicians to visualize severely damaged arteries, especially the carotid (head), coronary (heart), and femoral (leg) arteries.

Here's what to expect:

- You must be on a clear liquid diet before the procedure. Baseline lab tests will be performed.
- A local anesthetic is injected at the site where the catheter will be inserted.
- The catheter is inserted and a radiologic device helps guide the catheter to the artery under investigation.
- A contrast material is injected into the artery to highlight the damaged areas.
- Cost: $250–$800

4 **Arthrocentesis** is the placement of a needle into the space in a joint in order to remove fluid or blood or to inject medication. Most arthrocentesis procedures are done on the knee.

Here's what to expect:

- The doctor examines the joint and marks the spot for the placement of the needle.
- A local anesthetic is applied to the puncture site.
- A needle is inserted into the joint space. You may feel a "pop" when the needle reaches the space.
- The fluid is siphoned off.
- If medication is injected, a syringe is attached to the needle and the drug is injected.
- Cost: About $60

5 **Arthroscopy** is one of the most commonly performed procedures. It allows physicians to directly examine the space between and around a joint, and is useful in diagnosing arthritis and rheumatoid conditions, and in obtaining biopsies.

Here's what to expect:

- Depending on the site, a local, spinal, or general anesthesia is given.
- The incision site is sterilized.

- Small incisions are made and an endoscope is inserted into the joint. The endoscope allows the physician to see the joint, obtain specimens, or repair damaged cartilage.
- Cost: $750–$1,000

6 **Balloon angioplasty**, also known as percutaneous transluminal coronary angioplasty, is a procedure that attempts to improve blood flow by using a tiny balloon catheter to widen arteries that have narrowed because of plaque buildup. It is an alternative to coronary artery bypass surgery. More than 1 million balloon angioplasties are done around the world every year, with more than 300,000 of them in the United States.

Here's what to expect:

- If you are not allergic to aspirin, your doctor may tell you to take aspirin before the procedure to help prevent blood clots from forming.
- You will be lying on your back on a table during the procedure, wide awake but sedated.
- A guide wire will be inserted into an anesthetized site on your arm or in your groin.
- A dye is injected into an artery or vein. The dye helps identify the blockage on x-rays.
- The doctor uses x-rays to help guide the catheter into the coronary artery and to the blockage identified by the dye.
- Once the blockage has been found, the doctor passes a tiny balloon-tipped catheter through the guide wire to the blockage.
- At the blockage, the doctor inflates the balloon, which presses the buildup against the vessel wall and widens the artery.
- An x-ray is taken to confirm the success of the angioplasty.
- The catheter is left in place for up to 24 hours in case blockage recurs.
- Cost: $575–$800

7 **Blood transfusion** involves adding blood to the body, using either whole blood or one or more blood components, such as platelets or packed red blood cells. Depending on the condition being treated, a blood transfusion is performed in the hospital or in an outpatient facility.

Here's what to expect:

- Vital signs (heart rate, blood pressure) are checked before the transfusion begins.
- An intravenous line is placed into the receiving vein in the arm.
- If the transfusion is done on an outpatient basis, you will be observed for at least two hours before being discharged.
- After being discharged, be aware of symptoms of a delayed transfusion reaction and of hepatitis: fever, headache, nausea, vomiting, abdominal pain, and loss of appetite.
- After discharge, don't use aspirin if you received platelets. Acetaminophen can be used for pain relief or fever.
- Cost: $100+ per pint for a person's own donated blood; less for blood from a blood bank.

8 **Bone marrow aspiration and biopsy** is a procedure in which a sample of the soft tissue (marrow) found in the center of bone is taken for diagnostic purposes. Individuals who undergo aspiration and biopsy have a marked increase or decrease in red blood cells, white blood cells, or platelets. This procedure is used to diagnose leukemia, anemia, lymphoma, and other blood disorders.
Here's what to expect:

- A mild sedative may be given.
- The injection site is cleaned and prepared, and a local anesthetic is applied.
- The needle is inserted and either the fluid or core of marrow cells is removed.
- Cost: $150–$350

9 **Breast biopsy—fine needle aspiration** involves the use of a needle and a syringe to remove minute tissue fragments from the breast. These specimens are examined for abnormalities, including cancer cells.
Here's what to expect:

- A sedative may be given.
- A local anesthetic is injected near the biopsy site.
- A thin needle is attached to a syringe and a sample is drawn into the syringe using suction.
- Cost: $100–$250

10 **Bronchoscopy** is a procedure that allows a doctor to view the trachea and breathing tubes through a special flexible microscope called a bronchoscope. It is used to examine the upper airways and vocal cords; to evaluate suspected malignancies or infections; or to remove foreign objects, excess secretions, and tumors from the trachea and its branches (tracheobronchial tree).

Here's what to expect:

- A sedative is given before the procedure begins.
- You may either sit or lie down during the procedure.
- To suppress the gag reflex, a local anesthetic is sprayed into the mouth and nose.
- A bronchoscope is inserted through the mouth and down the airway to the lungs. Specimens are taken as needed.
- Cost: $1,000–$1,500

11 **Cardiac catheterization** is an in-hospital procedure used to evaluate heart valve and overall heart function, to assess the coronary arteries, and to detect pulmonary hypertension.

Here's what to expect:

- A sedative may be given.
- The incision site is cleaned and prepared and an anesthetic is given.
- An incision is made, usually in the upper thigh, and a long catheter is inserted through a vein and snaked through to the heart.
- The purpose of the procedure—injection of dye, sample collection, evaluation of function—is performed.
- Cost: $3,000–$4,000

12 **Cervical biopsy** is typically done when the results of a Pap smear (see Chapter 25) reveal cell abnormalities that warrant further evaluation. Such abnormalities include the human papilloma virus and cervical cancer cells.

Here's what to expect:

- A sedative may be given.
- You lie on your back on an examining table with your feet in stirrups.
- A speculum is inserted into the vagina to help open up the cervix for the procedure.

- A biopsy forceps instrument is inserted into the vagina and a piece of cervical tissue is removed for microscopic evaluation.
- The speculum is removed.
- Discomfort and bleeding may occur for a day or two.
- Cost $75–$150

13 **Colonoscopy** is a procedure used to do a visual examination of the large intestine using a flexible instrument called a fiber-optic endoscope. Colonoscopy helps to detect or evaluate inflammatory bowel disease and to confirm diagnosis of benign and malignant lesions. It is also useful for locating bleeding sites in the colon and for monitoring the colon for recurrence of polyps or lesions after surgery.

Here's what to expect:

- For 48 hours before the procedure, you must stay on a clear liquid diet, and laxatives must be taken to clear out the intestinal tract.
- For the procedure, a lubricant is applied to the anus and the tip of the scope.
- The scope is inserted into the anus and guided through the colon.
- Air is injected into the colonoscope, which expands the colon and allows for better visualization.
- Suspicious lesions or abnormalities can be photographed or a biopsy can be obtained.
- Cost: $700–$1,000

14 **Colposcopy** is the use of a binocular microscope (colposcope) to examine the cervix to diagnose potential abnormalities of the cervix and vagina. It is often used after abnormal results have been reported by a Pap smear (see Chapter 25) to determine if cancer is present.

Here's what to expect:

- You lie on your back on an examining table with your feet in stirrups.
- A instrument called a speculum is inserted into the vagina, which makes it easier for the doctor to see the cervix.
- Iodine may be applied to the surface of the cervix to make it easier to see any abnormal areas.
- The colposcope is inserted into the vagina.

- If the doctor sees an abnormality, she may photograph these sites, or she may insert a straw-like instrument and take a small tissue sample. Samples will be taken from all abnormal sites.
- The colposcope and speculum are removed.
- Cost: $150–$350

15 **Culdocentesis** is the use of a needle and syringe to pierce the space deep in the vagina behind and under the cervix. This is done to get a fluid sample to help detect possible ailments in the pelvis and abdomen, including pelvic inflammatory disease, ovarian cancer, and ruptured ovarian cysts.

Here's what to expect:

- You lie on your back on an examining table with your feet in stirrups.
- A speculum is inserted into the vagina.
- A local anesthetic is applied to the far back of the vagina (called the cul-de-sac).
- A needle and syringe are used to pierce the rear wall of the vagina in an effort to obtain fluid.
- If no fluid is obtained, further tests may be needed.
- Cost: $150–$400

16 **Cystoscopy** is a procedure in which a flexible scope (cystoscope) equipped with a fiber-optic light source is used to view the urethra and bladder. It is done to evaluate urinary tract disease, to obtain biopsies, or to remove small stones.

Here's what to expect:

- You must void before the procedure.
- A sedative may be given.
- The cystoscope is inserted through the urethra into the bladder. A visual examination is done and photographs are taken. Biopsies are taken if needed.
- Cost: $300–$700

17 **Dermabrasion** is the removal of the surface layer of skin using high-speed sanding instruments in order to improve minor imperfections in the skin. It can help remove acne scars, warts, tattoos, fine facial wrinkles, and superficial scars. It is usually performed by a dermatologic surgeon, a plastic surgeon, or a cosmetic surgeon in the office, but if the area to be done is large, it may be done in a hospital under general anesthesia.

Here's what to expect from an outpatient procedure:

- You will receive either an oral or injected sedative.
- After the area to be treated is cleaned with an antiseptic, a local anesthetic is given. Freezing the skin is preferred because it makes the skin firmer and thus easier for the doctor to work on.
- Deeply etched or wrinkled areas are marked with a dye that guides the doctor when matching the skin level with the surrounding area.
- Bleeding is controlled by applying pressure.
- A gauze dressing is applied to the treated area and should remain on for several days.
- Cost: $300–$3,000, depending on the size of the area treated.

18 **Endometrial biopsy** is a diagnostic procedure in which a small tissue sample is removed from the endometrium (the inner lining of the uterus) to diagnose abnormal bleeding.

Here's what to expect:

- You lie on your back on the examining table with your feet in stirrups.
- A speculum is inserted into the vagina to allow a view of the cervix.
- A small, straw-shaped instrument is inserted through the cervix into the uterus and a tissue sample is scraped from the side of the uterus.
- An alternative method is to use a suction instrument to collect the sample.
- The speculum is removed.
- Cost: $75–$150

19 **Endoscopy** of the upper digestive tract is one of the most common procedures performed using an endoscope. This specific technique allows a doctor to view the esophagus, stomach, and duodenum through a flexible hollow tube (endoscope). It is often used to detect bleeding due to cirrhosis or ulcers and to identify difficulty in swallowing, pain in the esophagus, and other abnormalities.

Here's what to expect:

- A local anesthetic spray is used to numb the back of the throat, and an intravenous sedative is given.
- The hollow, flexible tube is passed through the mouth, esophagus, stomach, and duodenum.
- The doctor views the digestive tract on a monitor and collects specimens of fluid and tissue. The procedure lasts about 15 minutes.
- Cost: $700–$900

20 **Face peel (chemosurgery)** is a procedure that chemically burns the skin in order to minimize wrinkles, brown spots, and other signs of aging of the skin. A chemical face peel can be either deep, medium, or light.

Here's what to expect from a light or medium peel:

- For several days before the procedure, the face should be washed with antibacterial soap daily.
- Depending on the size of the area to be treated and the depth needed, a local or general anesthetic will be given. If a local is given, a sedative is also administered.
- Before the chemical solution is applied to the designated area, the face is washed with surgical antiseptic and ether.
- As the chemical is applied, the skin is stretched so the solution will coat the skin uniformly.
- Cost: About $1,500

21 **Hemodialysis** involves filtering the blood of a person experiencing kidney failure to remove wastes and other impurities. Because hemodialysis requires access to a blood vessel and the procedure must be done indefinitely, several times a week, a permanent access site must be established in the arm or other convenient location. A plastic or Teflon catheter is placed in the chosen site using an artery and a vein: one for the blood to leave the body and the other for the filtered blood to return.

Here's what to expect during hemodialysis:

- You get into a comfortable position, usually partially reclining in a chair.
- The blood lines from the dialyzer (the filtering machine) are connected to the access site.

- The machine is turned on and the blood is filtered and returned to the body. The procedure takes from 3 to 6 hours, depending on the patient's condition.
- Before leaving the hemodialysis site, the patient's vital signs are checked to make sure he is well enough to be discharged.
- Cost: About $60,000 per year

22 **Hemorrhoids banding** is a procedure in which large hemorrhoids or those that protrude from the anus can be treated in the doctor's office.
Here's what to expect:

- You may need to use a laxative before the procedure to ensure the rectum is empty.
- The doctor may apply a spray anesthetic to the treatment area, although banding is usually relatively painless.
- A short viewing tube called a proctoscope is inserted into the anus.
- The doctor grasps the hemorrhoid with a pair of forceps and places a rubber band around its base, using a banding instrument.
- The hemorrhoid will shrink and fall off within a few days. The area may be sore for a few days as well.
- Cost: $200–$300

23 **Laparoscopy** is a procedure in which a small, lighted telescopic instrument called a laparoscope is used to examine various internal organs by inserting it through a small incision. It is useful in diagnosing the cause of pelvic pain, evaluating masses in the pelvic area, and in obtaining biopsies. Some minor surgical procedures, such as tubal sterilization (see Chapter 31), can also be performed using this approach.
Here's what to expect:

- A sedative is given and a local or general anesthetic is administered, depending on the procedure to be performed.
- A small (½ to 1 inch) incision is made below the navel, and a needle is inserted to inflate the abdomen with carbon dioxide.
- The laparoscope is inserted through the incision to examine the abdominal cavity and to perform the needed activity.
- Cost: $4,000–$5,000

24 **Lithotripsy (shock wave)** is the use of high-energy shock waves to break up kidney stones and allow them to leave the body. This procedure can be done as emergency treatment when a kidney stone has become lodged and is causing pain, or as a preventive measure for individuals with stones that have not yet caused an emergency situation. Stones of one inch or smaller are the best candidates for shock wave lithotripsy. This procedure usually eliminates the need for surgical removal of the stones.

Here's what to expect:

- You lie on a table covered by a water- or gel-filled cushion. You will get a local anesthetic, as the shock waves can cause discomfort.
- Electrocardiograph electrodes may be attached to the chest to monitor the heart.
- An x-ray is taken to locate the stone.
- A machine called a lithotripter, positioned under the table, focuses high-energy ultrasonic shock waves onto the stone through the cushion.
- Approximately 500 to 2,000 shocks will be applied.
- After the procedure is over, your vital signs will be monitored every 4 hours for the first 24 hours. Your urine output and fluid intake will also be monitored, and urine will be collected and analyzed for stone fragments.
- You may have some blood in your urine for a few days following the procedure.
- Cost: $5,000–$7,000

25 **Lumbar puncture** is a diagnostic procedure used to identify infection of malignancy or to evaluate pressure in the cranium (the skull chamber that houses the brain).

Here's what to expect:

- A sedative is usually given.
- A local anesthetic is applied to the insertion site.
- A long needle is inserted into a designated space between the vertebrae and cerebrospinal fluid is drawn out.
- Cost: $50–$150

26 **Paracentesis**, also known as a belly tap or abdominal tap, is a procedure done to obtain fluid from the abdominal cavity for either diagnostic (to detect cancer, inflammation, or rupture of blood vessels, for example) or therapeutic purposes.

Here's what to expect:

- You may be given a sedative.
- You lie on your back and your abdomen is sterilized with a cleansing solution.
- A long needle is inserted next to the navel and fluid is drawn out for evaluation.
- Cost: $100–$200

27 **Pericardiocentesis** is a procedure that removes excess fluid from around the heart, an area known as the pericardial sac. This is done to relieve pressure on the heart and to help it pump blood better, or to do an analysis for the presence of infection, inflammation, or cancerous cells. This is a controversial procedure; some physicians believe it should be done only in emergencies.

Here's what to expect if you do have it done:

- Hospital admission is required and all vital signs will be documented. Emergency cardiac equipment will be available.
- A sedative will be given and the procedure site will be cleaned and prepared.
- A long needle is inserted through the chest wall and guided to the pericardial sac, usually with the help of ultrasonography or fluoroscopy.
- Fluids and cells are drawn from the sac for evaluation.
- Cost: $250–$350

28 **Root canal treatment** is needed when decay in a tooth has penetrated the center, or pulp, of the tooth. When decay has reached that point, the individual is usually in pain, because the pulp contains nerves and blood vessels.

Here's what to expect:

- The dentist will take an x-ray to determine the extent of the damage.
- An anesthetic administered in a needle is given to numb the tooth and gum.
- The tooth is drilled out to remove the pulp, and the nerves and blood vessels are pulled out as well.

- An antiseptic solution is applied to sterilize the cavity. If an infection has set in, a temporary filling will be inserted until it is healed, then the cavity will be sterilized again.
- If there is no infection, the root canal and the cavity are filled in.
- Cost: $250–$750

29 **Sigmoidoscopy** is a procedure used to confirm a diagnosis of inflammatory bowel disease and to detect and diagnose abnormal growths, polyps, fissures, and abscesses within the rectum and anal canal. It is used as a screening tool for healthy older individuals to detect colorectal cancer and other disorders of the lower gastrointestinal tract.

Here's what to expect:

- An enema is administered before the procedure to allow good visualization.
- A sedative may be given if needed.
- A flexible endoscope measuring 35 to 60 cm (14 to 24 inches) is inserted into the rectum. The physician examines the rectum and colon and obtains a biopsy sample.
- Cost: $700–$900

30 **Thoracentesis** is the removal of fluid or air from the lungs using a needle or catheter. This procedure is done to relieve pressure on the lungs, to identify diseases of the lung, and to get medication to the lungs.

Here's what to expect:

- Before the procedure, you may get a sedative and undergo an ultrasound or chest x-ray to determine where the fluid is located.
- You may sit semi-upright in bed or sit leaning on a table during the procedure.
- After anesthesizing the puncture site, the doctor inserts a needle through the chest wall and into the membrane around the lungs.
- A catheter is introduced into the needle and a syringe or drainage tube is attached to the catheter to draw out the fluid.
- Once the fluid has been aspirated, the catheter is removed.
- Cost: $100–$200

31 **Tooth fillings** are done when a tooth decays. Few people have escaped the pain of a toothache and the sound of the dental drill. For some of you, it's been a while since you've had the "pleasure."

Here's what to expect:

- Local anesthesia delivered in a needle may be used to make the tooth and gum numb.
- An x-ray may be taken to determine if there is any additional damage below the tooth.
- The decayed area of the affected tooth is drilled away and the dentist shapes the hole in preparation for a filling.
- The soft filling material is placed into the hole, where it will completely harden within a few hours.
- Cost: Generally $50–$150, depending on the size of the filling

chapter twenty-seven

47 Medical Specialists and What They Do

Nowadays there seems to be a specialist for everything. That can be an advantage when you need a diagnosis or treatment for a difficult medical problem, because a specialist is likely to be more intimately familiar with your particular condition and aware of cutting-edge treatments that might benefit you.

If you ever need a specialist, and if your medical plan allows you to choose your own physicians, you can get a referral from your primary doctor, ask friends or relatives if they can recommend someone, or contact a medical specialists organization that provides referrals and information. Two general referral organizations are:

American Board of Medical Specialties: www.abms.org

Council of Medical Specialty Societies: www.cmss.org

The list presented here describes what each specialist does.

Specialists

1 Adolescent Medicine Specialists: Internists who specialize in the unique physical, psychological, and social characteristics of adolescents and their health care needs. By definition, such specialists handle a wide range of problems, from acne to sexually transmitted diseases.

2 Allergists and Immunologists: Treat rhinitis, asthma, hay fever, eczema, and certain skin disorders that are related to allergic reactions, as well as adverse reactions to foods, drugs, and insect bites. These specialists are also trained in the diagnosis and management of autoimmune diseases (for example, rheumatoid arthritis, lupus) and other problems with the immune system.

3 Anesthesiologists: Provide pain relief and restore a stable condition following surgery or a medical or obstetric procedure. Anesthesiologists evaluate the risk of patients about to undergo surgery; diagnose and treat chronic cancer and other pain; diagnose and treat patients who have critical illnesses; and supervise postanesthesia recovery.

4 Cardiologists: Focus on the prevention, diagnosis, and treatment of heart disease and other disorders of the heart, lungs, and blood vessels, and manage cardiac conditions such as abnormal heartbeat rhythms and heart attack.

5 Cardiovascular or Thoracic Surgeons: Operate on the heart, lungs, trachea, esophagus, major blood vessels, diaphragm and chest wall.

6 Child Psychiatrists: Psychiatrists who have additional training in the diagnosis and treatment of childhood and adolescent problems, including developmental, behavioral, emotional, and mental disorders.

7 Colon and Rectal Surgeons: Diagnose and treat diseases and disorders involving the large intestine (colon and rectum) and the perineal area. This means they treat hemorrhoids, abscesses in and around the anus, and anal fissures (painful tears in the anal lining), as well as problems with the intestinal tract, such as polyps, cancer, and inflammatory conditions.

8 Critical Care Physicians: Internists who diagnose, treat, and follow up on patients who have multiple organ dysfunction or failure. These specialists often have administrative responsibilities in intensive care units.

9 Dermatologists: Specialize in the diagnosis and treatment of benign and malignant skin disorders and disease. These conditions include skin cancers, moles, sexually transmitted diseases, contact dermatitis, and other allergic and nonallergic skin conditions. They also have training in surgical techniques and in the management of cosmetic skin problems, such as hair loss and scars.

10 **Emergency Medicine Specialists:** Provide immediate recognition, evaluation, care, stabilization, and disposition of patients who have an acute illness or injury. Emergency medicine specialists focus on preventing death or additional disability in and out of a hospital setting.

11 **Endocrinologists:** Internists who subspecialize in disorders of the endocrine glands; for example, the thyroid and adrenal glands. Endocrinologists deal with disorders such as diabetes, pituitary diseases, menstrual and sexual problems, and metabolic and nutritional disorders.

12 **Family Physicians:** Diagnose and treat a wide variety of ailments for patients of all ages. They have completed a broad training program that includes internal medicine, pediatrics, obstetrics and gynecology, psychiatry, and geriatrics, with emphasis on disease prevention and primary care of entire families.

13 **Gastroenterologists:** Diagnose and treat problems of the esophagus, stomach, liver, pancreas, gallbladder and intestines. Some of the conditions they treat include ulcers, diarrhea, cancer, jaundice, and abdominal pain, using various diagnostic and therapeutic approaches such as endoscopes to view internal organs.

14 **General Surgeons:** Manage a broad range of surgical possibilities in the body. General surgeons diagnose as well as provide preoperative, operative, and postoperative care to their patients and are expected to be familiar with other surgical specialties so they can recognize when to refer patients to other specialists.

15 **Gerontologists:** Diagnose and treat diseases and medical conditions that normally affect the elderly and have special skills in the preventive and rehabilitative aspects of care for the elderly. They are often called upon to visit long-term care settings as well as patients' homes.

16 **Hematologists:** Internists who diagnose and treat disorders of the blood, lymph glands, and spleen. Some of the conditions they handle include leukemia, sickle cell disease, clotting disorders, and anemia.

17 **Immunologists:** Treat allergic diseases and disease processes that affect the immune system.

18 **Infectious Disease Specialists:** Diagnose and treat infectious diseases, such as HIV/AIDS, measles, tuberculosis, and pneumonia, and fevers of unknown origin. Some are trained in subspecialties, such as tropical infectious diseases or conditions associated with travel.

19 **Internists:** Diagnose and treat (nonsurgically) diseases and disorders of the internal organs in adolescents, adults, and the elderly. Internists are trained to treat cancer, infections, and diseases of the heart, blood, joints, kidneys, and the digestive, vascular, and respiratory systems. They also have an understanding of disease prevention, mental health, and common disorders of the ears, eyes, skin, nervous system, and reproductive system.

20 **Medical Geneticists:** Diagnose and treat individuals who have genetically linked diseases. Medical geneticists work closely with other medical specialists and use various testing methods to assist them in specialized genetic counseling.

21 **Nephrologists:** Diagnose and treat conditions that affect the kidneys. These specialists treat kidney disease, high blood pressure, and fluid and mineral imbalances, and consult with surgeons if kidney transplantation is needed.

22 **Neurologists:** Diagnose and treat disorders of the nervous system, such as stroke, seizures, and multiple sclerosis.

23 **Neurosurgeons:** Diagnose, evaluate, and treat disorders of the central, peripheral, and autonomic nervous systems and provide preventive and rehabilitative services for these systems as well. Neurosurgeons treat patients who have disorders of the brain, skull, meninges (brain covering), pituitary gland, spinal cord, and vertebral column, including those who may need spinal fusion.

24 **Nuclear Medicine Specialists:** Use radioactive detection and imaging instruments to diagnose and treat disease. Such techniques often allow them to detect a wide variety of diseases before the structure of the involved organ can be seen to be abnormal by other techniques. They also use radioactive molecules to attack and kill cancer cells or to relieve severe cancer pain that has spread to the bone.

25 **Obstetricians and Gynecologists:** Diagnose and treat diseases of the female reproductive system and care for women throughout pregnancy, childbirth, and the postpartum period.

26 **Oncologists:** Diagnose and treat all types of cancer and other types of tumors. Oncologists usually select and administer chemotherapy and consult with surgeons and oncology radiologists concerning cancer treatments.

27 **Ophthalmologists:** Diagnose, treat (medically and surgically), and monitor diseases and disorders of the eye and its components. They prescribe corrective devices (glasses and contact lenses).

28 **Oral and Maxillofacial Surgeons:** Diagnose and treat diseases of the mouth, teeth, jaw, and facial structures.

29 **Orthopedic Surgeons:** Diagnose and treat (medically, physically, or surgically) diseases of the bones, muscles, and joints in children and adults. They treat individuals whose musculoskeletal problems include injuries, deformities, trauma, infections, and degenerative diseases of the hands, feet, spine, knee, hip, elbow, and shoulder.

30 **Osteopaths:** Focus primarily on the use of manipulation to restore structural and functional balance to the body, but are also trained in medical and surgical techniques.

31 **Otorhinolaryngologists (ENTs):** Diagnose and treat surgical and medical problems of the ears, nose, and throat.

32 **Pathologists:** Examine the body tissues, blood, and other body fluids for disease. Pathologists also perform autopsies to determine cause of death.

33 **Pediatricians:** Diagnose and treat medical problems and provide for the emotional and social health of children from birth to young adulthood. Pediatricians are concerned with the impact of social, environmental, and biological factors on a child's development.

34 **Physiatrists:** Evaluate patients to discover the causes of their disabilities and recommend individualized physical rehabilitation.

35 Plastic Surgeons: Restore, repair, or reconstruct body parts, including facial structures and skin, especially for burn victims, as well as hands, extremities, breasts, torso, and external genitals. They are trained in the management of complex wounds, in the use of implants, and in tumor surgery.

36 Podiatrists: Diagnose and treat conditions that affect the feet and ankles.

37 Preventive Medicine Specialists: Focus on the health and well-being of individuals and defined populations in an effort to protect, promote, and maintain health and to prevent disease and disability. They consider environmental and occupational factors that may adversely affect peoples' health. They also plan, implement, and direct population health and disease management programs.

38 Proctologists: Diagnose and treat diseases of the colon, rectum, and anus.

39 Psychiatrists: Medical doctors who specialize in the prevention, diagnosis, and treatment of psychiatric disorders, including mental, addictive, and emotional problems such as mood disorders, anxiety disorders, substance-related problems, sexual and gender identity disorders, and schizophrenia. Psychiatrists can prescribe medication and order diagnostic laboratory tests.

40 Pulmonologists: Internists who diagnose and treat diseases of the lungs and airways. Conditions managed can include cancer, pneumonia, asthma, bronchitis, sleep disorders, emphysema, pleurisy, and other lung disorders.

41 Radiation Oncologists: Radiologists who use radiant energy to treat patients, especially for malignant tumors.

42 Radiologists: Use x-rays, ultrasound, computerized axial tomography (CAT), and magnetic resonance imaging (MRI) to diagnose diseased or injured internal structures.

43 Rheumatologists: Internists who diagnose and treat diseases and conditions of the muscles, bones, tendons, and joints using nonsurgical methods. They commonly diagnose and treat arthritis, back pain, athletic injuries, and muscle strains.

44 **Sports Medicine Specialists:** Diagnose and treat diseases and conditions associated with participation in sports. They are trained in the areas of physical rehabilitation, injuries, exercise physiology, nutrition, psychology, and the role of exercise in promoting a healthy lifestyle.

45 **Undersea and Hyperbaric Specialists:** Treat conditions associated with decompression and diving accidents, and use hyperbaric oxygen therapy to treat bone infections, gas gangrene, non-healing wounds, carbon monoxide poisoning, and tissue damage from burns and radiation.

46 **Urologists:** Treat diseases and disorders of the genitourinary system and the adrenal gland.

47 **Vascular Surgeons:** Surgically correct disorders of the blood vessels, excluding those of the brain.

Medical Support People

Doctors aren't the only medical professionals who can be specialits. Some non-physician specialties are listed here.

Audiologists: Professionals who help individuals who have hearing problems by showing them how to adjust to hearing loss and how to prevent further loss.

Circulating nurses: Surgical nurses who, although not directly involved in surgical procedures, perform tasks such as retrieving wrapped surgical tools from cabinets and relaying information to others outside the operating room.

Dietitians: Individuals who counsel patients on healthy cooking and eating habits and develop special menus for people with specific nutritional needs.

Licensed practical nurses (LPNs): Nurses who have completed one year of nursing training and who assist RNs with nursing care. They can take vital signs, give medications, and dress wounds.

Nurse anesthetists: Registered nurses who are trained in the use of drugs given for anesthesia. These individuals either assist an anesthesiologist or give anesthesia under a doctor's supervision.

Nurse practitioners (NPs): Registered nurses who have advanced clinical and academic experience. NPs can diagnose common ailments and in some states can prescribe medications.

Nursing assistants: Aides trained to take vital signs and provide personal care, such as serving meals, bathing, grooming, and attending to toilet needs. Many states have a certification program.

Pharmacists: Individuals trained in the science of drugs and their benefits and side effects. Training includes five years of special studies, but does not result in a medical degree.

Phlebotomists: Technicians who draw blood and prepare samples for laboratory analysis.

Physical therapists: After surgery, an injury, or illness, physical therapists help patients maximize their mobility and independence. Physical therapists use exercise programs, massage, electrical stimulation, ultrasound, and hydrotherapy to accomplish their goals.

Physician's assistants: Nationally certified individuals who assist doctors with various duties, including administering therapy, giving physical exams, and educating patients.

Prosthetists: Individuals who make and adjust artificial limbs and who teach patients how to use them.

Registered nurses (RNs): Nurses with a minimum two-year degree who supervise other nurses and provide hands-on nursing care.

Respiratory therapists: These therapists use exercises and various equipment to help individuals who have difficulty breathing because of specific respiratory conditions (e.g., asthma, bronchitis) or cardiovascular disease.

Scrub nurses: Surgical nurses who assist surgeons during a surgical procedure.

Speech pathologists or therapists: Individuals who help patients who need assistance with language skills or in finding ways to communicate. People with stroke, brain disorders, and speech impediments can get help from these professionals.

chapter twenty-eight

24

Alternative Practitioners:
How They Can Help You

For the majority of people across the world, alternative medicine is standard health care—and not an "alternative." The World Health Organization estimates that globally, 65 to 80 percent of people rely on alternative medicine as their primary mode of medical treatment. Within the last few decades, Americans have also increased their interest in and use of alternative medicine. For example:

- A report in a 1998 issue of the *Journal of the American Medical Association* notes that the total number of visits to alternative medicine practitioners has surpassed the total visits to U.S. primary care physicians.

- Fifty-eight percent of people seek alternative medicine remedies to prevent future illness or to maintain their health.

- Although lots of people are going to alternative care providers, less than 40 percent of these people let their primary care doctors in on the secret. That may not be such a good idea, as sometimes conventional treatments may not jive well with alternative approaches. Some drugs and herbs, for example, can cause serious reactions when mixed. That's why it's important to let all of your health providers know about any therapies or treatments you are using, including nutritional supplements, herbs, prescription medications, and exercise programs.

- According to the *Journal of the American Geriatrics Society*, about 30 percent of people 65 years and older use at least one alternative medicine modality. Herbal medicine is the most popular choice among this age group.

Among the largest groups of people who turn to alternative medicine are those with serious or life-threatening diseases. A study by the *Journal of Clinical Oncology* (July 2000) found that 83.3 percent of the people receiving outpatient treatment for cancer had tried at least one alternative treatment approach. Some said they did so simply to improve their quality of life and to prolong it, but nearly 38 percent said they used complementary medicine to cure their cancer. The most common forms of treatment used were spiritual practices, herbal medicine, nutritional therapies, and movement and physical therapies.

If you decide that an alternative medical approach is for you, you may need some help in locating a qualified practitioner. You can start your search by asking for a referral from a conventional doctor. Getting a recommendation from a friend or relative who has used the services of a specific practitioner is another good resource. There are also dozens of professional health organizations that provide information and referrals.

Here we provide descriptions of some common alternative practitioners. Before becoming a patient or client of any health care provider, conventional or alternative, you should investigate the provider's background, experience, licensing, and certification.

When you meet with a practitioner, go with your gut feeling: If he seems reluctant to provide you with information about his experience or training, or if he promises miracles or cures, run—don't walk—away. Likewise, if she is stubbornly opposed to conventional medicine or if she's vague about the treatment you will receive, look for another practitioner.

In a commentary in the *Journal of the American Medical Association* (November 1998), Dr. Wayne Jonas of the Office of Alternative Medicine at the National Institutes of Health in Bethesda, Maryland, said he believes "the increasing popularity of complementary and alternative medicine . . . reflects changing needs and values in modern society in general." We agree, and we're sure alternative practitioners do, too.

1 **Acupuncturists** restore balance and harmony to the body by influencing the flow of the life force, or chi. Acupuncture is based on the theory that two energy forms—yin and yang— make their way through a series of pathways in the body called meridians, and along the meridians are approximately 800 locations known as acupuncture points. An acupuncturist can affect the flow of yin and yang and restore health by inserting needles at points specific to an ailment or need. Acupuncture has been successful in treating arthritis, tension headache, back pain, fibromyalgia, dermatitis, eczema, high blood pressure, depression, and asthma, among other medical complaints.

An acupuncture session usually lasts 30 to 60 minutes, although your first visit may be longer because the practitioner will need to diagnose the ailment and discuss treatment with you. Once the needles are placed, they may remain inserted for 20 minutes or longer. The acupuncturist may rotate the needles, burn an herb called mugwort over the sites (a practice called moxibustion), or apply low-voltage electrical stimulation to the needles (called electro-acupuncture). Once the needles are removed, the practitioner may recommend herbal remedies for you to use at home, depending on the condition being treated. Most states regulate acupuncturists and practitioners of Oriental medicine.

2 **Alexander Technique teachers** are individuals trained in the methods of F. Mathias Alexander (1869–1955), who developed a series of simple movements that allow people to develop increased awareness of and control over their daily activities. Alexander believed that people suffer from fatigue, pain, headache, and other physical ailments because they have gotten into a habit of poor posture. His techniques are designed to correct posture and thus restore energy, achieve flexibility, and improve overall health.

Each Alexander Technique session lasts 30 to 60 minutes, during which students learn nonstrenuous movements that will help them gain conscious control of their physical actions and maintain good posture during their daily routine. As with any new habit, physical poise comes with repetition and practice; thus the techniques must be practiced daily, in a particular order, for them to become fully integrated into a person's lifestyle.

Alexander Technique teachers (they prefer to be called teachers instead of therapists) receive certification through one of several training facilities. Training and certification takes a minimum of three years and includes at least 1,600 hours of instruction.

3 **Aromatherapists** are individuals who are trained in the art of using essential oils for therapeutic purposes. There are courses and certificate programs for aromatherapy; however, states do not require a license or certification for people to practice as aromatherapists. That means anyone can claim to be an aromatherapist, so caveat emptor: Let the buyer beware.

No definitive scientific basis has been established for the effectiveness of aromatherapy, although the fact that it does produce positive results in many people can't be disputed. Aromatherapists can counsel you on which essential oils may help you treat different conditions, such as headache, arthritis, depression, the common cold, sinus infections, menstrual cramps, insomnia, and stress. They can show you how to mix essential oils with carrier oils and different ways in which the oils can be used.

Aromatherapy is commonly practiced by naturopaths, massage therapists, chiropractors, psychotherapists, practitioners of Chinese medicine, and Ayurvedic practitioners.

4 Ayurvedic practitioners practice Ayurvedic medicine—a healing system that originated in India more than 5,000 years ago—and adhere to the principle that the mind and body are always in communication. To rid the body of disease, the mind needs to work with one or more of the five senses to restore harmony. Thus Ayurvedic practitioners prescribe and work with therapies that affect the senses; for example, diet and nutrition, herbs, aromatherapy, massage, music therapy, and sound therapy.

One of the first things Ayurvedic medicine practitioners do is to determine a person's mind–body type, or dosha. There are three doshas—vata, pitta, and kapha—and people can be dominant in one or be a combination of two or three. Once the dosha has been identified, specific treatments tailored to a person's mind–body type can be prescribed, such as certain dietary recommendations, aromatherapy, and massage.

Ayurvedic practitioners are not licensed in the United States, and no state or federal agencies regulate their practices. Individual schools that graduate students of Ayurvedic medicine set standards of competency.

5 Biofeedback clinicians help individuals learn to use the power of their minds to take control of certain conscious and autonomic bodily processes, such as pain, anxiety, hypertension, and teeth grinding. Specialists who typically seek certified training in biofeedback are usually psychiatrists, psychologists, nurses, internists, physical therapists, and dentists.

The most common type of biofeedback is electromyographic. During a session, a sensor is placed on a painful or tense area of your body. The sensor sends signals back to a recording device, which measures the amount of electrical activity at that site. The clinician may help you with visualization suggestions or guided imagery. With practice, you will learn to reduce or eliminate the pain or tension even without the machine, which means you can then practice biofeedback anytime, anywhere. You can also learn to identify the situations that trigger your symptoms and how to cope with stress-related pain, such as muscle spasms and migraines. The number of sessions it takes to achieve any of these goals varies depending on the condition being treated and how much practice you do.

6 **Chiropractors** reduce or eliminate problems caused by a misalignment of the vertebrae without the use of drugs or surgery. Instead they use spinal manipulation, craniosacral therapy (adjustment of the bones in the skull), herbal and nutritional therapy, hydrotherapy, reflexology, and breathing exercises.

Chiropractors believe that many medical problems can be alleviated or cured once the relationship between the nervous system and the spine is in harmony. Manipulations are effective in the treatment of neck and back pain, headache, migraine, and various conditions that affect the muscles and joints.

During your first visit, you will give your medical history, after which the chiropractor will conduct physical, orthopedic, and neurological examinations; do a postural and spinal analysis; and order x-rays or other diagnostic tests if they seem warranted. Once a diagnosis is made and a treatment course has been chosen, the practitioner may use hydrotherapy, massage, ultrasound, or heat therapy in addition to manipulations.

All states and the District of Columbia regulate and license chiropractors.

7 **Colon hydrotherapists** use water to flush out waste and toxins from the upper and lower portions of the intestinal tract. People who go to colon hydrotherapists believe that this form of detoxification is effective in relieving many physical conditions, including constipation, headache, digestive problems, and fatigue, and that it may help prevent colon cancer.

During a hydrotherapy session, you will lie in a comfortable position. A therapist will insert a tube into your rectum and water or an herbal solution (both at body temperature) will be sent into the upper colon, where it will flush impacted feces, bacteria, and other waste and toxins. A second tube transports the waste and water from the body. The therapist will massage your colon through your abdomen during the procedure to help loosen any impacted material. Some hydrotherapists use acupressure or reflexology to assist elimination. The entire process takes about 45 to 60 minutes and is generally not painful.

This is a procedure that should be done only by a professionally trained therapist. Some naturopaths and other health care professionals receive colon therapy training through continuing education programs at massage schools and offer colon hydrotherapy as part of their practice. Florida is the only state that currently licenses colon hydrotherapists.

8 Craniosacral therapists manipulate the bones of the head, face, and vertebral column as well as the membranes under the skull. The adjustments are very subtle but sufficient to affect the flow of cerebrospinal fluid and thus relieve stress and tension in the skull and spinal cord. Craniosacral therapy is used to treat headache, ear infections, stroke, pain related to the TMJ (temporomandibular joint), sinus conditions, back pain, and other conditions.

You could experience craniosacral therapy if you go to a chiropractor, acupuncturist, physical or occupational therapist, or osteopath who received training through continuing education or postgraduate training. Adjustments are brief and painless. Craniosacral therapy is effective for both adults and children. Adjustments should be made on infants only by a therapist specially trained in that technique.

9 Feldenkrais therapists have completed a three- to four-year professional program, which certifies them to teach gentle movements designed to re-educate the muscles and promote optimal physical functioning. The Feldenkrais Method, developed by Moshe Feldenkrais during the mid twentieth century, is effective in reducing pain and in the treatment of digestive disorders, problems with coordination and balance, sleep problems, multiple sclerosis, and cerebral palsy.

The Feldenkrais Method consists of two parts. In the portion called Functional Integration, you work one-on-one with a therapist to learn appropriate movements selected especially for you from more than 1,000 developed by Feldenkrais. The second part is Awareness through Movement, during which you follow exercises designed to increase your awareness of what your body is doing.

Each session generally lasts from 30 to 60 minutes, and in between sessions you can practice what you've learned at home. Feldenkrais therapists continually develop their skills in order to meet yearly certification requirements.

10 Herbalists in the United States are self-defined professionals who are either self- or professionally taught to use herbs for therapeutic purposes. Although there are no state or national licensing or certification programs for herbalists, some professional organizations grant certification to individuals who meet a set level of training. Some licensed medical professionals, including medical doctors, naturopaths, and osteopaths, are also trained as herbalists, and these individuals can prescribe herbs as part of their practice. Thus herbalists who do not have a medical license cannot legally "prescribe" herbal remedies but can consult and teach others about therapeutic herbs.

If you live in or visit the United Kingdom, you can consult a "medical herbalist," as herbalists are licensed in England. However, if you are looking for effective herbal remedies in the United States, it is best to consult a naturopath or other licensed professional who is also an herbalist.

11 Homeopaths are professionally trained in the principles and methods of homeopathy, a holistic form of medicine in which remedies are given to help the body heal itself. Homeopathy is based on the principle of "like cures like," which means that a minute amount of a given substance will treat symptoms caused by larger amounts of the same substance.

Your first visit to a homeopath will last at least an hour, during which time the doctor will develop a profile of your physical, emotional, spiritual, and social characteristics, review your personal and family history, and discuss your lifestyle habits, such as diet and exercise. Homeopaths believe a holistic picture of a person's mind and body is necessary before any treatment can be prescribed. Prescriptions are based on all the information and characteristics the homeopath has identified. If the first prescription does not bring results within a few days, you'll probably get another prescription. Your homeopath will also probably recommend specific lifestyle modifications as needed.

In the United States, most homeopaths also hold another medical degree—medical doctor, naturopath, chiropractor, osteopath—that allows them to diagnose and prescribe homeopathic remedies. More and more medical doctors are becoming trained as homeopaths; you may be fortunate enough to have such a professional in your city or town. Currently there is no legal licensing or governmental regulation of homeopaths in the United States. Some states have laws that govern how homeopaths can practice; check the laws for your state.

12 Hypnotherapists use hypnosis for therapeutic purposes. Hypnotherapy is taught in many medical schools and was approved by the American Medical Association in 1958. There are also certification programs available.

Hypnotherapists are often psychiatrists or medical doctors who have received training in this healing technique either at medical school or through one of dozens of training facilities in North America. During a session, a hypnotherapist will help you relax and enter an intently focused, altered state of consciousness, as if you were in a trance. Although you are "under," you are still in control and so will not do anything that violates your moral principles or conscience. A hypnotherapist can use various techniques to help you identify and analyze the root of a specific problem or rid yourself of negative behaviors, thoughts, or emotions. Hypnotherapy can treat stress-related disorders such as headache, stuttering, irritable bowel syndrome, and impotence; and addiction to alcohol, drugs, and nicotine. Depression, overweight, and mood disorders have also been successfully treated with hypnotherapy.

13 **Iridologists** analyze and evaluate the irises of the eye to determine the health of various systems of the body. Iridologists are not medical doctors (unless a medical doctor has received training in iridology) and so cannot diagnose disease. Iridology is the creation of a physician who developed a complex chart that notes the relationship between tissue changes in the body and markings on the iris. Iridologists are trained to read more than 180 different zones on the chart, which can detect areas of weakness, strength, or other possible abnormalities.

During an iridology session, the practitioner will take a photograph of your eyes and enlarge it. Then an iris chart is superimposed over your photo to identify areas of strength and weakness. An iridology reading can detect nutritional imbalances and areas of toxicity, and also render an early warning of potential diseases or other medical problems. Many iridologists are also trained in nutrition and herbal medicine and may suggest remedies based on what they have seen in your eyes.

Iridologists can receive their certification through approved national and international programs and associations.

14 **Kinesiologists** are involved with the study of muscles and muscle movements. They generally practice applied kinesiology, which is a method of muscle testing that allows individuals to use their intuition to uncover the source health problems and work on a solution.

A session with a kinesiologist will include a physical assessment of your muscles to discover the location of imbalances in your body. The tests are simple and painless; you may be asked, for example, to extend your arm and hold it as the kinesiologist gently presses down on it. Once imbalances are identified—

they may be emotional, chemical, or structural—a treatment plan can be developed that may include specific nutritional guidelines, herbal supplements, and movements.

Applied kinesiology can help relieve back and neck pain, depression, fatigue, digestion problems, food sensitivities, acne, headache, and eczema. Practitioners generally receive their postgraduate training through weekend workshops.

15 **Massage therapists** provide hands-on manipulation of the body. There are dozens of approaches to massage, each distinguished by the types of strokes used, the part of the body used to apply the massage (palms, elbows, knees, fingers, knuckles), and the degree of pressure applied. Swedish massage, which is believed to be the most popular technique practiced in the United States, induces relaxation, increases range of motion, promotes circulation, and removes toxins from the body. Some other common types are Rolfing, sports massage, shiatsu, and deep tissue massage.

What you will experience during a massage session will vary depending on the type of massage therapist you go to. Generally you will undress and be draped with a towel. You may lie on a padded massage table, although shiatsu practitioners often do their sessions on the floor (see Shiatsu practitioners). Sessions typically last from 30 to 90 minutes.

About half the states have licensing laws for massage therapists, and many cities have local regulations as well. These laws set the legal requirement for the education level of massage therapists. This can range from 330 to 1,000 hands-on hours of training. Look for a licensed therapist.

16 **Midwives** are trained professionals who offer education, personal care, counseling, and support for women and their newborns during pregnancy and after delivery. Although regarded as alternative practitioners in the United States, midwives are recognized throughout the world as experts in maternity care for normal births.

If you are looking for a midwife, you'll find that two main categories exist in the United States: nurse-midwives and direct-entry midwives. The former have a nursing education as well as midwifery training and can practice anywhere in the nation; the latter have midwifery training only and can practice in only about a dozen states. There are both national certification and state laws governing midwifery. To help you select a midwife, you might contact an organization such as Midwives' Alliance of North America (www.mana.org).

17 **Naturopaths** are individuals trained under specific guiding principles: 1) that the body has the ability to heal itself, and so all remedies and therapies used should enhance that ability rather than mask symptoms; 2) that symptoms are the way the body rids itself of toxins and signals that it is out of balance; 3) that health is based on clean food, air, and water, as well as exercise, adequate sleep, and other healthy lifestyle choices; 4) that all aspects of a person—physical, emotional, mental, spiritual, social—need consideration during diagnosis and treatment; and 5) that all treatments and remedies should be as natural as possible.

Licensed naturopathic physicians (N.D.s) attend a four-year graduate level naturopathic medical school and receive all the same basic science education as a medical doctor, but also study nontoxic and holistic approaches to healing. On top of a standard medical curriculum, the naturopathic course involves four years of training in clinical nutrition, acupuncture, homeopathic medicine, herbal medicine, counseling, and psychology. Currently, naturopaths are regulated and licensed in 11 states: Alaska, Arizona, Connecticut, Hawaii, Maine, Montana, New Hampshire, Oregon, Utah, Vermont, and Washington.

Your first visit to a naturopath will probably last 60 to 90 minutes to allow the practitioner to collect all medical and personal history and to get a complete record of your nutrition and lifestyle habits. Subsequent visits usually last about 30 minutes. Once a diagnosis is made, possible treatments, including lifestyle and dietary guidelines, herbal or homeopathic remedies, or other approaches will be discussed and dispensed. Naturopaths who are trained in other treatment modalities, such as acupuncture, hydrotherapy, or kinesiology, may do those treatments in the office.

18 **Osteopaths** (Doctors of Osteopathy or D.O.s) are fully licensed medical doctors who undergo specialized training in manual manipulation of the body. Osteopathy is based on the principle that this manipulation can alleviate pain, enhance the body's own natural healing powers, and restore freedom of motion. Osteopaths prefer to prevent disease rather than simply to treat symptoms. They often use craniosacral therapy, lymphatic techniques (massage of the lymph system to improve its ability to fight invading organisms), and deep tissue massage to help the body heal itself.

A visit to an osteopath will involve many of the same initial procedures as a visit to an M.D. Once a diagnosis has been made, however, the treatment approach will differ and may include manipulation of the joints, physical therapy, instruction in proper posture, and dietary guidelines. You might think of an osteopath as a cross between a medical doctor, a naturopath, and a chiropractor.

19 **Pilates Method teachers** are trained to teach a series of exercises that stretch and strengthen muscles, open up the joints, and release tension throughout the body. Joseph Pilates, who opened his first Pilates studio in New York City in 1926, developed the method, which uses more than 500 movements performed on a series of five pieces of equipment.

A Pilates teacher is like a personal trainer. He or she will work with you, usually 60 minutes at a time, to teach you how to do the movements on the various machines. All movements are done with controlled breathing and are designed to protect and strengthen the back. The main piece of equipment used in Pilates is called the Universal Reformer, a padded platform with a base that slides back and forth. Various springs and pulleys attached to the Reformer are used to do the movements. The movements are small and the repetitions are short.

Currently there are only a few facilities that train Pilates teachers, and none of the states regulate the programs.

20 **Polarity therapists** work with the vital life force, a concept, embraced by Eastern philosophies, that assumes an energy force exists in and surrounds all living things. These therapists use their hands to establish a connection between themselves and their client to restore and rebalance the client's flow of energy. Polarity therapists may help prevent illness and facilitate healing and have been successful in treating headache, back pain, digestive disorders, and emotional stress.

The polarity approach is fourfold: gentle hands-on bodywork to enhance energy flow; counseling on diet and nutritional habits; polarity yoga exercises; and psychological counseling. Each session, which typically lasts 45 to 60 minutes, usually incorporates these four elements to help bring about a balanced healing. The yoga exercises must be practiced daily at home. Polarity therapists believe that the special feature of polarity therapy—the psychological counseling in which clients verbalize their therapeutic journey—helps bring the other three elements together.

Polarity therapy is usually taught in massage schools, but special programs also exist that teach the methods separately. Look for a therapist who is registered or certified by the American Polarity Therapy Association.

21 **Reflexologists** manipulate specific sites on the feet, and occasionally on the hands and ears as well, by pressing, massaging, or stroking in order to relieve pain and tension and to improve circulation to a specified part of the body. To a reflexologist, the feet are like a road map on which specific points, called reflex zones, are associated with different body parts and organs. For example, pressing the specified zone on the foot will relieve a headache.

A reflexologist can teach you which reflex zones to press or massage to treat yourself. Reflexology has been successful in treating aches and pains, digestive problems, inflammatory skin conditions, stress, menstrual irregularities, constipation, and headache. Many reflexologists are self-taught and incorporate the treatments into their other healing practices, such as naturopathy and chiropractic. Reflexology is taught at more massage schools in the United States than any other form of bodywork.

22 **Reiki** is a healing system based on Tibetan practices that are at least 10,000 years old. Its practitioners use highly focused visualization and the laying of hands on a client's chakras (seven points of physical or spiritual energy in the body) to unblock any barriers to the universal life force, which, according to the principles of Reiki, is available to everyone. The practitioner then channels energy to the client to restore harmony and balance.

During a Reiki session, you will lie on your back on a massage table or other comfortable flat surface. You'll probably hear soft music playing in the background and perhaps smell the scent of incense, candles, or essential oils. The practitioner will move from one chakra site to another until all seven open to the flow of energy. A typical session takes 60 to 90 minutes, but shorter treatments can also be effective. Some Reiki practitioners give shorter sessions while clients are seated in a chair. Another approach is distance Reiki, in which energy is transmitted to a client from far away, with the client's permission.

Reiki practitioners can go through three levels of training: Levels I and II can be done over a weekend each, while the third level, Master, may take up to a year. Distance healing can be learned at the second level. Reiki can help relieve stress, depression, anxiety, and pain, and can treat injuries by speeding up healing.

23 **Shiatsu** practitioners perform a Japanese bodywork technique that applies pressure ("shiatsu" means "finger pressure") to points on the body that correspond to acupuncture points. Practitioners use their thumbs, fingers, and palms to apply varying amounts of pressure in a way that is usually more forceful than massage. The application of pressure is interspersed with massage and gentle stretches that help increase muscle flexibility and joint mobility.

Unlike massage therapists, a shiatsu practitioner usually works on clients as they lie on the floor on a padded mat. This allows them to use their own bodies to brace the client during certain stretches. A typical session lasts 30 to 60 minutes.

Some training programs license or certify their graduates. Check your state laws regarding any differences in regulations between massage therapists and shiatsu practitioners.

24 **Therapeutic Touch practitioners** evaluate a person's energy field and then help rebalance it to restore harmony to the body. Therapeutic touch was developed by a registered nurse, who based it on the principle that illness results when there is a blockage or imbalance in the energy field that both surrounds and penetrates a person's body.

During a therapeutic touch session, you will likely sit in a straight-backed chair or on a stool that allows the practitioner to move freely around you. Practitioners assess your energy field by passing their hands close to or lightly touching your body. Areas that radiate heat, cold, tingling, or other sensations to the practitioner are areas of congestion. The practitioner then focuses energy on removing the blockage.

Therapeutic touch is used to relieve anxiety, tension, stress, headache, and other stress-related pain, and to speed recovery from trauma. Practitioners usually receive their training at one of several workshop programs in North America.

chapter twenty-nine

The *100* Most Prescribed Drugs in the United States and What They're For

As a consumer, you have the right to be informed about any medication your doctor prescribes for you. Of course, you are not limited to the facts your doctor or pharmacist provides: There are many books, articles, and Web sites that offer reliable information (see Chapters 68 to 72). However, only your doctor will know the details of your particular problem, as well as your health history, so he or she remains your best resource.

With rights come responsibilities. It is your responsibility, for example, to tell all your health care providers, including alternative practitioners, about any medications—over-the-counter, prescribed, herbal, nutritional, or recreational—that you are taking, as any one of them might interact with a prescription drug and cause serious consequences.

Know Your Prescription

Research shows that 50 percent of consumers who buy prescription drugs fail to follow the accompanying instructions for use, and it's a rare individual indeed who asks questions of the doctor or pharmacist about prescribed medications. If you want your medicine to be safe and effective, however, it's important to know what you're taking and how you should be taking it.

When you pick up your prescription from the pharmacy, follow these simple tips:

- Say "Yes" when asked if you want a consultation, even if it's for a refill (and if it is a refill, check to make sure you've gotten the same medication you just ran out of). Ask questions at this time.

- Check to see that both the name of the drug and the condition it treats are on the bottle or package. There are many drug names that sound alike (Xanax and Zantac, for example), and if the prescription was called in over the phone, mistakes can occur. Listing the condition will help avoid those mistakes.

- Make sure the pharmacist gives you a printed product information sheet on the drug. This does not replace a consultation; it is in addition to it. Read the information (at home) and call your doctor or pharmacist with any questions.

- Use the same pharmacy for all of your medications. Most pharmacies have a computerized customer base that keeps information about everything you are taking or have taken in the past.

Common Prescriptions

Here is a list of the drugs most often prescribed in the United States. The drugs are listed by 1) brand name; 2) generic name; and 3) main indications for use, with 4) a brief comment about the drug.

The comments on some of the drugs in the list include a "limited use" rating by Sidney M. Wolfe, M.D., author of *Worst Pills, Best Pills* (New York: Pocket Books, 1999). The criteria for this rating include one or more of the following:

- Published studies say the drug should be used only as a second-line treatment if another drug fails.

- Published evidence suggests that the drug is widely used inappropriately and thus may be unsafe.

- Published evidence suggests that the drug is more dangerous than another, effective drug, but not dangerous enough to deserve the rating "Do not use."

- It is a combination drug that should be used only as a second line of defense.

Things to Know

NSAIDs. Nonsteroidal anti-inflammatory drugs. Used to treat inflammation and pain.

Hydrochlorothiazide: A diuretic (water pill).

"Do not use": This rating is given because 1) safer drugs are available; and 2) the drugs have a high rate of adverse effects.

"Do not use until ___": Dr. Sidney Wolfe, author of *Worst Pills, Best Pills*, maintains that people should wait at least five years from when a drug is released to the market before taking it, because an insufficient number of tests is usually done before drugs are released. Most of the dangers are detected within the first five years after a drug's release.

HEART DRUGS

1. Lipitor. Atorvastatin. For hypercholesterolemia (high cholesterol), hyperlipidemia (high triglycerides). Better tolerated and more effective than other cholesterol-lowering drugs.

2. Norvasc. Amlodipine. For angina (chest pain), hypertension (high blood pressure). Effective for all major types of angina.

3. Lanoxin. Digoxin. For atrial fibrillation, heart failure. Doctors should first try a thiazide diuretic and prescribe digoxin only if the diuretic fails.

4. Zestril. Lisinopril. For heart failure, hypertension. Rated "limited use."

5. Zocor. Simvastatin. For high cholesterol. Rated "limited use."

6. Coumadin. Warfarin. For arrhythmia (irregular heartbeat), myocardial infarction (heart attack). Severe side effects can occur if this drug is not taken exactly on schedule. Consult with your doctor.

7. Vasotec. Enalapril. For congestive heart failure, hypertension. Rated "limited use."

8 Lasix. Furosemide. For edema (water retention), hypertension. Rated "limited use."

9 Pravachol. Pravastatin. For hypercholesterolemia. Rated "limited use."

10 Atenolol. Atenolol. For hypertension and angina. Effective and well-tolerated.

11 Accupril. Quinapril. For heart failure, hypertension. Rated "limited use."

12 Cardizem CD. Diltiazem. For angina, atrial fibrillation. Rated "limited use."

13 Toprol-XL. Metoprolol. For angina, hypertension. Recommended only if diet and exercise don't bring down high blood pressure.

14 Dyazide. Triamterene. For edema, hypertension. Rated "limited use."

15 Cardura. Doxazosin. For hypertension, benign prostatic hyperplasia (benign growth of the prostate gland). Newest drug on the market for this prostatic condition.

16 Lotensin. Benazepril. For hypertension. Rated "limited use."

17 Procardia XL. Nifedipine. For hypertension. Rated "limited use."

18 Esidrix. Hydrochlorothiazide. For edema, heart failure.

19 Cozaar. Losartan. For hypertension. Diet and exercise should be tried first as treatment for hypertension before resorting to a drug.

20 Hytrin. Terazosin. For hypertension, benign prostatic hyperplasia. Use should be limited to treatment of hypertension.

21 Monopril. Fosinopril. For hypertension. Rated "limited use."

22 Calan. Verapamil. For angina, arrhythmia. Rated "limited use."

23 Ziac. Bisoprolol. For hypertension. Once-a-day dosing makes it easy. Rated "limited use."

24 Lescol. Fluvastatin. For hypercholesterolemia. Easy to take (once-daily dosing) and low side effects.

25 Furosemide. For edema. A powerful diuretic and should be taken only under medical supervision.

26 Metoprolol. For angina, hypertension. Diet and exercise and, failing that, hydrochlorithiazide are the first-choice treatments for hypertension.

27 Diovan. Valsartan. For hypertension. Rated "Do not use until 2003" (see Things to Know, page 214).

28 Hyzaar. Losartan. For hypertension. A combination drug. Diet and exercise and, failing that, hydrochlorithiazide are the first-choice treatments for hypertension.

MIND DRUGS

29 Prozac. Fluoxetine. For depression. Effective but may cause serious allergic reactions. Limited information on its use in older adults.

30 Zoloft. Sertraline. For anxiety, panic. Rated "limited use."

31 Paxil. Paroxetine. For depression, anxiety, panic disorder. Rated "limited use."

32 Xanax. Alprazolam. For anxiety, panic. Use should be limited to treatment of panic disorder.

33 Wellbutin SR. Bupropion hydrochloride. For depression. Rated "limited use."

34 Ativan. Lorazepam. For anxiety. Rated "Do not use" because of adverse effects and unproven long-term benefits (see Things to Know, page 214).

35 Risperdal. Risperidene. For psychosis. Rated "limited use."

36 Elavil. Amitriplyline. For depression. Rated "Do not use" because it has many adverse effects (see Things to Know, page 214).

37 BuSpar. Buspirone hydrochloride. For anxiety. A benefit is that it does not cause withdrawal when stopped. Rated "limited use."

38 Celexa. Citalopram. For depression. One of the newest drugs for depression on the market.

39 Effexor XR. Venlafaxine. For depression. Rated "limited use."

40 Zyprexa. Olanzapine. For psychosis. Rated "limited use."

41 Diazepam. For anxiety, alcohol withdrawal. Rated "Do not use" (see Things to Know, page 214).

42 Serzone. Nefazodone. For depression. Rated "limited use."

PAINKILLERS AND ARTHRITIS DRUGS

43 Hydrocodone with APAP. Hydrocodone bitartrate and acetaminophen. For pain. Has small potential for addiction.

44 Celebrex. Celecoxib. For arthritis pain. Less likely to cause gastrointestinal problems than nonsteroidal anti-inflammatory drugs given for arthritis.

45 Tylenol with Codeine. Acetaminophen with codeine. For pain. Effective, but often overprescribed.

46 Darvon. Propoxyphene with APAP. For pain. Rated "Do not use" (see Things to Know, page 214) because it is no more effective than aspirin or codeine but much more dangerous.

47 Ultram. Tramadol. For pain. Rated "Do not use" (see Things to Know, page 214) because it is no more effective than codeine along with acetaminophen or aspirin and much more dangerous.

48 Motrin. Ibuprofen. For pain and inflammation. Like all NSAIDs (nonsteroidal anti-inflammatory drugs), this drug can cause stomach bleeding.

49 Relafen. Nabumetone. For arthritis. Rated "limited use."

50 Naproxen. For arthritis, pain. Can cause gastrointestinal problems including stomach bleeding and gas.

51 Vioxx. Refecoxib. For osteoarthritis, acute pain. One of the newest COX-2 inhibitor drugs, reportedly causes fewer gastrointestinal problems than other drugs used to treat arthritis.

GASTROINTESTINAL DRUGS

52 Prilosec. Omeprazole. For ulcers, esophagitis, reflux. Drug of choice for short-term treatment of severe reflux esophagitis.

53 Prevacid. Lansoprazole. For peptic ulcers and acid disorders. A drug of choice for peptic ulcers.

54 Propulsid. Cisapride. For reflux, acid disorders. Rated "Do not use" because it has been associated with a high incidence of side effects, including death.

55 Ranitidine. For peptic ulcers. About equally effective as famotidine and nizatidine (two other generic drugs used to block stomach acid).

ASTHMA, ALLERGIES, RESPIRATORY TRACT

56 Albuterol. For asthma. Take only the inhaled form, as taking the oral form increases the risk of adverse effects.

57 Claritin. Loratodine. For rhinitis, seasonal allergies. Rated "limited use."

58 Zyrtec. Cetirizine. For rhinitis. Rated "Do not use until 2002."

59 Allegra. Fexofenadine. For rhinitis, seasonal allergies. Rated "Do not use until 2002."

60 Flonase. Fluticasone. For rhinitis, seasonal rhinitis. Usually begins to work in 12 hours, but it may take several days for the effects to be noticed.

61 Serevent. Salmeterol. For asthma. Not effective once an attack has started.

62 Flovent. Fluticasone. For dermatosis, rhinitis. The Food and Drug Administration has rated it as "little or no therapeutic advantage."

63 Atrovent. Ipratropium. For chronic bronchitis. Not effective for asthma because it takes about 15 minutes to work.

64 Nasonex. Mometasone. For rhinitis. One of the newest drugs for rhinitis on the market.

65 Allegra-D. Fexofenadine/pseudoephedrine. For rhinitis. Rated "Do not use until 2002."

INFECTIONS

66 Trimox. Amoxicillin. For infections. One of the newest antibiotics.

67 Zithromax. Azithromycin. For cervicitis, lower respiratory tract infection. Prescribed more than other antibiotics in its class (macrolides). Rated "limited use."

68 Augmentin. Amoxicillin. For infections (ear, respiratory, sinus, skin). Not prescribed as often as the newer amoxicillin, Trimox.

69 Cipro. Ciprofloxacin. For infections (gastrointestinal, bone, joint, diarrhea, skin). Rated "limited use."

70 Cephalexin. For infections (bone, ear, skin, upper respiratory). An expensive drug that is no more effective than many other, less expensive, antibiotics.

71 Amoxil. Amoxicillin. For infection. Always take the full course of prescribed treatment.

72 Trimethoprim and sulfamethoxazole. For infections. This combination of generic antibiotics offers more benefit than either drug alone.

73 Biaxin. Clarithromycin. For bronchitis, sinus infection, skin infections. Rated "limited use."

74 Diflucan. Fluconazole. For candidiasis, cryptococcal meningitis. All of the prescribed amount should be taken, even if you feel better before you are done, or symptoms may return.

75 Levaquin. Levofloxacin. For infections—bronchitis, upper and lower respiratory, sinus. Rated "Do not use until 2003."

76 Cefzil. Cefprozil. For respiratory infections, bronchitis. Rated "limited use."

77 Ceftin. Cefuroxime. For infection. Wolfe (see Things to Know, page 214) notes that the *Medical Letter* rarely lists cefuroxime as a drug of choice for infections.

78 Lotrisone. Clotrimazole. For fungal infections. One of the newest clotrimazole drugs.

DIABETES

79 Glucophage. Metformin. For type II diabetes. Drug of choice for elderly people with hyperglycemia.

80 Glucotrol XL. Glipizide. For diabetes. Rated "limited use."

81 Glyburide. Glyburide. For hyperglycemia. Rated "limited use."

82 Rezulin. Troglitazone. For hyperglycemia. Rated "Do not use." Has been removed from the market in Japan and Britain because of severe adverse effects.

83 Amaryl. Glimepiride. For diabetes. Rated "Do not use until 2002."

HORMONES

84 Premarin. Conjugated estrogens. For menopause, osteoporosis, vaginitis. Increases the risk of endometrial and breast cancers in some women. It is made from horse urine.

85 Synthroid. Levothyoxine sodium. For goiter, hypothyroidism (underactive thyroid). A drug of choice for hypothyroidism.

86 Prempro. Conjugated estrogens and medroxyprogesterone. For menopause, osteoporosis. The presence of progestins is believed to reduce the risk of endometrial cancer associated with unopposed estrogen.

87 Levoxyl. Levothyroxine. For goiter, hypothyroidism. Should be taken only by people whose thyroid does not produce a normal amount of thyroid hormones.

88 Ortho Tri-Cyclen. Norgestimate/ethinyl estradiol. For birth control. An apparent increased risk of breast cancer is associated with oral contraceptives.

89 Triphasil. L-norgestrel/ethinyl estradiol. For birth control. The magnitude of the risk of cancer is still unknown.

90 Medroxyprogesterone. For amenorrhea, contraceptive. Rated "limited use."

OTHERS

91 K-Dur. Potassium chloride. For hypokalemia (low potassium). Eating a potassium-rich diet is usually a more effective and less expensive way to correct hypokalemia.

92 Prednisone. For arthritis, asthma, shingles, colitis, inflammatory conditions. This steroid suppresses the immune system, making you more vulnerable to infection.

93 Ambien. Zolpidem. For insomnia. Rated "limited use."

94 Fosamax. Alendronate. For osteoporosis, Paget's disease. Rated "limited use."

95 Viagra. Sildenafil citrate. For erectile dysfunction. Risk of heart attack appears to exist when used by men with heart disease.

96 Xalatan. Latapoprost. For glaucoma. You may notice darkening of the iris and of the eyelid skin color with prolonged use.

97 Klonopin. Clonazepam. For epilepsy. Continuous use of Klonopin may lead to drug-induced dependence.

98 Imitrex. Sumatriptan. For migraines. Rated "limited use."

99 Neurontin. Gabapentin. For epilepsy. Most prescribed anticonvulsant drug.

100 Cyclobenzaprine. For muscle spasms.

chapter thirty

Homeopathic Remedies
for *71* Medical Conditions

Homeopathy (a Greek word derived from *homios*, meaning "like," and *pathos*, meaning "suffering") is a form of medicine in which the remedies prescribed allow the body to heal itself. Samuel Hahnemann (1755–1843), the father of homeopathy, based this method of healing on three principles:

1. *The Law of Similars*, which states that a substance that can cause symptoms in a person who is well can also, when given in minuscule amounts, eliminate or reduce those same or similar symptoms in individuals who are ill. Unlike allopathic medicine (from the Greek *allos*, meaning "different"), in which illness is treated by opposing the symptoms, homeopathy treats with like remedies. For example, eating the belladonna plant causes stomach cramps and throbbing headache, two symptoms for which the homeopathic remedy is effective.

2. *Minimum dose*, which states that repeatedly diluting a substance increases rather than decreases its ability to heal, while also eliminating the risk of side effects.

3. *Prescribing principle*, which states that remedies are prescribed based on people's unique needs, including their physical and emotional states, diet, personality, lifestyle, temperament, and other factors.

How to Take Homeopathic Remedies

Although there are thousands of homeopathic remedies, only about 200 are used routinely. Unlike conventional over-the-counter and prescription medications, which typically are dosed in milligrams (a 325 mg aspirin, for example), homeopathic remedies are commonly given based on the centesimal (hundreds) or "c" scale. The "c" indicates how the remedy was diluted. A 1c remedy is 1 part substance and 99 parts water or alcohol and water. The most commonly prescribed remedies in the United States are 6c and 30c. Homeopathic remedies are available in drops, granules, and pills.

In this chapter, we list 71 common medical conditions and a few typical homeopathic remedies for each one. The remedies and dosages given are suggestions only; please consult a professional homeopath who can help you choose the remedy and dosage that is best for your unique needs. Refer to the sidebar for an explanation of each of the remedies. See Part VII for referrals for homeopaths.

1 *Acne*

• For acne characterized by itchy outbreaks on the face, shoulders, and chest; when symptoms improve with exercise or mental stimulation and worsen during menstruation—take kali bromiatum, 6c four times daily for up to 14 days.

• For acne associated with hormonal changes; when symptoms improve in a cool, dry environment and worsen with heat and before menstruation—take pulsatilla nigricans, 6c three times daily for up to 14 days.

2 *Anemia*

• When anemia is caused by severe blood loss and is accompanied by nervous tension and fatigue; when symptoms improve with sleep and warmth and worsen in cold, drafty environments and at night—take china, 6c three times daily for up to 14 days.

• When anemia is accompanied by constipation, headache, and low spirits; when symptoms improve with fresh air and when sweating, and worsen in cold or thunderstorms and from overexertion—take natrum muriaticum, 6c three times daily for up to 14 days.

3 *Anxiety*

• For anxiety caused by overwork and accompanied by nervousness and edginess; when symptoms improve with massage, fresh air, and reassurance from others, and worsen with exercise and consumption of hot food and beverages—take phosphorus, 6c every 2 hours for up to 10 doses.

• For anxiety caused by lack of confidence and accompanied by sleeplessness and loss of appetite; when symptoms improve with consumption of hot food and beverages and with movement and worsen in stuffy rooms and from overeating—take lycopodium, 6c every two hours for up to 10 doses.

4 *Arteriosclerosis*

• For arteriosclerosis accompanied by a craving for salt, frequent fainting spells, and nervousness; when symptoms improve in fresh air, with sleep, and when lying on the right side and worsen in the morning and evening and when lying on the left side—take phosphorus, 6c twice daily for 1 month.

• For arteriosclerosis accompanied by fainting spells, confusion, and liver problems; when symptoms improve in fresh air and worsen in heat or when shaking your head—take glonoinum, 6c twice daily for up to 1 month.

5 *Arthritis*

• When you feel restless generally and very stiff when you first rise in the morning but less so as you move; when symptoms improve with application of heat but worsen in cold, wet weather—take rhus toxicondendron, 6c three times daily for up to 14 days.

• When there is much pain with the least movement and the joints are very tender; when symptoms improve with complete rest and worsen with any movement—take bryonia, 6c three times daily for up to 14 days.

6 *Asthma*

• For asthma attacks that come on suddenly, especially after exposure to a cold, dry wind; when symptoms improve with fresh air and warmth and worsen in stuffy rooms and when you're near music—take aconite, 6c every 10 to 15 minutes until there is significant improvement.

• For asthma attacks accompanied by restlessness and burning chest pains; when symptoms improve by drinking warm beverages and sitting up and worsen in cold air and with consumption of cold drinks—take arsenicum album, 6c every 10 to 15 minutes until there is significant improvement.

7 Back Pain

• For acute back pain that isn't bothersome while you're moving but is painful when you first get up or start to move; when pain improves with the application of heat—take rhus toxicodendron, 6c three times daily for up to 2 weeks.

• For acute back pain that comes on after you've had a cold or during wet weather and that improves with application of heat—take dulcamara, 6c three times daily for up to 2 weeks.

8 Bedwetting

• When bedwetting occurs during nightmares or dreams; when the child feels better after a nap and feels worse when lying on the right side or when touched—give equisetum, 6c at bedtime for up to 14 nights.

• When bedwetting occurs soon after the child falls asleep and is caused by emotional stress or coughing; when the child feels better in damp, warm weather and worse in cold, dry weather—give causticum, 6c at bedtime for up to 14 nights.

9 Bee Sting

• When the affected area is numb or cold and is accompanied by inflammation and pain—take ledum, 6c immediately after the sting and then every 10 minutes until the pain subsides or for up to 6 doses, then three times daily if necessary for up to 3 days.

• When the affected area is hot, red, and obviously swollen—take apis, 6c every 10 minutes until the pain subsides or for up to 6 doses, then three times daily, if necessary, for up to 3 days.

10 Bladder Infection

• When you have a sudden, urgent need to urinate but there is only a dribble, followed by a burning pain; when symptoms improve with warmth and at night and worsen with movement and with consumption of cold water and coffee—take cantharis, 6c hourly for three doses, then four times daily until symptoms are eliminated.

• When the infection begins quickly and is accompanied by feelings of urgency and burning and sometimes fever; when symptoms improve when sitting or standing and with application of hot compresses and worsen with movement, jarring, and noise—take belladonna, 6c hourly for three doses, then four times daily until symptoms are eliminated.

11 *Boils or Abscesses*

• For a boil in its early stages; when the skin is swollen, dry, burning, red, and throbbing; when symptoms improve at night and when you apply pressure to the boil and worsen when you place cold compresses on the boil—take belladonna, 30c every hour for up to 10 doses.

• For a boil in its later stages; when the boil is sensitive to touch; when symptoms improve with the application of warm compresses and worsen in drafts and cold air—take hepar sulphuricum, 6c every hour for up to 10 doses.

12 *Breast Cysts*

• When the area around the cyst is painful and hard and there is itching inside the breast; when symptoms improve with application of pressure and worsen with consumption of alcohol and from sexual excess or abstinence—take conium, 6c four times daily for up to 14 days.

• When the pain comes and goes suddenly and is so severe it can make you cry; when symptoms improve with fresh air and in dry, cool environments and worsen at night, in heat, and premenstrually—take pulsatilla nigricans, 6c four times daily for up to 14 days.

13 *Bronchitis*

• During the initial stages of the disease, if your symptoms include a high fever, anxiety, and a dry, tickly cough; when symptoms improve with fresh air and warmth and worsen in stuffy rooms and when near music—take aconite, 6c hourly for 3 doses, then four times daily until symptoms improve significantly.

• If the cough is painful and very dry, resulting in stabbing pain in the chest; when symptoms improve with rest and when pressure is applied to the chest and worsen when bending forward—take bryonia, 6c hourly for 3 doses, then four times daily until symptoms improve significantly.

14 *Bursitis*

• When the affected site is swollen, hot, and red and the pain may be stinging; when symptoms improve with cold compresses and in cool surroundings and worsen with heat and from touch and pressure—take apis, 6c three times daily for up to 14 days.

• When the affected site is stiff and swollen and there is tearing pain; when symptoms improve with heat and movement and worsen with cold and damp—take rhus toxicodendron, 6c three times daily for up to 14 days.

15 *Chicken Pox*

• When the blisters burn and are very itchy and the child is restless; when symptoms improve with a hot bath and movement and worsen at night and in windy, stormy weather—take rhus toxicodendron, 6c four times daily for several days.

• When the blisters burn and are very itchy and the child is irritable and cries easily; when symptoms improve with cold and worsen with heat—take antimonium crudum, 6c four times a day for several days.

16 *Chronic Fatigue Syndrome*

• When fatigue is accompanied by trembling caused by overwork, irritability, fear of losing control, and muscle fatigue; when symptoms improve with movement, heat, and eating and worsen with pain, cold, dry air, cold beverages, and with even slight mental excitement—take kali phosphoricum, 30c twice daily for up to 14 days.

• When fatigue is accompanied by constantly feeling cold, joint and muscle pain, and aching and burning from stiffness; when symptoms improve with movement and warmth and worsen with cold foods and beverages and between midnight and 2 A.M.—take arsenicum album, 30c twice daily for up to 14 days.

17 *Common Cold*

• Use this remedy for the beginning stages: When the infection begins suddenly after exposure to cold and there is high fever and restlessness; when symptoms improve with fresh air and warmth and worsen in stuffy rooms and when exposed to music—take aconite, 6c hourly for up to 24 hours, then three times daily as needed.

• For a cold that comes on slowly and is accompanied by a red, swollen throat and hot mouth, that improves in the evening and with warmth and sleep and worsens in cold, dry, windy weather and in the early morning hours—take nux vomica, 6c every 2 hours for up to 4 doses.

18 *Colic*

• When an infant is crying angrily and has its knees positioned under its chin; when symptoms improve when you apply gentle pressure on the stomach and worsen when fed—give colocynthis, 6c every 5 minutes for up to 10 doses.

• When an infant screams at the slightest movement and has a bloated stomach and dry stools; when symptoms improve in a cool environment and when cold compresses are applied and worsen with exposure to noise and bright light—give bryonia, 30c every 5 minutes for up to 30 doses.

19 *Conjunctivitis*

• When the infection comes on suddenly, the eye is very swollen and red and burns with pain, and the eye is sensitive to light; when symptoms improve with warmth and warm compresses and worsen at night, with pressure, and in light—take belladonna, 6c hourly for 3 doses, then four times daily.

• If the eye tears a lot and the tears burn but remain clear rather than yellowish; when symptoms improve with coffee consumption and when lying down in a dark room and worsen in bright light and when outdoors—take euphrasia, 6c hourly for 3 hours, then four times daily.

20 *Constipation*

• For constipation accompanied by soft stools that are difficult to eliminate and a feeling as if the stools are located in the upper left-hand side of the abdomen; if symptoms improve when you're warm or when you consume warm food and beverages and worsen in cold air, in the early morning, or when you eat starchy foods—take alumina, 6c every 2 hours for up to 10 doses.

• For constipation characterized by hard, dry stools that burn when you pass them; when symptoms improve in warm, fresh air and when lying on your right side and worsen in a damp, cold environment and in the morning and evening—take sulfur, 6c every 2 hours for up to 10 doses.

21 *Cough*

• For a dry, croaking cough, accompanied by great thirst and a sudden fever, that improves in fresh air and worsens at night or when you're in warm rooms or near tobacco smoke—take aconite, 30c every 4 hours for up to 10 doses.

• For a cough accompanied by a thick, green mucus and loss of appetite, that improves in fresh air and worsens in the evening and when you're in warm, stuffy rooms—take pulsatilla nigricans, 30c every 4 hours for up to 10 doses.

22 *Depression*

• For depression caused by grief and accompanied by inappropriate behavior and a tendency to hold your emotions in; when symptoms improve when you walk and when you eat and worsen when you are cold or consume coffee or other stimulants—take ignatia, 6c three times daily for up to 14 days.

• For depression caused by fluctuations in hormone levels and accompanied by crying at the slightest upset; when symptoms improve in fresh air and a cool, dry environment and worsen premenstrually and in hot, stuffy conditions—take pulsatilla nigricans, 6c three times daily for up to 14 days.

23 *Diaper Rash*

• When the rash is red, scaly, and dry; when symptoms improve in fresh air and when the infant is warm and dry and worsen when it is being bathed and is exposed to heat—give sulfur, 6c four times daily for up to 5 days.

• When the rash is composed of small blisters and the infant is restless; when symptoms improve when the infant is warm and dry and worsen when it is undressed—give rhus toxicodendron, 6c four times daily for up to 5 days.

24 *Diarrhea*

• For diarrhea caused by food intolerance or anger and accompanied by painful urination and much flatulence; when symptoms are improved in fresh air and from fasting and worsen in hot weather or when you eat or drink—take aloe, 6c every hour for up to 10 doses.

• For diarrhea accompanied by green stools and gas that is not relieved by burping; when symptoms improve in fresh air and in a cold environment and worsen at night or in warm places—take argentum nitricum, 6c every 30 minutes for up to 10 doses.

25 *Earache*

• For earache accompanied by an infection that improves when you are sitting or standing or when you apply cold compresses to your forehead and worsens at night or when you are exposed to noise, light, or jarring motion—take belladonna, 30c every 30 minutes until you see your doctor.

• For earache accompanied by sharp pain that improves when you apply warm compresses to your forehead and wrap your head warmly and worsens when you are exposed to cold and drafts and when you touch the affected ear— take hepar sulphuricum, 6c every 30 minutes until you see your doctor.

26 *Eczema*

• For eczema that especially affects the palms of the hands and behind the ears, is moist with a gooey discharge, and is accompanied by rough, dry skin; when symptoms improve with sleep and worsen when you eat cold or sweet food or seafood—take graphite, 6c four times daily for up to 14 days.

• For eczema characterized by itchy, red bumps or fluid-filled blisters; that improves with hot water compresses and worsens when you rest and scratch—take rhus toxicodendron, 6c three times daily for up to 10 days.

27 *Eyestrain*

• For eyes that ache when you move them, that improve when you are in fresh air and when you apply cold compresses over the affected eye, and worsen in cold, stormy weather and from exertion or emotional stress—take natrum muriaticum, 6c four times a day for up to 7 days.

• For eyes that burn and feel strained, that improve when you move them and worsen in cold, damp weather and when you lie down or drink alcohol—take ruta graveolens, 6c four times a day for up to 7 days.

28 *Fear*

• For a strong fear of death and fear of open spaces, accompanied by restlessness; when symptoms improve in fresh air and worsen in warm rooms or when exposed to music or tobacco smoke—take aconite, 30c every 30 minutes for up to 10 doses.

• For a fear of failure and of crowds accompanied by a feeling that something terrible is going to happen; when symptoms improve in fresh air and worsen from consumption of sweet foods and at night—take argentum nitricum, 6c every 30 minutes for up to 10 doses; then four times a day for up to 14 days.

29 *Fever*

• For high fever accompanied by red cheeks, glassy eyes, and mental dullness; when symptoms improve with warmth and when sitting or standing and worsen at night and with noise and movement—take belladonna, 30c every hour or two for 3 doses or until the fever is reduced.

• For a high fever that comes on quickly but without affecting your mental capacity, and is accompanied by anxiety or fear; when symptoms improve in fresh air and with warmth and worsen in stuffy rooms and when near music—take aconite, 30c every hour or two for 3 doses or until the fever subsides.

30 *Flatulence*

• When bloating and gas occur after eating and you have a tendency to get full quickly; when symptoms improve with cool, fresh air and hot foods and worsen when eating onions and garlic and in stuffy rooms—take lycopodium, 6c every 30 minutes for several doses, then three times daily for up to 14 days if necessary.

• When even mild foods cause bloating and slow digestion; when symptoms improve with fresh air and when passing gas and worsen in warm, wet weather and when lying down—take carbo vegitabilis, 6c every 30 minutes for several doses, then three times daily for up to 14 days if necessary.

31 *Flu*

• For flu accompanied by restlessness, high fever, and sore throat; that improves in fresh air; and that worsens in the evening and when you're in warm rooms or near tobacco smoke or music—take aconite, 30c every 2 hours for up to 10 doses.

• For flu accompanied by weakness, chills, splitting headache, and sore throat; that improves in fresh air, after urinating, and when bending forward; and worsens in the early morning and late at night, when it's humid, and in the sun or fog—take gelsemium, 6c every 2 hours for up to 10 doses.

32 *Gingivitis*

• For bleeding gums accompanied by bad breath that improves when you rest or are dressed warmly and worsens when you are exposed to extremes in temperature—take mercurious solubilis, 6c every 4 hours for up to 3 days

• For bleeding, swollen, or ulcerated gums that improve when you are in fresh air and are fasting and worsen when exposed to warmth, sunlight, and noise—take natrum muriaticum, 6c every 4 hours for up to 3 days.

33 *Hayfever*

• For hayfever that is accompanied by swollen, photosensitive eyes discharging a thick substance and improves when you lie down in a dark room and worsens in warm, windy weather and in bright light—take euphrasia, 6c as needed for up to 10 doses.

• For hayfever that is accompanied by a burning nasal discharge and pain in the forehead, and that improves in fresh, cool air and worsens in warm rooms or in cold, damp weather—take allium, 6c as needed for up to 10 doses.

34 *Headache*

• For pain caused by emotional stress that improves when you eat, walk, or rest and worsens when you drink coffee or are in fresh air—take ignatia, 30c every 10 to 15 minutes for up to 10 doses.

• For pain caused by muscular tension, especially in the neck and shoulders; that improves with warmth and when you eat and worsens in the cold, in a draft, and during menstruation—take cimicifuga, 6c every hour for up to 6 doses.

Homeopathic Remedies: What You're Taking

Most people are unfamiliar with the origins of homeopathic remedies. Unlike herbal remedies, which naturally come from plants and are usually identifiable by name, homeopathic remedies can be made from minerals, animal parts, or plants. In most cases, the names are in Latin, which adds to the confusion. This list will help you know what you're taking.

Aconite (aconitum napellus): fresh flowers, leaves, and root of the monkshood plant

Allium (allium cepa): the fresh bulb of the red onion

Aloe (aloe socotrina): the juice, which is then powdered, of the aloe plant

Alumina: aluminum oxide

Antimonium crudum: the black sulfide of the element antimony

Apis (apis mellifica): the whole, live honeybee

Argentum nitricum: silver nitrate extracted from the mineral acanthite, the main ore of silver

Arnica (arnica montana): the whole, fresh leopard's bane plant in flower

Arsenicum album (white arsenic): prepared from the mineral arsenic

Belladonna (atropa belladonna): the fresh flowers and leaves of the deadly nightshade

Bryonia (bryonia alba): the fresh root of the white bryony plant

Calcarea carbonica: calcium carbonate derived from mother-of-pearl from oyster shells

Cantharis (lytta vesicatoria or cantharis vesicatoria): the whole, live beetle (Spanish fly)

Capsicum (capsicum fruitescens): dried capsules and seeds from the mature chili pepper

Carbo vegitabilis: charcoal, made from beech, poplar, or silver birch trees

Causticum: potassium hydrate—a mixture of lime and potassium sulfate

Chamomilla: whole, fresh chamomilla plant

(continued)

China (china officinalis): dried bark of the cinchona tree

Cimicifuga: the fresh root and rhizome of the cimicifuga racemosa plant (also called bugbane, black snakeroot, and black cohosh)

Coffea (coffea arabica): unroasted coffee beans

Colocynthis (citrullus colocynthis): dried fruit minus the seeds of the bitter apple

Conium: juice derived from the flowering stems and leaves of the hemlock

Drosera (drosera rotundifolia): the whole, fresh plant in flower

Dulcamara (solanum dulcamara): the young, green shoots and leaves of the fresh plant (woody nightshade) in flower

Equisetum (equisetum hiemale): whole, fresh horsetail plant

Euphrasia (euphrasia officinalis): the whole, fresh plant (eyebright) in flower

Gelsemium (gelsemium sempervirens): the fresh root of the jasmine plant

Glonoinum: nitroglycerine

Graphite (graphite): a form of carbon

Hamamelis (hamamelis virginiana): the fresh bark of twigs and the outer root layer of the witch hazel plant

Hepar sulphuricum: the impure calcium sulfide prepared by heating oyster shell powder and flowers of sulfur

Ignatia (ignatia amara or strychnos ignatii): the seeds from the St. Ignatius bean

Iodum: iodine

Ipecac (cephaelis ipecacuanha): dried root of the ipecacuanha plant

Kali bichromicum: potassium dichromate, prepared by mixing yellow potassium chromate in solution

Kali bromatum: potassium bromide, prepared from the salt

Kali phosphoricum: potassium phosphate, prepared by mixing dilute phosphoric acid and a solution of potassium carbonate

(continued)

Ledum (ledum palustre): the fresh plant (wild rosemary) in flower, dried and powdered

Lycopodium (lycopodium clavatum): the spores and pollen from the wolfsclaw (also known as club moss or stag's horn moss)

Mercurious solubilis: mercury derived from cinnabar, the most important ore of mercury

Natrum muriaticum: sodium chloride, derived from rock salt

Nux vomica: strychnine, derived from the seeds of the poison nut plant

Phosphorus: derived from the mineral phosphorus

Pulsatilla nigricans: the fresh plant (pasqueflower) in flower

Rhus toxicodendron: the fresh leaves of poison ivy

Ruta graveolens: juice from the whole, fresh plant (rue) before it flowers

Sabal serrulata: from the herb saw palmetto

Sanguinaria: from the root of the bloodroot plant

Sepia officinalis: the pigments in the ink of the cuttlefish

Silica: once derived from quartz or flint, but now prepared in the laboratory

Staphysagria (delphinium staphysagria): seeds of the stavesacre (larkspur) plant

Sulfur: derived from the mineral, also known as brimstone

Urtica (urtica urens): whole, fresh plant (dwarf stinging nettle)

35 *Heartburn*

• For heartburn accompanied by a burning feeling behind the breast-bone and extreme thirst; when symptoms improve when you eat but worsen after you eat and when you're in fresh air—take capsicum, 6c four times daily for up to 7 days.

• When heartburn is particularly bad at night; when symptoms improve when sipping warm beverages and placing warm compresses on the stomach and worsen with cold foods and when lying on the right side—take arsenicum album, 6c every 15 minutes until you get relief, then three times daily as needed for up to 7 days.

36 *Hemorrhoids*

• When hemorrhoids are accompanied by a bruised, sore feeling and symptoms are worse in warm, humid weather—take hamamelis, 6c four times daily for up to 5 days.

• For hemorrhoids accompanied by constipation, a sedentary lifestyle, and irritability; when symptoms improve with warmth and humidity and in the evening and worsen in cold, dry, windy weather and when eating spicy foods—take nux vomica, 6c every 15 minutes for severe pain until you get some relief, then three times daily or as needed for up to 7 days.

37 *Hepatitis*

• When even slight movement causes sharp pain; when symptoms improve with rest and pressure and worsen with movement and when bending forward—take bryonia, 6c three times daily for up to 14 days.

• When inflammation comes on suddenly and is accompanied by high fever, anxiety, and restlessness; when symptoms improve with fresh air and warmth and worsen in stuffy rooms or when near music—take aconite, 6c three times daily for up to 14 days.

38 *Hiccups*

• When hiccups are the result of excessive intake of food or irritating substances or associated with a digestive disorder; when symptoms improve with humidity and warmth and in the evening and worsen in cold, dry, windy weather and when eating spicy foods—take nux vomica, 6c every 10 to 15 minutes for 3 or 4 doses.

• When hiccups are the result of emotional upset or after eating or drinking; when symptoms improve with warmth or changing position and worsen with cold air or when near the smell of tobacco—take ignatia, 6c every 10 to 15 minutes for 3 or 4 doses.

39 *Hives*

• When the skin is burning, swollen, and red and the hives especially affect the eyelids and lips; when symptoms improve in fresh air and after a cold bath and worsen with sleep or in the heat—take apis, 30c every hour for up to 10 doses.

• When the skin has itchy, severe, slightly raised blotches, especially on the fingers and hands; when symptoms improve when lying down and worsen in cold, damp air and from scratching—take urtica, 6c every hour for up to 10 days.

40 *Indigestion*

• For indigestion caused by overeating or eating too late in the evening, and accompanied by a burning sensation in the stomach and excessive flatulence; that improves in cold, fresh air and after burping and worsens at night and in warm, wet weather—take carbo vegitabilis, 30c every 10 to 15 minutes for up to 7 doses.

• For indigestion that begins about two hours after eating and is accompanied by nausea and vomiting; if symptoms improve when you raise your hands over your head or if you're in fresh air and worsen in the evening or when you're in a hot, stuffy room—take pulsatilla nigricans, 6c every 10 to 15 minutes for up to 7 doses.

41 *Insomnia*

• For insomnia brought on by unexpected news and accompanied by an overactive mind; if symptoms improve when you're lying down or sucking on ice and worsen when you've been exposed to noise or strong odors and you're using sleeping pills—take coffea, 30c 1 hour before bed for 10 nights. Repeat the dose if you wake up and cannot return to sleep.

• For insomnia caused by exhaustion or stress and accompanied by a tendency to fall asleep easily but wake up around 3 A.M. and have trouble getting to sleep again; if symptoms improve with warmth and worsen from overeating and in windy, cold weather—take nux vomica, 30c 1 hour before bed for 10 nights. Repeat the dose if you wake up and cannot go back to sleep.

42 *Irritability and Anger*

• For irritability caused by overwork or exhaustion and accompanied by a tendency to lose your temper quickly; when symptoms improve with sleep and in the evening and worsen when you are cold and consume spicy foods or stimulants—take nux vomica, 6c every 30 minutes for up to 10 doses.

• For anger accompanied by insecurity, sometimes accompanied by violent behavior; when symptoms improve with sympathy and in a cool environment and worsen in stuffy rooms and when wearing tight clothing—take lycopodium, 6c every 30 minutes for up to 10 doses.

43 *Labor Pain*

• When labor progresses slowly and is accompanied by a great deal of crying, chills, and restlessness; when symptoms improve with crying, fresh air, and raising the hands above the head and worsen with heat and in the night—take pulsatilla nigricans, 30c every 5 minutes for up to 10 doses.

• When labor is extremely painful and causes involuntary screaming; when symptoms improve with warmth and when sucking ice and worsen when you're exposed to strong smells, noise, cold, or fresh air—take coffea, 30c every 5 minutes for up to 10 doses.

44 *Laryngitis*

• When there is hoarseness and loss of voice accompanied by high fever and restlessness; symptoms improve in fresh air and worsen when you're in a warm room or near music or tobacco smoke—take aconite, 30c four times a day for up to 7 days.

• When laryngitis results from too much shouting or singing; improves in fresh air and worsens around noon or if someone touches your skin—take argentum nitricum, 6c four times a day for up to 6 days.

45 *Mastitis*

• When the breasts are swollen and hard and the pain is severe; when symptoms improve with applied pressure to the breasts and worsen with movement—take bryonia, 6c hourly for 4 doses, then four times daily until you get relief.

• When breast pain is throbbing, the skin is hot, and inflammation is intense; when symptoms improve with warmth and sitting or standing and worsen with movement—take belladonna, 6c hourly for 4 doses, then four times daily until you get relief.

46 *Measles*

• When measles are accompanied by anxiety and a high fever that comes on suddenly; when symptoms improve in fresh air and worsen in a warm room or when you're near tobacco smoke or music—take aconite, 6c hourly for 3 doses, then four times daily until symptoms subside.

• When measles develop slowly and are accompanied by drowsiness; if symptoms improve when you're perspiring or bending forward and worsen in the sun or in damp, heat, or humidity—take gelsemium, 6c hourly for 3 doses, then four times daily until symptoms subside.

47 *Menopause*

• For menopause accompanied by vaginal pain during sexual intercourse, anxiety about sex, left-sided headache, and hot flashes; if symptoms improve when you sleep and exercise and worsen before menstruation and when in hot, damp places—take sepia officinalis, 30c every 12 hours for up to 7 days.

• For menopause accompanied by weight gain, panic attacks, and noises in the ear; when symptoms improve in the morning and worsen in cold, damp, windy weather—take calcqrea carbonica, 30c every 12 hours for up to 7 days.

48 *Menstrual Cramps*

• When cramps appear suddenly, become severe, and disappear quickly; when bleeding is heavy; when symptoms worsen with jarring movements—take belladonna, 6c every 15 minutes for 3 doses, then four times daily, if needed, until the pain subsides.

• When cramps are severe and make you irritable; when symptoms improve while you're fasting and in warm, wet weather and worsen when you're angry or exposed to fresh air—take chamomilla, 6c every 15 minutes for 3 doses, then four times daily, if needed, until the pain subsides.

49 *Migraine*

• For migraine that is worse on the left side and improves with rest or when your eyes are closed, but worsens when you move, vomit, cough, or eat rich foods—take ipecac, 6c every 15 minutes for up to 10 doses.

• For migraine located over the right eye that improves when you take in acidic beverages or foods and when you sleep but worsens in the sunlight or when someone touches your skin—take sanguinaria, 6c immediately at the first sign of pain and then every 15 minutes for up to 10 doses.

50 *Morning Sickness*

• When you are irritable and moody and the mere thought or smell of food makes you nauseated but eating actually helps; when symptoms improve with fresh air and warmth and worsen in the early morning and evening—take sepia officinalis, 6c every hour for up to 4 doses. If you get relief but the nausea returns, you can repeat the dosage, but do not use sepia for more than a few days.

• When morning sickness is worse upon waking and is accompanied by irritability; when symptoms improve with warmth and worsen in cold, dry, windy weather and from eating spicy foods—take nux vomica, 6c every hour for up to 4 doses. If you get relief but nausea returns, repeat the dosage, but do not use nux vomica for more than a few days.

51 *Mumps*

• When mumps are accompanied by night sweats, bad breath, and sensitivity to hot and cold; when symptoms improve with rest and in moderate temperatures and worsen with dampness and at night—take mercurious solubilis, 6c every 30 to 60 minutes for 3 doses.

• When mumps are accompanied by restlessness and aching muscles; when symptoms improve with continuous movement and dry warmth and worsen with rest and in windy, stormy weather—take rhus toxicodendron, 6c every 30 to 60 minutes for 3 doses.

52 *Neuralgia*

• When the pain is sudden, sharp, and begins after exposure to a cold draft; when symptoms improve with fresh air and worsen with exposure to tobacco smoke and in a warm room—take aconite, 6c hourly for several hours, then four times daily for up to 10 days.

• When the pain feels stabbing or cutting; when symptoms improve with pressure or warmth applied to the affected side, and worsen in damp, cold weather—take colocynthis, 6c hourly for several hours, then four times daily for up to 10 days.

53 *Pneumonia*

• When onset of pneumonia is sudden, especially in dry, cold weather, and is accompanied by chest pain, fever, and anxiety; when symptoms improve with fresh air and worsen with exposure to tobacco smoke and in a warm room—take aconite, 30c every 2 hours for up to 10 doses.

• When pneumonia is accompanied by sharp chest pains; when symptoms improve as you lie on the affected side and worsen with the slightest movement—take bryonia, 30c every 2 hours for up to 10 doses.

54 *Premenstrual Syndrome (PMS)*

• When PMS is marked by moodiness, the need for reassurance, a stomach that is sensitive to rich foods, and indecisiveness; when symptoms improve with fresh air and when walking slowly and worsen at night—take pulsatilla nigricans, 6c twice daily for up to 14 days.

• When PMS is marked by impatience, spasms, cramping, and feeling cold; when symptoms improve with warmth and pressure and worsen with cold, dry, windy weather and when eating spicy foods—take nux vomica, 6c twice daily for up to 14 days.

55 *Prostate Problems*

• When there is an urgent need to urinate and urination is difficult or painful, and the area around the prostate is cold; when symptoms improve with warmth and worsen with cold—take sabal, 6c four times daily for up to 21 days.

• When the prostate is hard, the testes are shrunken, and there is loss of potency; when symptoms improve with movement and fresh air and worsen in hot rooms—take iodum, 6c four times daily for up to 21 days.

56 *Psoriasis*

• When the skin is dry and scaly and there is a burning sensation; when symptoms improve with heat and movement and worsen in cold, dry, windy weather or at times close to midnight—take arsenicum album, 6c four times daily for up to 14 days.

• When the skin is thick and dry, especially at the fingertips and behind the ears, and may crack and itch; when symptoms improve with sleep, warmth, and fresh air and worsen with cold, damp air and in the morning and evening—take graphite, 6c four times daily for up to 14 days.

57 *Rosacea*

• When the skin on the face is dry, flaky, and burning; when symptoms improve with movement and heat and worsen in cold, dry, windy weather and around midnight—take arsenicum album, 6c three times daily for up to 21 days.

• During the early phases when the face is dry, hot, and red; when symptoms improve with warmth and when standing or sitting and worsen with movement, noise, and the sun—take belladonna, 6c three times daily for up to 21 days.

58 *Sciatica*

• When severe, cramping pains travel down the leg accompanied by occasional numbness; when symptoms improve with pressure on the affected side and worsen in cold, damp weather—take colocynthis, 6c three times daily for up to 14 days.

• When the muscles are stiff and painful, especially upon rising in the morning; when symptoms improve with heat and movement and worsen with rest and in stormy weather—take rhus toxicodendron, 6c three times daily for up to 14 days.

59 *Shingles (Herpes zoster)*

• When blisters are painful and very itchy; when symptoms improve with warmth and movement and worsen at night and with rest—take rhus toxicodendron, 6c four times daily until symptoms improve.

• When swelling and stinging pain are the main symptoms; when symptoms improve with cold and worsen with heat—take apis, 6c four times daily until symptoms improve.

60 *Sinus Infection*

• For sinus congestion that is accompanied by green-yellow, stringy mucus and severe sneezing, and improves when hot compresses are applied to the face and worsens in hot weather and in the morning—take kali bichromicum, 6c every 2 hours for up to 2 days.

• For sinus congestion that is accompanied by a tender face and copious amounts of yellow mucus; that improves when you're in a warm environment and worsens if touched or when in a draft—take hepar sulphuricum, 6c every 2 hours for up to 2 days.

61 *Sore Throat*

• For sore throat that comes on suddenly and is accompanied by hot, dry skin, great thirst, and swollen tonsils; that improves with fresh air and worsens when you are in a warm room or near music or tobacco smoke—take aconite, 30c every 2 hours for up to 10 doses.

• For sore throat accompanied by a raw, burning feeling in the throat, a hoarse voice, and thick saliva; that improves with movement and when you are warm and worsens at night and in damp or cold weather—take dulcamara, 6c every 2 hours for up to 10 doses.

62 *Sprains and Strains*

• When the injury is caused by overuse and there is bruising, pain, and swelling; if symptoms improve when you keep your head lower than your feet and worsen with continued movement—take arnica, 6c every 15 minutes for 3 doses, then three times daily until the injury has healed or for up to 10 days.

• When muscle injuries are painful and stiff; when symptoms improve with movement and warmth and worsen with rest and in stormy weather—take rhus toxicodendron, 6c every 15 minutes for 3 doses, then three times daily until the injury has healed or for up to 10 days.

63 *Sties*

• For a sty that is accompanied by red, inflamed eyes, itchy eyelids, and a head of pus on the eyelid and that improves with heat—take pulsatilla nigricans, 6c every hour for up to 10 doses.

• For a sty that begins as a boil and then develops pus, and that improves with heat—take staphysagria, 6c every hour for up to 10 doses.

64 *Stomach Flu (Gastroenteritis)*

• When you experience diarrhea and vomiting at the same time, accompanied by chills, restlessness, and a preference for cold beverages; if symptoms improve when you keep warm or consume hot drinks and worsen when you see or smell food or consume cold drinks—take arsenicum album, 6c every hour for up to 10 doses.

• For stomach flu accompanied by severe stomach cramps, diarrhea, and irritability; if symptoms improve when you stay warm and sleep or lie sideways with your knees tucked under your chin and worsen when you eat or drink or are exposed to cold, damp weather—take colocynthis, 6c every hour for up to 10 doses.

65 *Teething*

• When the infant is irritable and has one hot, red cheek and one pale; when symptoms improve as you carry the infant and worsen in heat and fresh air—give chamomilla, 30c every 30 minutes or more often if needed, for up to 10 doses.

• When the infant has a hot, flushed face accompanied by restlessness, staring pupils, and high fever; when symptoms improve with warmth and worsen with exposure to light, noise, or jarring motions—give belladonna, 30c every 30 minutes or more often if needed, for up to 10 doses.

66 *Tonsillitis*

• When the throat is very tender and sore, the right tonsil is more affected, and your neck is stiff; if symptoms improve when you sit or stand and worsen at night or when you're exposed to light or noise—take belladonna, 30c every 2 hours for up to 10 doses.

• When there is stabbing pain in the throat accompanied by hoarseness and bad breath; symptoms improve when you eat or wrap up your neck and worsen in cold air or if the throat is touched—take hepar sulphuricum, 6c every 2 hours for up to 10 doses.

67 *Toothache*

• For toothache that is accompanied by severe shooting pain, that improves when you place ice cold water in your mouth and worsens when you apply heat or eat hot foods—take coffea, 6c every 5 minutes for up to 10 doses.

• For toothache with throbbing pain, that improves after you eat even though it is painful to do so and worsens at night and in the fresh air—take belladonna, 30c every 5 minutes for up to 10 doses.

68 *Urinary Incontinence*

• When incontinence is caused by weakened muscle control triggered by coughing, sneezing, or laughing—take causticum, 6c three times daily until relief is apparent, or for up to 10 days.

• When the bladder is irritated or infected and there is dribbling of urine; when symptoms improve with warmth and sleep and worsen in dry, cold, wintry weather—take nux vomica, 6c three times daily until relief is apparent, or for up to 10 days.

69 *Warts*

• For warts on the back of the hand that are smooth and hard and may be large—take dulcamara, 6c daily for 14 days.

• For warts that are close to the nail or on the face and are accompanied by pain and possibly bleeding; when symptoms improve with warmth and worsen in dry, cold winds—take causticum, 6c daily for 14 days.

70 *Whooping Cough*

• See remedies under "Common Cold" for early stages of whooping cough. Once the whoop appears and the coughing has become violent and painful or has caused a nosebleed; when symptoms improve while you're walking and breathing in fresh air and worsen when lying down and when talking—take drosera, 6c four times daily or every few minutes during an attack.

• When the cough is accompanied by thick, stringy mucus that is yellow or green; when symptoms improve with heat and movement and worsen at night and when first awakened—take kali bichromicum, 6c four times daily or every few minutes during an attack.

71 *Yeast Infection (Candidiasis)*

• For candidiasis caused by stress or pregnancy and accompanied by an itchy, milky discharge; when symptoms improve in the morning and worsen before and after menstruation and in cold, damp weather—take calcarea carbonica, 6c six times daily for up to 5 days.

• For candidiasis caused by a hormone imbalance and accompanied by vaginal itching and a sore, burning vagina; when symptoms improve with sleep and exercise or heat applied to the vulval area and worsen with cold and in the early morning and evening—take sepia officinalis, 6c six times daily for up to 5 days.

chapter thirty-one

The *64* Most Common Surgical Procedures and Their Likely Outcomes

An estimated 23 to 25 million surgical procedures are performed in the United States each year. Most of those are simple outpatient procedures, but going under the knife, even for something as mundane as having a wart removed, can be stressful and frightening for the patient.

If you or a member of your family will be undergoing surgery, you have the right to ask questions and to receive clear, honest answers to them. Your surgeon and his or her staff should explain the surgery to you and your family and address your concerns. You may be understandably nervous or anxious; it may help to write down your questions so you won't forget anything.

Here are some questions you might consider asking your surgeon:

- What is the exact cause of the problem I am having now?
- Will this surgical procedure eliminate or cure the problem?
- Are there any alternative treatments we can consider that do not involve surgery?
- What can I expect if I decide not to have this surgical procedure?
- Where will the incision be made?
- How long will the surgery take?
- How many of these surgeries have you performed?
- Is this a standard procedure or is it new or experimental?

The Three Levels of Surgery

When you think of surgery, what sort of picture do you conjure? Lots of blood and an exposed heart or brain? In fact, most surgery isn't so spectacular. It involves procedures that fall into three general categories: minimally invasive, minor, and major.

"Minimally invasive" refers to the size of the incision. Gallbladder and appendix removal, for example, are considered minimally invasive surgical procedures when they are performed using the laparoscopic approach. In this technique, which is also known as keyhole or pinhole surgery, a small (about one-quarter inch) incision is made in the patient's navel. A thin wand with a tiny camera attached—a laparoscope—is inserted into the incision. Other surgical tools are inserted through other small incisions to complete the procedure.

Naturally, if you're the one going "under the knife," both minimally invasive and minor surgery, which includes procedures such as vasectomies, wart removal, and biopsies, probably seem major to you. Those classified as major, which include procedures such as mastectomy, heart surgeries, and transplantations, are undergone by 1 in 14 Americans each year. Regardless of the type of surgery you may need, you probably have lots of questions about the surgery and what to expect afterward. Be sure to ask your surgeon all those questions.

- How much pain can I expect after the procedure?
- When I wake up after the procedure, will I be hooked up to monitors, an IV, or other instruments?
- What are the possible complications associated with this procedure?
- How often do such complications occur?
- What are my chances of experiencing any of these complications?
- What are the consequences of these complications?
- How long will I be in the hospital after the procedure?
- What medications will I be taking after the procedure?
- Will I need any specialized care?
- When can I go back to work or school? Drive? Exercise? Have sex?
- Will I need physical therapy?

Questions like these are being asked every day by people who are about to undergo surgical procedures. Some of those surgeries are probably in this list, which includes the most common operations performed in the United States.

1   **Abdominoplasty (tummy tuck):** Removal of excess skin and fat from the abdomen, with best results experienced by people who are of relatively normal weight but who have weak abdominal muscles and excess skin.

Prognosis: Complete healing is expected, but it's slow. Depending on the extent of the tuck, scarring can be considerable.

2   **Amputation:** Removal of a limb or appendage, usually because of extensive injury to blood vessels that cannot be repaired or reconstructed. Impaired blood circulation associated with diabetes is one of the most common reasons for amputation.

Prognosis: If gangrene (tissue death caused by an inadequate blood supply or infection) sets in, the sooner amputation is done, the better the chances of recovery. One in five people with gangrene die, usually because of infection in the blood.

3   **Aortic aneurysm:** Removal of an aneurysm (an enlargement of a portion of the aorta caused by a weakness in the artery wall) from the aorta.

Prognosis: Chances of recovery are good if the aneurysm has not ruptured or caused the inner artery wall to tear away (dissect) from the outer artery wall. If a rupture or dissection has occurred, chance of survival is between 15 and 50 percent.

4   **Appendectomy:** Removal of the appendix, a small tubular organ with no known function, which is attached to one end of the large intestine. An appendectomy is minimally invasive and is usually done through a tiny incision with the use of an endoscope. It can also be done with conventional open surgery.

Prognosis: Complications are rare. Recovery normally takes 3 to 4 days.

5   **Blepharoplasty:** Removal of excess skin and fat from the lower eyelid to reduce or eliminate wrinkles and bags under the eyes.

Prognosis: The results usually last about 5 years.

6 **Brain tumor removal:** Procedure typically done to remove an abnormal growth on the brain.

Prognosis: Depends on whether the tumor is benign or malignant, size and location of the tumor, and at what stage it was discovered and treated. Radiation therapy may be necessary.

7 **Breast augmentation:** The implantation of a prosthesis, typically a saline-filled implant, inside the female breasts to enlarge them or to change their appearance.

Prognosis: Severe complications are rare but can include a rupture of the implant. Adhesions near the scars can cause discomfort.

8 **Breast reduction:** Removal of excess breast tissue, fat, and overlying skin from the female breasts.

Prognosis: Severe problems are rare. Postoperative pain can be significant, but the instant relief from back pain previously caused by excessively heavy breasts is a relief to most women.

9 **Bunion removal:** Removal of a bony, fibrous outgrowth (bunion, also known as hallux valgus) near the big toe. A bunion causes the big toe to curve inward; the operation allows the big toe to be straightened.

Prognosis: Complete recovery expected.

10 **Carotid endarterectomy:** Removal of an obstruction in the carotid artery (in the neck), caused by cholesterol buildup in the arteries.

Prognosis: Complete recovery expected. Possible complications include infection and, very rarely, stroke or injury to facial nerves.

11 **Carpal tunnel syndrome:** Cutting of the transverse carpal ligament, which is the fibrous tissue that crosses the wrist, to relieve pain and numbness in the hand and a weakened grip.

Prognosis: Complete recovery expected. Most people don't experience a return of symptoms.

12 **Cataract surgery:** Removal of the lens of the eye and replacement with an artificial lens. The procedure is done using a local anesthetic and the patient can usually go home the same day.

Prognosis: Complete recovery expected and vision should improve significantly.

13   **Cervical conization:** A minor surgical procedure that involves removal of a cone-shaped piece of the cervix because previous test results (a Pap smear) showed a precancerous or cancerous condition.
Prognosis: Complete recovery expected from the surgery; if the specimen is malignant, further tests will be needed to determine whether the cancer has spread.

14   **Cesarean section:** Removal of an infant through an incision in the mother's abdomen and uterine wall rather than via vaginal delivery.
Prognosis: Complete recovery expected.

15   **Cholecystectomy (laparoscopic):** Removal of the gallbladder using laparoscopy and tiny incisions.
Prognosis: Complete recovery expected, and recovery time is less than that associated with conventional surgery.

16   **Circumcision:** Removal of the foreskin of the penis, most often done on infants.
Prognosis: Complete recovery expected.

17   **Cleft lip repair:** Correction of an abnormal split in the upper lip, a common birth defect. It is usually performed on infants but can be done later in life.
Prognosis: Full recovery expected. Infrequently, excess scar tissue forms, which can be removed during an outpatient procedure.

18   **Colectomy:** Removal of a portion of the colon, mainly done because of cancer, abnormal growth, or a disease such as Crohn's disease.
Prognosis: If done for colorectal cancer and the disease is caught at an early stage, 90 percent of people live at least five years cancer-free. Chances drop to about 75 percent if it is done at a later stage, and the prognosis is poor if the cancer has spread.

19   **Cornea transplant (keratoplasty):** Removal of a diseased cornea and implantation of a healthy cornea from a donor.
Prognosis: Complete recovery expected. Vision improves within a few days for some patients; others get no improvement for months or a year or more.

20 **Coronary artery bypass:** Use of blood vessels from the leg or chest to bypass one or more narrowed or blocked coronary arteries.

Prognosis: Angina is usually cured, and the probability of a future heart attack is reduced.

21 **Craniotomy:** For removal of a blood clot, aneurysm, or tumor, or to drain a brain abscess.

Prognosis: Complete healing expected; stroke, excessive bleeding, or brain swelling are possible complications.

22 **Dilatation and Curettage (D&C):** Scraping the lining (endo-metrium) and the contents of the uterus. A D&C is done for various reasons; for example, to diagnose abnormal bleeding, as an elective abortion, or to treat minor diseases of the uterus.

Prognosis: Complete recovery expected.

23 **Ectopic pregnancy:** A pregnancy that develops outside the uterus, typically in the fallopian tubes, occasionally on the ovary or on the outside of the abdominal cavity or the cervix. About 1 percent of pregnancies are ectopic.

Prognosis: An ectopic pregnancy cannot come to term. Rupture is an emergency situation that requires immediate surgery. Full recovery is likely and subsequent pregnancies are usually normal.

24 **Episiotomy:** An incision at the exterior of the vaginal opening to create an enlargement to allow easier passage of the infant or to prevent dam-age to the mother's vagina, rectum, and bladder during childbirth.

Prognosis: Complete recovery expected.

25 **Esophagectomy:** Removal of the esophagus, usually done because of cancer.

Prognosis: If the procedure is done to treat early-stage cancer, chances of five-year survival are good. Complete recovery is expected for esophagectomies performed for other reasons.

26 **Hair implants:** Relocation of segments of hair-bearing skin, usually taken from the back of the head. Because many procedures are needed with healing time in between, the entire process may take up to two years or longer.

Prognosis: It may be several months before it can be determined whether the transplant is successful.

27 **Heart transplant:** Replacement of a diseased heart with a healthy one.

Prognosis: Rejection of the heart is a risk indefinitely. If rejection of the transplant can be controlled with immunosuppressive medication, life expectancy can be 10 years or longer.

28 **Heart valve replacement:** Replacement of one or more diseased heart valves with a mechanical or porcine (derived from pigs) valve.

Prognosis: Complete recovery expected. Possible complications include heart attack, stroke, and infection.

29 **Hemorrhoidectomy:** Removal of hemorrhoids (varicose veins that occur inside or on the outside of the anus).

Prognosis: Surgery is successful in most people regardless of age. Infection and severe pain when defecating are possible complications. Patients often need stool softeners for a few months.

30 **Hernia repair:** There are two main types of hernias. *Incisional:* The intestine extends through a weak area in the abdomen, especially near a previously repaired hernia or an abdominal incision. *Inguinal:* An intestine protrudes through an internal weakness or defect in the muscular layer of the abdomen.

Prognosis: Complete recovery expected, but hernias often recur. Heavy lifting should be avoided for several months.

31 **Hip fracture repair (hip nailing):** A surgical procedure to reattach the broken pieces of a fractured femur, the bone in the thigh that connects the hip joint to the hip bone. More than 200,000 hip fractures occur in the United States every year, and about half of them happen to people who are 80 years old or older.

Prognosis: Recovery can be expected if rehabilitation is followed.

32 **Hip replacement:** Replacement of the ball-and-socket joint with metal or plastic parts, typically because of a fractured hip or severe pain and stiffness that hinders movement.

Prognosis: Complete recovery expected if physical therapy and precautions are followed carefully during the first 6 weeks after surgery, although care still needs to be taken after that time.

33 **Hysterectomy:** Removal of the uterus, cervix, and often the fallopian tubes and ovaries, through an incision in the abdomen. Hysterectomy may be performed because of known or suspected cancer, endometriosis, chronic pelvic infection, severe menstrual pain, or ovarian disorders.
Prognosis: Complete recovery expected.

34 **Kidney removal (nephrectomy):** Removal of a kidney due to cancer or kidney failure. A kidney transplant may be done at the same time if a donor is available.
Prognosis: Complete recovery expected.

35 **Kidney stone removal:** Removal of a kidney stone from the ureter.
Prognosis: Complete recovery expected. However, more than 50 percent of people who are treated for a kidney stone develop another one within about 7 years.

36 **Kidney transplant:** Removal of a diseased kidney and implantation of a healthy kidney.
Prognosis: The 10-year survival rate is about 50 percent if the kidney was taken from a cadaver and 80 to 85 percent if it was from a live donor. Transplant patients will need to take immunosuppressive drugs for the rest of their lives.

37 **Knee replacement:** Replacement of the knee joint with metal or plastic parts. Typically done for people with arthritis that has severely worn the knee or when knee pain significantly affects movement.
Prognosis: Good results expected if intensive physical therapy is followed. The long-term durability of the replacement parts is uncertain.

38 **Laminectomy:** Removal of an intervertebral disk that is protruding from its normal position (a ruptured disk) in the spine.
Prognosis: Healing is slow, and discomfort and weakness may continue.

39 **Laryngectomy:** Removal of the larynx (voice box), usually because of cancer. During this operation, a hole (called a tracheostomy) is made in the front of the neck to allow the patient to breathe. If the cancer has affected the lymph nodes, they are removed as well.

Prognosis: Complete recovery expected from the procedure. Larynx cancer can be cured if it is caught early enough. However, life expectancy depends on the extent of the disease at the time of surgery and whether it has spread to other parts of the body.

40 **LASIK:** Laser-assisted in-situ keratomileusis is a surgical procedure in which a laser is used to reshape the cornea to correct nearsightedness. Scarring is minimal.

Prognosis: More than 90 percent of people achieve better than 20/40 vision, usually within 1 week of surgery. Occasionally a second procedure is needed.

41 **Liposuction:** Use of suction equipment to permanently remove deposits of fat from the hips, buttocks, abdomen, thighs, or chin. The fat is sucked out through an incision.

Prognosis: Although this procedure is often thought to be permanent, it is reported that about one-third of patients have a return of fat to the treated site. Touch-ups are often necessary to remove additional fat.

42 **Liver transplant:** Removal of a diseased liver and replacement with a healthy one.

Prognosis: Transplants are successful in 70 percent of adults and 90 percent of children. If a liver transplant fails, another transplant can be done when a liver is available.

43 **Lobectomy:** Removal of a portion of a lung, usually performed because of cancer. If the entire lung is removed, the surgical procedure is called pneumonectomy.

Prognosis: In some cases, lobectomy may cure the underlying lung disease. For other patients, quality of life may improve.

44 **Lumpectomy:** Removal of a lump, known to be or suspected of being cancerous, from the female breast.

Prognosis: Complete recovery expected from the procedure. Radiation therapy may be needed to help prevent recurrence of the cancer.

45 **Mastectomy:** Removal of the female breast because of the presence of breast cancer. A radical mastectomy involves removal of the breast, the lymph nodes under the arm, and the pectoral muscles. A modified radical mastectomy does not remove the pectoral muscles, and a simple mastectomy leaves both the lymph nodes and the pectoral muscles.

Prognosis: Complete recovery expected from the procedure. Chemotherapy or radiation therapy may be needed to prevent recurrence of the cancer.

46 **Meniscectomy:** Removal of damaged cartilage from the knee. Most injuries are the result of a torn ligament.

Prognosis: Complete recovery expected; weakness in the knee is a possible complication.

47 **Myomectomy:** Removal of fibroid tumors from the uterus through incisions made in the lower abdomen.

Prognosis: Complete recovery expected.

48 **Orchiectomy:** Removal of one of the testicles because of cancer or gangrene.

Prognosis: Complete recovery expected. Removal of one testicle should not affect sexual function or the ability to have children.

49 **Ovarian cyst removal:** Removal of a cyst from the ovary.

Prognosis: Complete recovery from the surgery. If cancer is diagnosed, chemotherapy or radiation therapy may be prescribed.

50 **Pacemaker implant:** Insertion of a temporary or permanent pacemaker into the chest wall.

Prognosis: A pacemaker may successfully restore normal heart rate, but the overall prognosis depends on the presence of underlying disease, such as coronary artery disease. After surgery, patients are usually asked to wait 6 weeks before participating in strenuous activities.

51 **Polypectomy:** Removal of one or more polyps from the rectum.

Prognosis: Complete recovery expected.

52 **Prostatectomy:** Removal of a portion or all of an enlarged prostate gland. It can be done with a cystoscope, a thin instrument that is inserted through the urethra; or through an incision in the lower abdomen.

Prognosis: Complete recovery expected. Possible complications include sterility and impotence.

53 **Radical neck dissection:** Procedure to remove cancerous growths from the lymph nodes in the neck.

Prognosis: Expect complete healing. Some disfigurement of the neck may be unavoidable, but some cancers are completely cured following this surgery.

54 **Rhinoplasty:** Reconstruction of the nose, performed for cosmetic or therapeutic (blocked nasal passages) reasons.

Prognosis: Complete healing expected, but it is slow. Minor changes occur during the 18 months after the surgery while the scar tissue matures, and patients must be very careful not to injure the nose during that time. Rhinoplasty has a higher degree of dissatisfaction from patients than most other cosmetic surgery procedures.

55 **Rhytidectomy:** Commonly known as a face-lift. Removal of excess skin, tissue, and fat from the face in order to eliminate wrinkles, tighten sagging skin, and remove double chin.

Prognosis: Nothing lasts forever. Depending on age, skin condition, general health, and many other factors, touch-ups or another face-lift may be elected.

56 **Small-bowel resection:** Removal of a diseased section of the small intestine because of blockage, trauma, or a tumor.

Prognosis: Complete recovery expected

57 **Splenectomy:** Removal of the spleen, usually due to injury or trauma, infection, or tumors.

Prognosis: Complete recovery expected. Possible complications include infection, blood clots, pneumonia.

58 **Sterilization (female):** Cutting and tying the fallopian tubes to prevent sperm from traveling up the tubes to fertilize eggs. This procedure is usually performed using laparoscopic technique or following a cesarean section.

Prognosis: Complete recovery expected. Most cases are not reversible. Failure rate (accidental pregnancy because the procedure was not done successfully) is about 0.4 percent.

59 **Strabismus (wandering eyeball) correction:** Procedure that strengthens or weakens the muscles that regulate the horizontal movement of the eyeball.

Prognosis: More than one operation may be needed, depending on the extent of the problem.

60 **Thyroidectomy:** Partial or complete removal of the thyroid gland due to a cancerous tumor, malfunction of the gland, or a benign growth (goiter).

Prognosis: Complete recovery expected. Lifetime thyroid hormone therapy may be needed. For thyroid cancer, radiation therapy may be needed.

61 **Tonsillectomy and adenoidectomy:** Removal of the tonsils, usually after several bouts of tonsillitis, and the adenoids. These two procedures are often done together.

Prognosis: Complete recovery expected. Nasal congestion, sore throat, and earaches are common for a few days postsurgery.

62 **Trabeculectomy:** Procedure that relieves the buildup of pressure in the eye associated with chronic glaucoma.

Prognosis: Usually succeeds in eliminating the symptoms of glaucoma (loss of peripheral vision and blurred vision) and preventing vision loss.

63 **Varicose vein surgery:** Removal of varicose (swollen, distorted, painful) veins just below the skin's surface in the thigh or calf.

Prognosis: Recovery is expected but is slow. Varicose veins can recur after surgery but they are often scattered and can usually be removed with a minor in-office procedure under local anesthesia.

64 **Vasectomy:** Cutting and tying the vas deferens (the sperm channels inside the scrotum), which stops the flow of sperm. A vasectomy provides an effective and safe form of birth control with little or no physical impact on sexual performance or desire.

Prognosis: If done correctly, 100 percent successful as a birth control method. It can be reversed in some cases.

chapter thirty-two

15 Secrets of the Shamans

When native peoples around the world need medicine, they usually turn to nature's drugstore: medicinal plants. Many people are not aware that conventional medicine has often taken advantage of the healing secrets from these traditional cultures. The result is that about 25 percent of the prescription drugs we use today have components that were derived from plants, and about three-quarters of these plant-based drugs were developed because of native folklore claims.

One common drug is quinine, a derivative of cinchona bark, which is used to treat malaria. The aboriginal peoples of Ecuador were using the bark when a physician in the 1620s heard about it and used it to treat the Countess of Chinchon in Peru. She had malaria, and the Countess recovered with the treatment. The rest, as they say, is history. Today, approximately 10,000 tons of cinchona bark are harvested each year to yield 500 tons of quinine and related drugs.

Among other prescription drugs with "roots" in the botanical world is rauwolfia, which is an extract of the snakeroot plant. It was used for centuries in the Far East as a sedative. Today, doctors use it for people with high blood pressure. A derivative of rauwolfia, reserpine, is prescribed by psychiatrists for people with severe mental disorders. Among Native Americans, foxglove was used to treat dropsy, a condition in which fluid accumulates in the legs because of a heart disorder. Researchers found that foxglove contains the ingredient known as digitalis, which is often used today to stimulate a weak heart.

In some cultures, keepers of the secrets of medicinal plants are known as shamans. In others, they are referred to as priests, mystics, yogis, or healers. All are teachers and keepers of healing wisdom that has been passed down from generation to generation for centuries.

Here, revealed to you, are 15 secrets from these healing traditions. Many of the listed remedies are now under investigation to determine their medicinal value, and a few are already available on the American market. This may be only the beginning of a whole new world of plant-based medicines.

1 Andiroba (*Carapa guianensis*). The oil pressed from the seed of this large (130 feet or taller) tree from the Amazon region is used by Amazonian peoples to reduce aches and pains, rashes, and skin tumors. It can also be used to repel insects, a definite advantage in the Amazon jungle.

2 Aripari (*Macrolobium acaciaefolium*). Native peoples of the Amazon use this tree not only to make boats, but also to brew a strong tea from the bark to relieve diarrhea. The powdered leaves are also used to treat ulcerated wounds.

3 Ashwagandha (*Withania somnifera*). Ashwagandha is the most widely used medicinal plant in India. For more than 2,000 years, Indians have taken it to improve health, enhance sexual desire, relieve fatigue, reduce inflammation, and combat stress. It contains a large number of alkaloids and many unique compounds. Scientists have yet to identify the components that give ashwagandha its healing abilities. Ashwagandha is available in the United States.

4 Babassu (*Orbignya martiana*). The kernels of the hard nuts that grow on this tall palm tree are the source of babassu oil, which is similar to coconut oil. The oil is very high in fatty acids and makes an effective natural skin and hair cleanser.

5 Cat's Claw (*Uncaria tomentosa*). The Peruvians call this herb the "vine of life," una de gato, or cat's claw. It was first used by the Riberenos Indians to treat arthritis and to detoxify the liver and kidneys. When people in the United States heard about cat's claw, it was used secretly by individuals with AIDS because it helps strengthen the immune system. Today, cat's claw is widely available in the United States and is used to treat arthritis, reduce blood pressure, relax blood vessels, and enhance immunity. Its immune-boosting qualities have been credited to six alkaloids (organic substances found in plants that react with salts) that are found in the inner bark of the plant.

6 **Catuaba (*Erythroxylum catuaba*).** In the Amazon, aboriginal peoples use the bark of the catuaba tree as an aphrodisiac. Apparently, they have had much success with it. In Brazil, there is a saying that if a man younger than 60 becomes a father, it happened because of him; if a man older than 60 becomes a father, it was the catuaba. Scientists have examined the catuaba bark and found that it contains large amounts of minerals and trace elements, including calcium, potassium, and magnesium. Catuaba is available in the United States in powder, tea, and capsules.

7 **Chyawanprash.** This potion comes from the Ayurvedic tradition and is a formula that reportedly fights aging and senility, rejuvenates the cells, and maintains youthfulness and vigor. It can be made up of anywhere from 20 to 80 natural herbs, and has the consistency of jam. Its main ingredient, amla (tropical gooseberry, *Embellica officinalis*) is said to be the richest natural source of vitamin C in the world. Indian legend has it that in ancient times, an old wise man named Chyawan was meditating in the forest when a young princess came by and accidently touched the old man's hair. According to custom, a woman could touch only one man during her lifetime, so the king asked that the old man marry the princess. Because of the great age difference, Chyawan developed a recipe for long life. Ever since then, for 2,000 years or more, his formula (or variations of it) has been the most popular tonic in India. Regardless of the other herbs added to the formula, amla is always the main one.

8 **Copaiba (*Copaifera officinalis*).** This is the name of an oil that is gathered from the copaifera trees that grow mainly in the South American rainforests. Local aboriginals collect the oleoresin that accumulates in cavities in the tree trunk, and traditional healers use it to treat rashes and skin abrasions. In Europe and Latin America, it has been used for centuries to treat bronchitis, diarrhea, and hemorrhoids. Among some tribes, the resin is used to treat skin gonorrhea, syphilis, urinary incontinence, and psoriasis. Peruvian traditional healers recommend it for stomach ulcers, and they mix it with andiroba oil to treat herpes. Copaiba oil is believed to be an effective disinfectant and diuretic and to have stimulant properties.

9 **Cowhage seed (*Mucuna pruriens*).** The seeds inside the furry pod of this perennial shrub are used in Ayurvedic medicine as an aphrodisiac and also to treat impotence and urinary conditions. The cowhage plant, which grows throughout India, Southeast Asia, and Malaysia, is under investigation for its possible use in treating Parkinson's disease and other brain disorders. That's because the seeds contain many substances, including nicotine, lecithin, and levodopa, a substance given to people with Parkinson's disease to help stop their rigidity and tremors.

10 **Jurubeba (*Solanum paniculatum*).** Hangovers can happen anywhere, including the Amazon. The local aboriginal people use infusions of jurubeba to cure their overindulgences, as well as to relieve indigestion and reduce inflammation of the liver and spleen. Scientists have identified several components of the plant that may explain these abilities.

11 **Maca (*Lepidium meyenii*).** In the Andean plateaus of Peru, the maca plant is believed to have been cultivated for about 2,000 years. The harsh conditions there—freezing temperatures, high winds, and intense sunlight— seem to suit maca just fine. This root vegetable is the subject of many legends that report that the plant has strong nourishing powers and that it promotes sexual desire and increases sexual energy. The native Peruvian Indians still grow and eat maca, which is rich in many minerals such as calcium, magnesium, phosphorus, iron, zinc, and many vitamins. Peruvians regard this plant highly for its fertility powers. Couples who have trouble conceiving eat maca every day until the woman gets pregnant. Maca has been shown to increase fertility in animals.

12 **Mastruco (*Chemopodium ambrosoides*).** This plant has the nickname "wormseed" because it contains a substance that kills ascaris, a nematode (parasitic worm) that lives in the large intestine. Infusions of mastruco are used to kill other types of parasites as well, including hookworms, tapeworms, and roundworms, and to cure dysentery. Native women use mastruco to relieve menstrual cramps and as a contraceptive.

13 **Muira-Puama (*Ptychopetalum olacoides*).** Another Amazon aphrodisiac is muira-puama, also known as potency wood. It has been compared to yohimbine (see Chapter 12) because it causes similar effects, although the adverse reactions are said to be milder. This small tree has slightly pink bark and roots, and both parts contain a resin purported to be the source of the libido-enhancing powers of this plant. One study of muira-puama in men with erectile dysfunction found that 51 percent of the men improved after treatment and 62 percent had an increase in libido. Muira-puama is available in the United States.

14 **Quebra pedra (*Phyllanthus niruri*).** This plant is referred to as shatter stone, because infusions of the leaves are used to eliminate gallstones and kidney stones. Scientists have found evidence that quebra pedra can inhibit the hepatitis B virus and that it contains anticancer substances. Quebra pedra is available in the United States.

15 **Tayuya (*Cayaponia tayuya*).** We reach for the aspirin; Amazon aboriginal peoples reach for tayuya, which reportedly relieves headache, backache, sciatica, gout, arthritis and rheumatism, and other types of pain. The Amazonians have used this plant since prehistoric times, often with some stevia (an extremely sweet herb) or honey to help take away the bitter taste. Tayuya is used outside the rain forest as well. Indians in Colombia use a derivative of the plant to treat sore eyes, and tribes in Peru like it for skin problems. Researchers have found that tayuya may also inhibit the Epstein-Barr virus and that it has cancer-inhibiting characteristics. Some natural health practitioners in the United States use tayuya to treat headache, gout, sciatica, neuralgia, indigestion, severe acne, eczema, herpes, and irritable bowel syndrome.

Part III

Where to Go for Good Health

No matter how much we want to be able to take care of ourselves and avoid doctors, dentists, medications, hospitals, and clinics, on occasion we need to turn to them for help. But we aren't always allowed the luxury of time when decisions need to be made about who to see or where to go, especially in a crisis or an emergency situation. When we are under stress, it is difficult to think clearly. It's always better to be prepared and to have an idea in advance about where we would go for medical care or other types of healing.

In this part of the book, we help you choose a hospital, a dentist, an alternative practitioner, and an alternative health facility to meet your needs. We provide you with the questions, criteria, and guidelines you need to make informed decisions in each of these areas.

We also consider a few other places that can help you care for your health. Where you live and where you work, for example, can have a significant impact on your physical, mental, emotional, and spiritual well-being. Have you ever thought about where some of the healthiest or safest places to live in the United States might be? We introduce you to what some people say are the best—and the worst—places to be when it comes to health and safety. Is your job safe? You may be surprised at some of the jobs that are considered to be the most dangerous in America.

If you have the means to try some alternative approaches to healing, you might consider visiting one of the 33 healing sites for the body, mind, and spirit around the United States and the rest of the world—sites that are identified as having healing powers.

33 Healing Sites for the Body, Mind, and Spirit

According to a poll conducted by *Newsweek* in 2000, 84 percent of adults in the United States believe that God performs miracles, and 48 percent say they have personally witnessed or experienced a miracle themselves. Among non-Christians and people who report they have no faith at all, 43 percent say they have asked for God's help.

What are people asking for? Although some may be praying to win the lottery, most say they ask for cures for themselves or for loved ones. They want to be healed, to be whole, to be in harmony with themselves and with the world. Often these people seek physical, emotional, or spiritual wholeness at specific healing or sacred sites. To paraphrase a Tibetan saying: Spending one day at a sacred site is like spending a thousand days at meditation.

That said, let's look at some healing sites around the world. We've tried to find some of the most fascinating and unusual ones, as well as ones that may be familiar to you.

By the way, whether or not you believe in the power of these places doesn't really matter. There's an old Hassidic saying that goes, "He who believes all these tales is a fool, but anyone who cannot believe them is a heretic."

Healing Sites from Around the World

1 *The island of Oita, Japan*, is home to many healing springs and spas. One group of nine springs is located at the foot of the Kuju mountain

chain. Sujiyu, one of the nine hot springs, was so named because its healing powers are reportedly effective for illnesses that affect the tendons, or "suji" in Japanese.

2 *The Western Wall in Israel* is all that remains of the temple built by Herod, destroyed in 70 CE. The Wall is visited by thousands of people each year, many of whom place prayers on the Wall in hope of an answer from God. In March 2000, Pope John Paul II placed the following prayer among the many already there: "God of our fathers, you chose Abraham and his descendants to bring your name to the nations. We are deeply saddened by the behavior of those who, in the course of history, have caused these children of yours to suffer."

3 *The tomb of Saint James the Great* lies in the medieval city of Compostela in the northwest corner of Spain. Saint James is credited with converting the Iberian peninsula to Christianity. About 10,000 people a year travel to Compostela to ask God for special favors, to give thanks for prayers that have been answered, or to heal spiritually.

4 *The Shrine of Saint Thomas Becket of Canterbury* was, in its day, said to be the richest in the world. Within 10 years after Saint Thomas died in 1170, a total of 703 miracles were recorded and attributed to the act of visiting his shrine. However, none of that splendor remains today, as the tomb was plundered during the reign of Henry VIII. Some people claim miracles still happen to those who come to pay their respects to this martyr.

5 *Bodh Gaya (or Bodhgaya)*, the holy site in India where Gautama Buddha reached Supreme Enlightenment, is a field held sacred both by Buddhists and by people of any faith who wish to awaken their spirituality. It is the site of the Bodhi Tree, or the Tree of Awakening, where Gautama spent 49 days meditating before he became the Enlightened One. There is a temple on the site, the Mahabodhi Temple, built nearly 2,000 years ago. Thousands of people visit the temple each day.

6 *The Jamkaran Mosque* in Iran, located outside the holy city of Qom, has been a popular pilgrimage site for a thousand years. It is also a site for miracles. Although no one kept track of the reported miracles before 1998, officials at the mosque have begun to investigate and validate miraculous cures. So far, at least 6 miracles out of 270 claims have been verified by the Registry of the Divine Acts of Mercy in Iran.

7 A visit to the British Isles would not be complete without a trek to *Saint Winefride's Holy Well*, also known as the Lourdes of Wales. The well's origins go back to around 660 CE, when a young maiden named Winefride refused the advances of a chieftain. He became enraged and cut off her head. When her head fell to earth, a spring of water reportedly rose out of the ground. Then Winefride was restored to life by her uncle, Saint Beuno. Since that time, people have regularly come to the well to bathe (legend has it that you must do so three times), to pray for physical and spiritual healing, and to give thanks. In 1415, King Henry V reportedly traveled 45 miles on foot to the well to give thanks for his victory at Agincourt.

8 *The Temple of the Tooth*, or Dalada Maligaw, at Kandy, Sri Lanka, is the home of what is believed to be a tooth of the Buddha. The tooth was brought to Sri Lanka from India when Buddhism lost favor to Hinduism there. The temple is the holiest temple in Sri Lanka and a popular pilgrimage site. In January 1998, terrorists conducted a suicide bombing at the temple, which killed eleven people, including the two suicide bombers. Although the temple suffered some damage, the main structure was unharmed.

9 Visiting the *88 sacred places of Shikoku* in Japan should keep anyone busy for quite a long time. This pilgrimage is considered to be the most important one an individual can make in Japan. The target of a pilgrim's prayers for healing and thanks is Kobo Daishi, one of the most famous Japanese who ever lived. He was born in 774 and lived his life as a priest, poet, educator, and engineer. He founded a sect of Buddhism and a monastic center on Mount Koya. He was raised to the level of saint and is still revered by both Buddhists and non-Buddhists. A total of 88 temples have been attributed to him on the island of Shikoku. The traditional pilgrimage is done by walking around the circumference of the island, which takes about 50 to 60 days, in a clockwise direction, stopping to visit each temple. An additional 20 temples are also considered important to the pilgrimage, but apparently it's not necessary to visit them to have your prayers answered.

10 If you can't get to France to visit the original grotto where Our Lady of Lourdes appeared to Bernadette in 1858, you might go to *Euclid, Ohio*, where you can see the Shrine and Grotto to Our Lady of Lourdes. The shrine sits on property originally owned by a Mr. Harms, whose wife was a devout Catholic. The land became the property of the Good Shepherd Sisters in 1920. After some of the sisters visited the famous shrine at Lourdes in France, they decided to create a similar grotto on their property in Ohio. The crowning touch of the Ohio grotto was a piece of stone from the rock on which the Blessed Virgin reportedly stood when she spoke to Bernadette. The stone was broken into three pieces: Two were placed in the grotto and the third is kept in the gift shop on the property. The grotto was blessed and dedicated on May 30, 1926, by Most Reverend Bishop Scrembs. Since that time, thousands of people have come to the grotto to place their petitions, and hundreds of them have reportedly been granted.

11 In *Copacabana, Bolivia*, high in the mountains, is a sacred site that has its roots in mystical South American Indian gods, which the locals believe live in the natural features of the land. When the conquering Spanish Catholics came to the land, they built the Stations of the Cross on the site, monuments to Christ's life and death. Today, pilgrims of all beliefs come to the location for prayer.

12 In *Sedona, Arizona*, red rock formations rise in the land that originally was populated by the Yavapai Indians. These rocks—Cathedral Rock, Bell Rock, Airport Mesa, and Boynton Canyon—are believed to be power vortexes, sites where energy fields emanate from the earth. Yavapai legends say this area is a healing place where the goddess of creation appeared on the earth and gave birth to their nation. Many who visit these sites—and tens of thousands do every year—report feeling a renewal and healing that they cannot explain.

13 People from around the world have been drawn to *Mount Shasta* in northern California because of what is reported to be an incredibly vibrant energy that comes from the mountain. Streams on the mountain have been used in purification rituals by local Indians for centuries. People who live near Mount Shasta say they experience a loss of awareness when they are away from the mountain, a feeling that is regained once they return home.

14 *The Monastery of Saint Catherine's*, located at the foot of Mount Sinai in Egypt, contains the Chapel of the Burning Bush. This is believed to be the site where God spoke to Moses out of a burning bush and told him to return to Egypt to bring the Children of Israel to the Promised Land. The monastery has stood since the fourth century and was named after Saint Catherine a few centuries later, after she was beheaded for her religious beliefs.

15 *The Dome of the Rock* is one of the holiest places of Islam. This mosque, located in Jerusalem, was built at the summit of Mount Moriah, a site Muslims hold sacred because it is where Muhammad ascended from earth to make his way through the seven heavens to speak with Allah. It was during that journey that Muhammad is said to have received the words of the Koran, but the site is also special to Jews and Christians. Reportedly, King Solomon built the first temple on this spot, which some say is where Abraham prepared to sacrifice his son Isaac around the year 2000 BC. Thus, although it is an important place of worship for Muslims, it is open to people of all faiths.

16 Not far from the ancient walls of Jerusalem in Israel is the *Garden of Gethsemane*, where Christ is said to have prayed before he died. Located on the lower slopes of the Mount of Olives (see number 31), it is sometimes referred to as the Garden of Agony.

17 More than six million pilgrims a year visit the holy waters of the Kami at the *Ise Shrine* in Japan. These sacred waters are revered by those of the Shinto faith. When pilgrims visit the well, they dip a bamboo cup into the sacred water and take a sip. It is said that those who do so receive an abundance of life from the Kami, gods that come to humans in the form of the wonders of nature.

18 In addition to the holy waters of Ise, there are the *Jingu shrines at Ise*, which have been revered as the holiest of all Shinto sanctuaries since medieval times. Today there are 30 wooden shrines scattered throughout this forested area. The Uji Bridge spans the sacred Isuzi River, where visitors can purify themselves before they enter one of the shrines, the Naiju Grand Shrine. People of the Shinto faith maintain that Ise is the earthly home of the sun goddess and the founder of the nation, Amaterasu.

19 *Glastonbury, England* is the home of what is believed to be the Holy Grail, the chalice from which Christ drank at the Last Supper. Today the chalice resides at the Chalice Well Gardens in Glastonbury, where the waters of the well, which is also known as the Blood Spring, are said to have magical powers.

20 *The Taj Mahal* was built during the early seventeenth century by order of Shah Jahan in memory of his wife, Mumtaz Mahal. It took 20,000 laborers more than 22 years to complete the structure. It is located in Agra, India, and is a popular pilgrimage site for people of all faiths. About 100,000 people visit the monument and the surrounding grounds every day seeking tranquillity, healing, and perhaps just a photograph or two.

21 *The Bighorn Medicine Wheel* can be found on a ridge near a 10,000-foot summit in Wyoming's Bighorn Mountains. Very little is known about the people who built the wheel, which is constructed of rough stones that form a circle 70 feet in diameter. There are 28 spokes that extend from a center hub, which is about 12 feet in diameter. The structure is estimated to be about 700 years old. Some archaeologists believe the rocks were placed to provide a link with the heavens, because one of the cairns on the wheel's outer edge aligns perfectly with the point of sunrise at the summer solstice, and some of the other cairns align with the risings of major stars. The Medicine Wheel is considered to be a place for spiritual renewal.

22 *The Canyon de Chelly* in the northeast corner of Arizona is the tradtional home of the Navajo Indians. This is no new area for pilgrims: It is believed that this red-rock canyon has been visited by people seeking spiritual guidance and energy since 300 CE, when the Anasazi people were in the region. Even today, the canyon maintains its reputation as a place with tremendous healing powers.

23 In Colorado, the *Great Pagosa Hot Spring* may have been discovered by white explorers in 1859, but the Utes and other Indian tribes had been using the waters for countless years because of their healing powers. The natives said that bathing in the hot spring brought relief from rheumatism and other joint and health problems, and people today still go to Pagosa Springs for those reasons. Many claim that drinking the water brings the same results.

24 *Mount Fuji* in Japan has been revered since ancient times as a sacred peak. Known to the Japanese as Fuji-san, the mountain has ties to the Shinto religion; however, people of all faiths and nationalities visit the area, and about 300,000 people climb the mountain every year. The climb can take from 5 to 9 hours, and the goal is to experience goraiko, the sunrise, which reportedly is an extraordinary spiritual experience—if the weather is right.

25 *The Grotto of Massabielle at Lourdes* in France is perhaps one of the best-known healing sites in the world. More than 6,000 claims of miracles and healings associated with the shrine have been made, but only about 66 have been verified. The grotto is the site of the Virgin Mary's appearances to Bernadette Soubirous at the age of 14, between February 11 and July 16, 1858. The Virgin appeared to Bernadette 18 times, and crowds of people assembled even then. Ever since that time, millions of people have flocked to the site. The town of Lourdes itself has about 15,300 inhabitants, but more than 5 million people from 150 countries, many of them ill or handicapped, visit the Grotto every year.

26 On the island of Bali in Indonesia, you will find the sacred waters of *Air Panas*. This holy spring is an important pilgrimage site for Bali's Hindus, and for people of other faiths as well. The spring is reported to be sacred because the Batukau, the great spirit and god, lives there. Visitors swim in the water to experience its healing effects.

27 Another sacred healing site in Indonesia is *Dieng Plateau*. This lush highland in central Java was a place of pilgrimage from the eighth to the twelfth centuries, and is still visited by pilgrims. There are several small Hindu temples scattered around the area, which offers a little bit of something for everyone: a meadow, a forest, a plateau, hot springs, babbling brooks, and small ponds. Lake Warna, a volcanic pool on the plateau, is said to change color to reflect the mood of those who sit on its banks to meditate.

28 *The Ganges River* is India's most sacred waterway. Its name comes from the Hindu goddess of purification, Ganga, and it is said that those who bathe in the river will be healed of their disease, relieved of their fatigue, and lifted to spiritual tranquility. However, although the living flock to the river for life-giving purposes, the greatest purpose of the river is to transport the souls of the dead. That's why approximately 35,000 bodies are cremated near the river each year and the ashes sprinkled on the water.

29 *Angel Falls*, the world's tallest waterfall, drops 3,212 feet from the Auyantepuy Mountain in the Canaima wilderness of Venezuela. Outsiders didn't know of the existence of the falls until 1935, when

Jimmy Angel, an American bush pilot, discovered them while he was searching for gold. The spirits of the Inca gods are said to resonate from the cliffs, and some visitors say they have heard sounds of a city near the falls.

30 *The ancient ruins of Sarnath* in India lie in the city where the Buddha delivered his first sermon after he had attained Enlightenment. The Mulgandh-Kuti Vihar, a temple erected on the spot, contains relics of the Buddha. The temple and the surrounding area are of great importance to Buddhists and to anyone seeking enlightenment.

31 *The Mount of Olives* on the outskirts of the Old City of Jerusalem in Israel is where Christ is said to have spent some of his last hours on earth and to have wept over Jerusalem before he went to the city on Palm Sunday. It is regarded as a place of meditation and reflection.

32 To the native people of New Zealand, the Maoris, *Mount Tongariro* is tapu, or "sacred." Spirits and fairies reportedly live in the fog and mist near the mountain's peak, while evil spirits are said to live at the summit, where they send rain fire upon the landscape. A native tribe has buried its nobility in the mountainside and claim that the mountain itself is one of their ancestors.

33 A mountain range sacred to both Hindus and Buddhists is *the Himalayas*, which means "abode of the gods" in Sanskrit. This mystical range in Nepal is said to hide Mount Meru, a peak that the Hindus and Buddhists say was at the center of the earth and was populated by the gods.

chapter thirty-four

Hospitals: Some of the Best in Their Fields

We know that going to the hospital can be scary for children. You know the drill: "How long will I be in the hospital?" "Will I have to take medicine?" "Is it going to hurt?" "What kind of food will I get?"

Going to the hospital can be scary for adults too, and we have some of the same questions children do, but with one addition: "Am I going to a hospital that has a great track record for the procedure I need?"

Virtually all hospitals can handle routine problems, such as fractures, gallbladder removal, and tonsillectomies. But if you have a critical health problem, such as cancer or another potentially life-threatening disease, or if you need a transplant, chances are you're much more concerned about the reputation of the hospital and the quality of care than you are about the hospital food.

Studies show that when it comes to surgical procedures, "practice makes perfect"—or at least it makes for much better results. Hospitals that do a high volume of certain procedures, such as heart transplants, pancreatic surgery, coronary artery bypass surgery, treatment of HIV/AIDS, and surgery for esophageal cancer, have better survival rates than hospitals that treat a lower number of these same types of cases.

Where should you go if you need treatment for a serious health problem? An analysis conducted by the National Opinion Research Center at the University of Chicago may help you make that decision if the time should come. The Center evaluated 6,247 hospitals in 18 categories using various criteria, including mortality rates, quality of nursing care, and available technology. Of the more than 6,000 hospitals, 173 made the grade. The top 5 hospitals in each of the 18 categories are listed here. If you want to see the complete list, go to www.usnews.com/usnews/nycu/health/hosptl/tophosp.htm.

If you don't see one of your local hospitals on the list, don't panic. It does not mean your hospital provides poor service; it just means it has not been rated as one of the very best. If you want to see how specific hospitals in your area rate, you can check out a service called Health Grades, available at www.healthgrades.com.

Best Hospitals Overall

Johns Hopkins Hospital, Baltimore, MD

Mayo Clinic, Rochester, MN

Massachusetts General Hospital, Boston, MA

Cleveland Clinic, Cleveland, OH

University of California Los Angeles Medical Center, Los Angeles, CA

Best for Cancer

Memorial Sloan-Kettering Cancer Center, New York, NY

University of Texas, MD Anderson Cancer Center, Houston, TX

Johns Hopkins Hospital, Baltimore, MD

Dana-Farber Cancer Institute, Boston, MA

Mayo Clinic, Rochester, MN

Best for Ear, Nose, Throat

Johns Hopkins Hospital, Baltimore, MD

University of Iowa Hospital & Clinics, Iowa City, IA

Massachusetts Eye & Ear Infirmary, Boston, MA

Mayo Clinic, Rochester, MN

University of Michigan Medical Center, Ann Arbor, MI

Best for Digestive Disorders

Mayo Clinic, Rochester, MN

Johns Hopkins Hospital, Baltimore, MD

Cleveland Clinic, Cleveland, OH

Massachusetts General Hospital, Boston, MA

Mount Sinai Medical Center, New York, NY

Best for Eyes (by reputation only)

Johns Hopkins Hospital, Baltimore, MD

University of Miami Bascom Palmer Eye Institute, Miami, FL

Wills Eye Hospital, Philadelphia, PA

Massachusetts Eye & Ear Infirmary, Boston, MA

University of California Los Angeles Medical Center, Jules Stein Eye Institute, Los Angeles, CA

Best for Geriatrics

University of California Los Angeles Medical Center, Los Angeles, CA

Johns Hopkins Hospital, Baltimore, MD

Mount Sinai Medical Center, New York, NY

Duke University Medical Center, Durham, NC

Massachusetts General Hospital, Boston, MA

Best for Gynecology

Johns Hopkins Hospital, Baltimore, MD

Mayo Clinic, Rochester, MN

Brigham & Women's Hospital, Boston, MD

University of California Los Angeles Medical Center, Los Angeles, CA

University of Texas, M.D. Anderson Cancer Center, Houston, TX

Best for Heart

Cleveland Clinic, Cleveland, OH

Mayo Clinic, Rochester, MN

Massachusetts General Hospital, Boston, MA

Johns Hopkins Hospital, Baltimore, MD

Brigham and Women's Hospital, Boston, MA

Best for Hormonal Disorders

Mayo Clinic, Rochester, MN

Massachusetts General Hospital, Boston, MA

Johns Hopkins Hospital, Baltimore, MD

Brigham & Women's Hospital, Boston, MA

Beth Israel Deaconess Medical Center, Boston, MA

Best for Kidney Disease

Massachusetts General Hospital, Boston, MA

Brigham & Women's Hospital, Boston, MA

Mayo Clinic, Rochester, MN

Cleveland Clinic, Cleveland, OH

New York Presbyterian Hospital, New York, NY

Best for Neurology

Mayo Clinic, Rochester, MN

Massachusetts General Hospital, Boston, MA

Johns Hopkins Hospital, Baltimore, MD

New York Presbyterian Hospital, New York, NY

University of California San Francisco Medical Center, San Francisco, CA

Best for Orthopedics

Mayo Clinic, Rochester, MN

Hospital for Special Surgery, New York, NY

Massachusetts General Hospital, Boston, MA

Johns Hopkins Hospital, Baltimore, MD

Cleveland Clinic, Cleveland, OH

Best for Pediatrics (by reputation only)

Children's Hospital, Boston, MA

Children's Hospital of Philadelphia, Philadelphia, PA

Johns Hopkins Hospital, Baltimore, MD

Children's Hospital, Pittsburgh, PA

Children's Hospital, Denver, CO

Best for Psychiatry (by reputation only)

Massachusetts General Hospital, Boston, MA

New York Presbyterian, New York, NY

CF Menninger Memorial Hospital, Topeka, KS

McLean Hospital, Belmont, MA

Johns Hopkins Hospital, Baltimore, MD

Best for Respiratory Disorders

National Jewish Center, Denver, CO

Mayo Clinic, Rochester, MN

Johns Hopkins Hospital, Baltimore, MD

Barnes-Jewish Hospital, St. Louis, MO

University Hospital, Denver, CO

Best for Rehabilitation (by reputation only)

Rehabilitation Institute of Chicago, Chicago, IL

The Institute for Rehabilitation and Research, Houston, TX

University of Washington Medical Center, Seattle, WA

Kessler Institute for Rehabilitation, West Orange, NJ

Mayo Clinic, Rochester, MN

Best for Rheumatism

Mayo Clinic, Rochester, MN

Johns Hopkins Hospital, Baltimore, MD

Hospital for Special Surgery, New York, NY

Brigham & Women's Hospital, Boston, MA

Cleveland Clinic, Cleveland, OH

Best for Urology

Johns Hopkins Hospital, Baltimore, MD

Cleveland Clinic, Cleveland, OH

Mayo Clinic, Rochester, MN

University of California Los Angeles Medical Center, Los Angeles, CA

New York Presbyterian Hospital, New York, NY

chapter thirty-five

Dentistry: How to Choose a Dentist and Dental Care

Your smile is like a handshake: It makes people feel welcome and tells a lot about you without your having to say a word. Naturally, you want it to be the best it can be. That's one of the reasons Americans handed over more than $54 billion for dental care in 1998. And it's a good reason to take special care when you choose the dentist who will help brighten and shape that smile.

Types of Dentists

Dental school lasts for four years, after which graduates can take their national and state board examinations and become general dental practitioners, the most common type of dentist. These professionals fill cavities, clean teeth, extract teeth, and replace damaged or lost teeth. Most also do simple root canal work, but refer difficult cases out to specialists. The initials D.D.S. (Doctor of Dental Surgery) or D.M.D. (Doctor of Dental Medicine) appear after the name of a general practitioner. According to the American Dental Association (ADA), these two titles are interchangeable and reflect exactly the same education and training.

Dentists who want to specialize in one of the eight categories recognized by the ADA can take two or more years of advanced training. To become board certified in one of the categories, a candidate must pass an examination given by a specialty board sanctioned by the ADA. Those eight recognized dental specialties are:

- **Endodontics:** The prevention and control of diseases that affect the root pulp and associated structures. These specialists do root canal therapy.
- **Oral and maxillofacial pathology:** The diagnosis of tumors and other dental diseases, and treatment of injuries of the head and neck.
- **Oral and maxillofacial surgery:** Tooth extractions, including wisdom teeth, that are too difficult for a general dentist to perform, as well as removal of cysts and tumors and surgical treatment of injuries, diseases, and defects of the jaw, mouth, and face.
- **Orthodontics and dentofacial orthopedics:** The diagnosis and treatment of tooth abnormalities and facial deformities, and the use of braces.
- **Pediatric dentistry:** Dental diagnosis and treatment of infants and children.
- **Periodontics:** The care of the gums and supporting tissues.
- **Prosthodontics:** Treatment of oral abnormalities through the use of prosthetic devices such as bridges, dentures, and crowns.
- **Public health (dental):** Prevention and control of dental disease and the promotion of community dental health.

Some dentists who have not completed ADA-sanctioned training in these areas still call themselves specialists. Many of them have indeed performed a lot of work in their specialty area and are very competent. However, some practice unscientific or unorthodox dentistry. They may have a diploma with an impressive-sounding name from a diploma mill or an unaccredited correspondence school. Always check the credentials of any dentist before you make your first visit. (See "How to Find a Dentist.")

Do You Want a Holistic Dentist?

The subject of holistic dentistry is controversial among those in the dental community. Marvin J. Schissel, D.D.S. and John E. Dodes, D.D.S., authors of *Healthy Teeth: A User's Manual*, reflect the opinion of many dentists when they say that holistic dentists "seem to be more interested in medical than dental procedures, and health claims made by holistic dentists seem clearly beyond the boundaries or competence of dental practice."

Dentists who consider themselves to be holistic or biologic, however, disagree.

Holistic dentists:

- Don't use toxic substances when treating patients, such as mercury in fillings or nickel in crowns.

- Only perform surgery as a last resort.

- Recognize the intimate connection between the teeth and the rest of the body. It's been shown, for example, that bacteria in the mouth can contribute to stomach ulcers and adversely affect the heart.

- Generally check for misalignment of teeth, muscles, and jaw, especially the temporomandibular joint (TMJ).

- Usually recommend natural products for dental cleaning and treatment, such as mixing baking soda and peroxide for teeth cleaning. Fluoride is generally avoided because they believe it is a toxic substance.

The primary difference between conventional and holistic dentists, however, is in the use of silver–mercury amalgams, or fillings. Holistic dentists believe that the toxins in amalgam fillings—primarily the mercury, which is known to be highly poisonous—gradually leak into the body and can cause cancer, multiple sclerosis, insomnia, chronic headache, and other ailments. Conventional dentists believe amalgams are safe.

The field of holistic dentistry is constantly evolving, and questions continue to arise about the toxicity of different materials used in dentistry. To keep up with the latest news and findings on both sides of the issue, consumers are encouraged to visit the following Web sites:

- Dental Amalgam Mercury Syndrome Support Group: www.icnr.com/uam/DAMSIntro.html

- The Holistic Dental Association: www.holisticdental.org

- International Academy of Oral Medicine and Toxicology: www.sukel.com/iaomt.htm

- International Association for Dental Research: www.iadr.com/

- The Mercury Page: http://vest.gu.se/~bosse/Mercury/default.html

- National Institutes of Health Technology Assessment: Dental Restoratives: http://text.nlm.nih.gov/nih/ta/www/09.html

How to Find a Dentist

The procedure for finding a dentist is much like that for finding a physician. Here are some guidelines:

- Call your local or statewide dental referral service (look in the yellow pages under "Dentist Referral").
- Call, write, or check out the Web site for the American Dental Association (www.ada.org).
- Ask friends, family, coworkers, and neighbors to recommend a dentist. Then check out the dentist's credentials with the American Dental Association or a dental referral service.
- Question faculty members of any dental schools in your area. Check credentials.
- Ask your family doctor or pharmacist to recommend someone. Check credentials.
- Call a local hospital that has an accredited dental service. Check credentials.
- Do you want a holistic dentist? Contact the Holistic Dental Association (www.holsticdental.org).

How to Rate your Dentist

You've chosen a dentist and had your first appointment and perhaps a treatment. Did you get quality care? Here are some things to consider when you rate your dentist.

- During the full examination, did the dentist inspect your teeth, gums, tongue, lips, inside of the cheek, palate, and the skin of your neck and face, as well as feel the neck for abnormal swelling?
- Does your dentist have a full mouth study (x-rays) of your mouth? (Did you have them transferred from your other dentist or have a new set taken?)
- Is any of the dental work irritating your gums or cheeks?
- Does the treated tooth look like a tooth?
- Did the dentist take the time to polish your fillings?
- Is your bite okay?

- Do you feel any pain when you drink cold or hot liquids?

- Does your tongue catch on the treated tooth?

- Were the office and treatment areas clean and orderly?

- Did the dentist and assistants always wear gloves and masks?

- Were the instruments sterile? There are several ways to ensure sterile instruments: Use of disposable instruments, or use of autoclaves (pressurized steam), chemical vapor sterilizers (a mixture of chemicals and water), or dry heat sterilizers (use of high temperatures). Although some experts say disposable instruments are preferred, all three methods of sterilizing instruments are perfectly safe when used correctly.

- Does the dentist use a "dental dam" for fillings and root canals? A dental dam is a square piece of rubber sheeting that allows the treated tooth to be exposed while preventing loose particles from falling into the throat or preventing contamination of the pulp chamber when doing a root canal. Because it can take a few minutes to position a dam, some dentists don't use them. They should be used during a root canal, and you can request that they be used for fillings.

- Did the dentist and assistants seem genuinely concerned about your needs and concerns? Because many people associate going to the dentist with pain and fear, a caring attitude is important.

- Did the dentist take the time to answer your questions? Were the answers presented in a clear and understandable manner?

- Does the dentist have a convenient location and office hours?

- How does the dentist handle emergencies? Is there a colleague or a referral source to help when the dentist is unavailable?

- How is payment handled? Does the dentist honor your insurance coverage?

Facts about the ADA Seal of Acceptance

We see it on toothpaste packaging, mouthwash bottles, and electric toothbrushes—the ADA Seal of Acceptance. What does it mean? Here's what's behind that seal.

- The purpose of the Seal of Acceptance is to help the public and dental professionals make informed decisions about safe and effective dental products.

The ADA will answer questions about the Seal and the products that bear it. See the ADA Web site: www.ada.org.

- The first statement on the safety and effectiveness of a dental product was prepared by the ADA in 1866. The product was toothpaste.

- The ADA established strict guidelines for testing and advertising dental products by 1930, and the first Seal of Acceptance was awarded in 1931.

- The Seal of Acceptance program is voluntary, but about 350 companies participate.

- Companies that participate in the program dedicate resources to evaluate, test, and market products in the program.

- About 1,300 dental products display the Seal of Acceptance. The majority, about 70 percent, are products prescribed or used by dentists, such as drugs and tooth restorative materials. The remaining 30 percent are consumer products such as toothpaste, mouthwash, manual and electric toothbrushes, and dental floss.

- For a product to qualify for the Seal, manufacturers must conduct clinical trials that follow strict ADA guidelines, provide evidence and data on the product according to ADA standards, and submit all advertising and patient education materials for review and approval by the ADA.

- An ADA Seal is granted for three years only; after that a manufacturer must reapply.

- Any time a product's ingredients change, the manufacturer must resubmit the product for review and approval before it is given the Seal.

chapter thirty-six

How to Choose a Health Care Provider

When it came time for Cheryl to replace her old car, she didn't simply drop into the nearest dealership and let a salesperson talk her into buying the most expensive sedan on the floor. She did her homework. Several models interested her, so she scoured the Internet for reports about their performance, reliability, estimated repair costs over a lifetime, and safety. Using this information, she narrowed her choice down to two cars, then asked recent buyers of each model about their level of satisfaction with their purchases. Finally, she made a list of options she wanted and started to do comparative price shopping, over the Internet and in her hometown. Why did she go to so much trouble? "Because I need a dependable car for work," she said. "I don't want to buy a lemon."

How much more important are our bodies than the cars we own, yet how many of us take even half that much time when we look for a physician? When we choose a health care provider, we are entrusting our wellness to that individual. Yet many people choose doctors or other practitioners randomly out of the telephone book, or based on their convenience to home or work. Although location is a consideration, there are many more factors to think about when selecting a health care provider for yourself or your family.

The list of different possible health care providers today is much longer than it was even 30 years ago. Not only are there dozens of specialists within conventional medicine (see Chapter 27), but there are also many types of alternative practitioners. Some of the criteria to consider when choosing a provider from either category are the same, but there are some clear differences, too.

The guidelines presented here can help you when selecting your next health care practitioner, whether that individual is an Eastern medicine doctor, a cardiologist, a massage therapist, or an osteopath.

How to Choose a Physician

Here are some general questions and issues to consider when choosing a personal physician or a family doctor.

- Where did this doctor attend medical school?
- When and where did the doctor do residency?
- Did the doctor pursue any training beyond that?
- Is this doctor board certified?
- How many years has this doctor been practicing?
- If you are interested in a particular procedure or treatment, how many times has this doctor done the procedure or treatment?
- If a doctor's sex, religious affiliation, age, or other personal information is important to you, check this out through the doctor's office or through one of the organizations listed under "How to Do a Doctor Checkup."
- With which hospital is this doctor associated?
- What hospital emergency department does he or she recommend?
- Does this doctor practice alone or in a group? If this particular doctor is not available, will one of the other doctors in the group see you?
- Does this doctor respond to calls on the weekends or at night?
- What are the office hours?
- What is this doctor's patient population? Does he or she typically treat more women than men, older or younger patients?
- What health insurance does this doctor accept?
- Will the doctor treat other members of your family?
- Does this doctor have lab or x-ray facilities in the office?
- Are the offices conveniently located?

- Does this doctor continue to see patients who are hospitalized or moved to a nursing facility?

- Ask friends, family members, and coworkers for recommendations.

- Get physician referrals from other health care professionals you trust.

- Contact organizations that offer physician referrals; see Chapter 70 for examples.

- Compare costs between physicians.

- Check up on whether there have been any disciplinary actions against your candidates (see "How to Do a Doctor Checkup").

How to Do a Doctor Checkup

If you want to check up on your doctor's training and credentials, there are several avenues you can take.

- You can begin with the most obvious places first for basic information on training and credentials: the doctor's office, the hospital where he or she is on staff, or the HMO to which the doctor belongs. None of them, however, are likely to tell you about any disciplinary actions.

- You can find out whether a doctor is truly certified in a specific field by contacting the American Board of Medical Specialties Certified Doctor Verification Service, available at www.abms.org/newsearch.asp. This is a free service. Disciplinary information is not available.

- You can check the training and certification status of more than 650,000 medical and osteopathic physicians licensed in the United States at the American Medical Association's Physician Select, at www.ama-assn.org/aps/amahg.htm Once again, the service is free, but there is no disciplinary information.

- The most comprehensive source of information, including any concerning disciplinary action, is Medi-Net (www.askmedi.com/), which has access to information on more than 900,000 physicians licensed in the United States. Medi-Net also has data on doctors who have been convicted of Medicaid or Medicare fraud and have had any actions taken against them by state disciplinary boards. There is a fee for this service ($14.75).

• The state medical boards of each state (except Alaska, Arkansas, Delaware, Hawaii, Louisiana, Montana, New Mexico, North Dakota, South Dakota, and Wyoming) list the names of disciplined doctors on their Web pages. Rather than look for your specific state's medical board, you can access the Public Citizen Research Group's Web site, which has links to the states' sites: www.citizen.org/hrg/publications/1506.htm.

How to Choose an Alternative Practitioner

Choosing an alternative practitioner is a little different from selecting a conventional medical doctor. We've provided two examples—Eastern medicine and naturopathy—to show you how to go about it. However, you can still use many of the guidelines for choosing a physician to help you make your selection. After all, what you want in any case are competent, understanding, accessible professionals who do what they are trained to do with your best interests in mind.

• Check out the practice requirements in your state. If you live in a state that requires a license for a particular alternative profession, it seems best to select a practitioner who has a license.

• Similar to conventional medicine, some alternative practices have national certification processes. Acupuncture, chiropractic, massage, and osteopathy have such certification; Ayurvedic doctors, herbalists, homeopaths, and yoga instructors do not. If there is a national certification for the practice you want, your practitioner should have it.

• Get referrals from a trusted physician or another alternative practitioner, or from a college or training facility. An acupuncture school, for example, should be able to recommend practitioners in your area. Get referrals from several different places; people who appear on more than one list should be winners.

• If there is an alternative medicine college or training facility in your area, it may have a clinic where you can get care or referrals. (See Chapter 37.)

• You can also get recommendations from professional associations, state licensing associations, and illness-specific groups. (See Chapter 70.)

• Ask questions of the practitioner before you start treatment. Any practitioner who makes extraordinary claims ("miracle cures"), requests payment up front for long-term treatments, refuses to discuss treatment costs, or won't take the time to answer a reasonable number of basic questions or refer you to another staff member who will answer your questions is likely not an individual you want handling your health care.

CHOOSING AN ACUPUNCTURIST OR CHINESE HERBOLOGIST

• Every state handles the licensing of acupuncturists and doctors of Eastern medicine in a different way. At least 33 jurisdictions have passed acts that require acupuncturists to be fully trained to practice. You need to check with the licensing entity in your state to find out your state's requirements. Depending on the licensing procedure in your state, you will need to contact either the state board of acupuncture, the department of health, licensing, or education, or the board of medical examiners.

• The licenses granted by states also differ. A practitioner can go by the title of Licensed Acupuncturist (L.Ac or Lic.Ac), Registered Acupuncturist (R.Ac), Certified Acupuncturist (C.A.), Doctor of Acupuncture (D.Ac), or Doctor of Oriental Medicine (DOM). An individual with any of these titles has met the requirements of his or her state to practice acupuncture and, again depending on the state, Chinese herbology, *tui na* (a type of massage), and other Eastern medicine practices.

• If you live in a state or jurisdiction that has regulations for Eastern medicine practitioners, look for a licensed individual.

• If you live in an unregulated area, it is best to look for a practitioner who has been board certified by the National Certification Commission for Acupuncture and Oriental Medicine (NCCAOM).

• For additional help, contact the Acupuncture Alliance or the NCCAOM for assistance in locating a professional in your area.

CHOOSING A NATUROPATH

• There are currently only five schools in North America licensed to train individuals for a Doctor of Naturopathy degree, which requires three years of standard premedical education followed by four years of naturopathic medicine training in acupuncture, botanical medicine, counseling, homeopathic medicine, clinical nutrition, and psychology. They are: National College of Naturopathic Medicine (Portland, OR); Bastyr University (Seattle, WA); Southwest College of Naturopathic Medicine (Tempe, AZ); Canadian College of Naturopathic Medicine (Toronto); and University of Bridgeport College of Naturopathic Medicine (Bridgeport, CT).

• If the naturopath you're considering has a degree from another facility, go to another naturopath. Some people who pass themselves off as naturopaths earned their degree through a correspondence course or workshops. A naturopath who is reluctant to show you any credentials is probably hiding something.

• Naturopathic medicine is not regulated in most states, which means some people call themselves "naturopaths" but do not meet the standards of the profession. As of July 1999, the states that licensed naturopaths were Alaska, Arizona, Connecticut, Florida, Hawaii, Maine, Montana, New Hampshire, Oregon, Utah, Vermont, and Washington. Puerto Rico also has a licensing law.

• If you live in a state that does not regulate naturopaths, ask for the credentials of the doctor you wish to see. Unlicensed states do not verify the education or qualifications of anyone who claims to be a naturopath, so you cannot expect the state to help you.

• Some naturopaths specialize in one or two areas, such as nutrition or herbal medicine. If you have a specific problem, say, nutritional concerns, you might look for a naturopath who focuses in this area.

• Be aware of the limitations of naturopaths: 1) They rarely have hospital privileges, but usually can make referrals for patients who need such care; 2) not all states grant naturopaths prescription privileges, so check your state's guidelines; and 3) naturopaths do not handle trauma, such as broken bones, burns, heart attacks, and serious wounds.

Rating Your Health Care Provider

These guidelines can apply to any health care practitioner and can be used to assess your practitioner after your first visit. That's when they should be on their best behavior.

• Did your appointment start on time?

- Does the practitioner appear to practice an unhealthy lifestyle? For example, was he or she smoking, overweight, depressed, or stressed?

- Were the office personnel friendly and helpful?

- Is the office environment pleasant?

- Did the practitioner seem rushed or impatient?

- Did the practitioner prescribe medications or treatments that you do not understand or that you believe are unnecessary?

- Did you feel pressured at any time during your visit to make decisions or to answer questions you were not comfortable with?

- Did the practitioner seem genuinely interested in you as a person?

- Is the practitioner open to the use of other therapies? (If a conventional doctor, is he or she open to alternative approaches? If an alternative provider, has a good relationship with conventional practitioners?)

- Overall, how did the visit make you feel? Confident? Relaxed? Reassured? Confused? Trust your instincts.

"HEY, DOC . . . LET'S TALK"

Some people feel intimidated by their doctors or are afraid they are "bothering" a health care provider if they ask questions. Nonsense. You should be able to communicate your concerns and needs to your health care practitioners, and they should listen and respond in a professional manner. If a practitioner won't take time to address your concerns or belittles you for having them, it's time to find another provider. Here are some ways to communicate better with health care practitioners.

- If you have had problems in the past communicating with your doctor, schedule an appointment to discuss your concerns. It is usually best to give your current practitioner another chance before you decide to switch to another doctor.

- When you do have an opportunity to talk with a practitioner, be prepared. Have a written list of questions or concerns. Many patients now have access to much more medical information than they did in the past, especially from the Internet. If you find research or information about your condition that you do not understand, ask questions.

- Communication is a two-way street. You may perceive resistance or reluctance from a practitioner to talk about certain issues, such as sexual problems or emotional issues; however, you will not know for certain until you ask. If the practitioner is not comfortable talking about your concerns, then you have reason to switch doctors.

- Don't feel obligated to keep going to a certain health care provider just because you don't want to hurt his or her feelings. You have the right to take your business elsewhere. Professionals will not take it personally—you are not responsible if they do.

chapter thirty-seven

Alternative and
Complementary Medicine:
41 Clinics to Serve You

W e often use words like "alternative," "complementary," and "unconventional" with regard to some types of health care, but the fact is, many of these modalities have become more mainstream than conventional medicine—at least if you go by the numbers. A Harvard University study in 1997 found that 40 percent of Americans had tried alternative medicine, compared with 33 percent in 1993. In fact, according to Dr. David M. Eisenberg, Director for Alternative Medicine Research and Education at Harvard/Beth Israel Deaconess Medical Center, in 1997 patients in the United States visited complementary providers nearly 200 million more times than they visited primary care physicians.

As Interest Grows, So Do Clinics

This rapid growth in public interest is spurring universities and hospitals to set up programs to study alternative and complementary medicine. In some cases, they're also establishing clinics where patients can receive alternative as well as conventional care. "Patients do not want only complementary care or only conventional care, but want a judicious evidence-based integration of the best of both," says Dr. Eisenberg.

To meet the demand, more and more medical schools are offering courses in complementary medicine. Reportedly, about 50 percent of schools now include at least a few such courses in their roster, and according to Martin Sullivan, M.D., director of the Duke Center for Integrative Medicine in Durham, North Carolina, five years from now it will be common for medical schools to have complete integrative medicine programs.

Integrative or Complementary Medicine Clinics, by State

The list of clinics given here is not exhaustive. In this rapidly changing area of medicine, new programs are evolving and becoming available all the time. Check the yellow pages in your area, and call local hospitals, medical schools, and other medical teaching facilities to ask if they have an integrative or complementary clinic open to the public.

Many of the complementary medicine clinics listed here offer a wide range of services. Most are associated with a teaching facility, so the services may be provided by student interns, under the supervision of licensed professionals.

If you visit a teaching clinic for health care, your provider may show up along with several students. Although some people are not comfortable with this arrangement, most find that teaching situations are handled very professionally and don't interfere with good care. And remember: Teaching clinics generally offer lower rates, or charge fees based on a sliding scale.

Arizona

1 Department of Integrative Medicine, Arizona Health Science Center, University of Arizona, P. O. Box 245099, Tucson, AZ 85724. Call 520-694-6555 or 520-626-7222.

A maximum of 12 new patients are seen each week. There is a waiting list of more than 1,000. Patient preference has been for Tucson residents. To get on the list, write to: Department of Integrative Medicine, University of Arizona, Attn: Wait List, P.O. Box 245153, Tucson, AZ 85724-5153.

2 Desert Institute of the Healing Arts, 639 N. Sixth Avenue, Tucson, AZ 85705. Call 800-733-8098.

A teaching clinic. Offers massage and Zen shiatsu.

California

3 Academy of Chinese Culture and Health Services, 1601 Clay Street, Oakland, CA 94612. Call 510-763-1299.

A teaching clinic. Offers acupuncture, acupressure, herbal medicine.

4 American College of Traditional Chinese Medicine, 455 Arkansas Street, San Francisco, CA 94107. Call 415-282-7600.

The college sponsors clinics in three neighborhoods: Potrero Hill, Fillmore, and Van Ness. Call for information. Offers acupuncture, tui na, herbal medicine, nutritional counseling.

5 California College of Ayurveda Healthcare Clinic, 1117A East Main Street, Grass Valley, CA 95945. Call 530-274-9100.

The Healthcare Clinic offers diet, herbs, sound therapy, aromatherapy, yoga, massage, meditation, Pancha Karma (a special herbal detoxification program), and lifestyle counseling.

6 China International Medical University (2 clinics), 822 S. Robertson Boulevard, Suite 300, Los Angeles, CA 90035. Call 310-289-8394.

One teaching clinic, one professional clinic. Offers acupuncture, herbal medicine, nutritional counseling.

7 The Chopra Center for Well Being, 7630 Fay Avenue, La Jolla, CA 92037. Call 888-424 6772 or 619-551 7788.

The center has a mind–body medical group that offers Ayurvedic consultations, diet counseling, stress management, exercise, emotional healing, nutritional supplements, herbal medicine; also massage services, herbal steams, and a Return to Wholeness Cancer Program.

8 Emperor's College Clinic, 1870B Wilshire Boulevard, Santa Monica, CA 90403. Call 310-453-8300.

A teaching clinic. Offers acupuncture, herbal medicine, massage.

9 Five Branches Institute of Traditional Chinese Medicine Clinic, 200 7th Avenue, Santa Cruz, CA 95062. Call 831-476-9424.

A teaching clinic. Offers acupuncture and other services. Have staff that specialize in neurology, internal medicine, gynecology, pediatrics, oncology, dermatology, rheumatology, and cardiology.

10 Meiji College of Oriental Medicine, Meiji College Clinic, 2550 Shattuck Avenue, Berkeley, CA 94704. Call 510-666-8234.

A teaching clinic. Acupuncture, electroacupuncture, herbal medicine.

11 UCSF Stanford Health Care Complementary Medicine Clinic, 1101 Welch Road, Palo Alto, CA. Call 650-498-5566.

Offers biofeedback, hypnosis, acupuncture, therapeutic massage, meditation, and yoga.

12 Pacific College of Oriental Medicine has three clinic locations:

7445 Mission Valley Road, San Diego, CA 92108. Call 619-574-6932.

915 Broadway, 3rd Floor, New York, NY 10010. Call 212-982-4600.

3646 N. Broadway, 2nd Floor, Chicago, IL 60613. Call 888-729-4811.

Offers acupuncture, moxibustion, tui na, qi gong, and herbal medicine.

13 Samra University of Oriental Medicine, 3000 S. Robertson Boulevard, 4th Floor, Los Angeles, CA 90034. Call 310-202-7555.

Usually open 7 days a week, offering acupuncture, herbal medicine, and other traditional Chinese medicine treatments.

14 Santa Barbara College of Oriental Medicine, 1919 State Street, Suite 207, Santa Barbara, CA 93101. Call 800-549-6299.

A teaching clinic. The Santa Barbara College of Oriental Medicine Clinic operates several community health care projects, including ones for HIV/AIDS, chronic pain, and hepatitis C. Plans are to expand to include drug detoxification and addiction care. Offers acupuncture, herbal medicine, and other services.

15 South Baylo University's Acupuncture and Herbal Medicine Center, 1126 North Brookhurst Street, Anaheim, CA 92801. Call 714-535-3886. Also, 2727 West 6th Street, Los Angeles, CA 90057. Call 213-738-1974.

Teaching clinics. Offer acupuncture, acupressure, herbal medicine, cupping, moxibustion, electroacupuncture, tui na, massage, nutritional counseling.

16 Yo San University Clinic, 13315 Washington Boulevard, Los Angeles, CA 90066. Call 310-577-3006.

A teaching clinic. Services include acupuncture, cupping, moxibustion, and herbal medicine.

Florida

17 Academy of Chinese Healing Arts, 513 S. Orange Avenue, Sarasota, FL 34236. Call 800-883-5528.

Both student and professional clinics. Call for information.

18 Florida Institute for Traditional Chinese Medicine, Community Health Medical Clinics. Two teaching clinics: 5335 66th Street N., St. Petersburg, FL 33709, call 727-541-2666; and 1802 E. Busch Boulevard, Tampa, FL 33612, call 813-932-2610.

Offer acupuncture, herbal medicine, tui na.

19 National College of Oriental Medicine, 710 Lake Ellenor Drive, Orlando Fl 32809. Call 407-888-8689.

A teaching clinic. Offers acupuncture, herbal medicine, nutritional counseling, tui na.

Illinois

20 Block Medical Center for Integrative Cancer Care, 1800 Sherman Avenue, Suite 515, Evanston, IL 60201. Call 847-492-3040.

Integrates conventional cancer treatments with alternative approaches such as vitamin infusions, bodywork therapies, mind–body stress management, and dietary assistance, as well as Total Approach to Cancer Recovery, a three-day program of small-group and individual sessions to empower people during their recovery.

Maryland

21 Maryland Institute of Traditional Chinese Medicine, 4641 Montgomery Avenue, Bethesda, MD 20814. Call 800-892-1209.

A teaching clinic. Offers acupuncture.

Massachusetts

22 The Mind/Body Medical Clinic and Institute, Division of Behavioral Medicine, Beth Israel Deaconess Medical Center, 110 Francis Street, Suite 1A, Boston, MA 02215. Call 617-632 9530.

Offers relaxation therapy, nutritional management, exercise therapy, cognitive and behavioral therapy.

Minnesota

23 Northwestern Health Sciences University in Minnesota is affiliated with all of the following teaching clinics:

Minnesota Institute of Acupuncture and Herbal Studies Teaching Clinic, 2501 W. 84th Street, Bloomington, MN 55431. Call 952-885-5450.

Provides acupuncture and Eastern medicine treatments.

24 The Natural Care Center at Woodwinds, Woodwinds Health Campus, 1875 Woodwinds Drive, Suite 100, Woodbury, MN 55125. Call 651-232-6830.

Offers acupuncture, chiropractic, massage therapy, Eastern medicine, naturopathy, and health and wellness assessments.

25 Bloomington Clinic, 2501 W. 84th Street, Bloomington, MN 55431. Call 952-885-5444.

Offers acupuncture, aquatics, maternal and child health care.

26 St. Paul Clinic, 621 S. Cleveland Avenue, St. Paul, MN 55116. Call 651-690-1788.

Offers acupuncture and chiropractic.

27 Eastside Natural Care Center, 1030 Payne Avenue, St. Paul, MN 55101. Call 651-776-2854.

Offers acupuncture and massage.

New Mexico

28 International Institute of Chinese Medicine. Two teaching clinic locations: 4600 Montgomery Boulevard, N.E. 1-1, Albuquerque, NM 87109, call 505-837-9778; and P.O. Box 29988, Santa Fe, NM 87592, call 505-438-7238

Offer acupuncture and herbal medicine.

29 Southwest Acupuncture College. There are three campuses and clinics:

2960 Rodeo Park Drive West, Santa Fe, NM 87505; call 505-438-8880.

4308 Carlisle N.E., Suite 205, Albuquerque, NM 87107. Call 505-888-8868.

6658 Gunpark Drive, Boulder, CO 80301; call 303-581-9955.

Provide acupuncture, herbal medicine, nutrition and patient education. Clinic days and hours vary each term.

New York

30 The Center for Holistic Urology, Columbia-Presbyterian Medical Center, Atchley Pavilion, 11th Floor, 161 Ft. Washington Avenue, New York, NY 10032. Call 212-305-0347.

Offers complementary treatment for men and women with disorders of the urinary tract. Nutritional therapy, acupuncture, herbal medicine, immunologic therapy, mind–body therapies, exercise therapy.

31 Memorial Sloan-Kettering Cancer Center, Integrative Medicine Service (3 separate clinics):

Integrative Medicine Outpatient Center, 303 E. 65th Street, New York, NY; call 212-639-4700.

Rockefeller Outpatient Pavilion, 160 E. 53rd Street, New York, NY; call 212-639-4700.

Memorial Hospital, 1275 York Avenue, New York, NY; call 212-639-8629.

The Outpatient Center offers massage, spiritual healing, art and music therapy, acupuncture, hypnotherapy, meditation, guided imagery and visualization, tai chi, nutritional counseling, yoga, and more. The Pavilion offers relaxation and massage. Memorial Hospital offers massage, relaxation, music therapy, and other services upon request. Services are available to cancer patients and their families and to the general public.

32 New York College for Wholistic Health Education and Research

Two health centers:

Wholistic Health Center at Syosset; 6801 Jericho Turnpike, Syosset, NY 11791; call 516-496-7766.

Wholistic Health Center at Stony Brook, 97 Main Street, Stony Brook, NY; call 631-941-3232.

Teaching clinics. Provide acupuncture, amma therapeutic massage, biofeedback, chiropractic, European massage therapy, herbal medicine, holistic nursing.

Oregon

33 National College of Naturopathic Medicine. Two main clinics:

11231 S.E. Market Street, Portland, OR 97216; call 503-255-7355.

4444 S.W. Corbett, Portland, OR 97201; call 503-224-8476.

The College also has 14 satellite clinics, each of which serves a special population, such as the homeless, mothers, children, the elderly, addicts, single mothers, students, and migrant workers.

34 Oregon College of Oriental Medicine Acupuncture and Herbal Clinic, 10541 S.E. Cherry Blossom Drive, East Portland, OR. Call 503-253-3443 for an appointment.

The clinic is a teaching facility and is affiliated with the Oregon College of Oriental Medicine.

Pennsylvania

35 Shadyside Center for Complementary Medicine, University of Pittsburgh Medical Center, 5230 Centre Avenue, Pittsburgh, PA 15232. Call 412-623 3023.

Offers acupuncture, reflexology, herbal medicine, massage.

Texas

36 American College of Traditional Chinese Medicine, 9100 Park West Drive, Houston, TX 77063. Call 713-780-9786.

A teaching clinic. Offers acupuncture, herbal medicine, tui na.

37 Dallas Institute of Acupuncture and Oriental Medicine Student Clinic, 2947 Walnut Hill Lane, Suite 101, Dallas, TX 75229. Call 214-351-6464.

A teaching clinic. Offers acupuncture, herbal medicine, nutritional counseling.

38 Texas College of Traditional Chinese Medicine, 4005 Manchaca Road, Suite 200, Austin, TX 78704. Call 800-252-5088 or 512-444-8082.

Traditional Chinese medicine approaches to the treatment of allergies, arthritis, weight control, nicotine withdrawal, back pain, TMJ, stress, premenstrual syndrome, and other conditions.

Washington

39 Bastyr Center for Natural Health, 1307 N. 45th Street, Seattle, WA. Call 206-834-4100.

Offers primary care from a naturopathic team or acupuncture and Eastern medicine team; also homeopathy, nutritional consulting, physical medicine, psychological counseling, hydrotherapy.

40 King County Natural Medicine Clinic, 403 E. Meeker Street, Suite 200, Kent, WA. Call 253-852-2866.

This clinic is managed by Bastyr University. King County offers acupuncture, naturopathy, nutritional counseling, chiropractic, and massage.

41 Northwest Institute of Acupuncture and Oriental Medicine, The Acupuncture Clinic, 701 N. 34th Street, Suite 300, Seattle, WA 98103. Call 206-633-5581.

A teaching clinic. Provides acupuncture, maternity care, trauma medicine, and women's health care.

chapter thirty-eight

The Healthiest Places to Live in the United States

Would you like to live in the healthiest city in the United States? Would you hide in shame if the city you live in was picked as the fattest city in America? Should you really make a life decision based on the results of a list published in a magazine? And just who makes up these lists, anyway?

How Do We Rate?

Consider the category "Healthiest Cities in the United States." If four different organizations were to create such a list, would all of their criteria be exactly the same? Most likely not. Some researchers include categories such as smoking and eating habits, some don't; some include crime, unemployment, divorce, and welfare figures; others don't. Every study not only uses different criteria but may also organize results differently. Some ratings list cities from best to worst; others separate them by region: best in the west, the south, and so on. As you can see, we're never comparing apples with apples when we look at any two lists that claim to have the "best" of anything.

In January 2000, *Self* magazine published the results of its study of the healthiest places for women to live in the United States. The study lists Nassau and Suffolk counties in New York among the healthiest places for women to live—number 2, in fact, right below Provo, Utah. Why? Because statistics show that women in those New York counties eat a higher percentage of fruits and vegetables than women elsewhere. (Among 24 other factors considered were crime rate, deaths from HIV and sexually transmitted diseases, and air quality.) Yet another list, appearing in the same issue of *Self*, listed the metropolitan areas showing the highest cancer rates for women. Can you guess which location was number 8 on that list? Nassau and Suffolk counties. So much for eating your veggies.

The truth is, it's not so much *where* you live but *how* you live that determines how healthy you are. If you move to a city that's rated as one of the healthiest in the nation but continue to practice an unhealthy lifestyle, your location isn't going to save you. Still, living in a healthy environment can't hurt.

HEALTHIEST PLACES TO LIVE IN THE UNITED STATES

As proposed by *Kiplinger's Personal Finance Magazine*, September 1996 (the first 10 on their list):

1. Rochester, MN
2. Iowa City, IA and Charlottesville, VA (tie)
3. Columbia, MO
4. La Crosse, WI
5. San Francisco, CA
6. Roanoke, VA
7. Sioux Falls, SD
8. Asheville, NC
9. Greenville, NC

BEST PLACES TO LIVE IN THE UNITED STATES

Now, according to *Money* magazine, the best in 1998 (but not comparing apples with apples):

Best in the Midwest:
- Large: Minneapolis, MN
- Medium: Madison, WI
- Small: Rochester, MN

Best in the West:
- Large: Seattle, WA
- Medium: Boulder, CO
- Small: Ft. Collins, CO

Best in the Northeast:
- Large: Washington, DC
- Medium: Trenton, NJ
- Small: Manchester, NH

Best in the South:
- Large: Norfolk, VA
- Medium: Richmond, VA
- Small: Charlottesville, VA

BEST PLACES TO RETIRE

With baby boomers approaching retirement age, finding the perfect place to spend their golden years is on the minds of many people. But the perfect place is not necessarily a tranquil, planned community with lots of rocking chairs and canned music. Why? Because instead of retiring to a front porch rocking chair, more and more people are taking up second careers, pursuing hobbies with a vengeance, going back to school, and becoming active in the community. Where they spend their retirement must appeal to those needs.

With those thoughts in mind, *Modern Maturity* magazine (June 2000) published its list of the 50 most active places for people to retire, and they give the results in five categories. Here are the top three results from each category:

- Tops in fresh air, health care, and leisure activities: Boulder, CO; Bend, OR; and Annapolis, MD
- Tops in exercising the mind (college towns): Austin, TX; Charlottesville, VA; Columbia, MO
- Top Big Cities: Boston, MA; San Francisco, CA; and Sarasota, FL
- Top Small Towns: Asheville, NC; Ashland, OR; Silver City, NM
- Top alternative health care, "quirky" places: Sonoma County, CA; Key West, FL; Reno, NV

Money magazine has a list, too, but no categories. Here are its top five picks:

- Ft. Collins, CO
- Bradenton, FL
- Asheville, NC
- Brunswick, ME
- Bend, OR

COMPARISONS: FATTEST OR UNHEALTHIEST AND FITTEST OR HEALTHIEST

Men's Fitness magazine (January 2000) published a list of the fattest cities in the United States. Here are the top 10:

1. Philadelphia, PA
2. Kansas City, MO
3. Houston, TX
4. Indianapolis, IN
5. New Orleans, LA
6. Chicago, IL
7. Detroit, MI
8. Columbus, OH
9. Memphis, TN
10. Omaha, NE and El Paso, TX (tie)

Unhealthiest places for women, according to *Self*, starting with the least healthy:

1. Beaumont–Port Arthur, TX
2. Bakersfield, CA
3. Flint, MI
4. Memphis, TN
5. Atlantic City, NJ
6. Modesto, CA
7. Stockton, CA

8. Lafayette, IN

9. Rockford, IL

10. Baton Route, LA

Now, a comparison between the "Fittest Cities," as listed by *Men's Fitness* magazine; and the healthiest cities for women, according to *Self*. As you'll see, it seems the fittest men will meet the healthiest women only in San Francisco or Honolulu.

Fittest cities for men:

1. San Diego, CA

2. Minneapolis, MN

3. Seattle, WA

4. Washington, D.C.

5. San Francisco, CA

6. Portland, OR

7. Denver, CO

8. Honolulu, HI

9. Colorado Springs, CO

10. Los Angeles, CA

Healthiest places for women:

1. Provo, UT

2. Nassau and Suffolk Counties, NY

3. Stamford, CT

4. Portland, ME

5. San Francisco, CA

6. Appleton, WI

7. Burlington, VT

8. Honolulu, HI

9. Boston, MA

10. Boulder, CO

And finally, the metropolitan areas with the highest cancer death rates for women. Remember, Nassau–Suffolk, New York, was also rated the second healthiest location. Go figure.

1. Jersey City, NJ
2. New York, NY
3. Bergen–Passaic counties, NJ
4. Newark, NJ
5. Middlesex–Somerset–Hunterdon, NJ
6. Monmouth–Ocean City, NJ
7. Atlantic City–Cape May, NJ
8. Nassau–Suffolk, NY
9. Philadelphia, PA
10. Newburgh, NY

chapter thirty-nine

The 20

Most Dangerous Jobs . . .

and a Few of the Safest

What's your first thought when you wake up in the morning. (The one right after you plead with the alarm clock, "Please, just another 5 minutes?") "Is the coffee ready?" "Will there be enough hot water?" "Will I have time to go to the dry cleaner's before work?" "Will I die on the job today?"

Believe it or not, people whose jobs are among the most dangerous in the world, who risk their lives every workday, usually don't think about the danger. They realize the risk is there, they accept it, and they take whatever precautions are necessary to help ensure they don't get injured or killed. If they allowed fear to take over, they would be more likely to get hurt or killed, or at least they would be too terrified to do their jobs.

It's Not Just Race Car Drivers

When you look at statistics provided by the U.S. Department of Labor, you'll see that the job listed as most dangerous in the United States is driving a truck. That's right. Due to accidents of various kinds, truck drivers suffer more fatal injuries than do people in any other occupation.

What about being in a work environment that is inherently dangerous? Occupations like police officer and firefighter may come to mind, but they're not number two or even number three or four on the list. Farm workers come in at number two because of the dangerous equipment they work with. Sales supervisors and proprietors get the number three slot. Why? Armed robbery. Robbery is the main motivation for workplace homicide and is the second leading cause of job-related fatalities. If you are or know someone who is a convenience store clerk, you should also know that about 31,000 of them are shot every year. Fortunately, most of them survive, which is the reason they reached only number 10 on the list.

Here are just a few facts about job-related safety from the National Safety Council. All figures are for 1998.

- There were 5,100 workplace deaths caused by unintentional injuries.
- There were an additional 1,200 deaths (approximately) that resulted from homicides and suicides at the workplace.
- A total of 3.8 million Americans experienced a disabling injury on the job.
- A disabling injury occurred at the workplace every 8 seconds.
- For women, homicide was the main cause of workplace death.
- Farm workers had 780 deaths and about 140,000 disabling injuries—the second highest death rate among the major industry groups.
- Job-related injuries cost Americans $125.1 billion.

Most Dangerous Jobs in the United States

According to the U.S. Department of Labor and the Occupational Safety and Health Administration (OSHA), these are the 20 most dangerous jobs in the United States. This list is a compilation of the data from both agencies. The top two occupations have kept their positions for several years. The exact order of the remaining jobs shifts slightly from year to year.

1 Truck driver

2 Farm worker

3 Sales supervisor or proprietor

4 Construction worker

5 Police detective

6 Airplane pilot

7 Nonconstruction laborer

8 Electrician

9 Security guard

10 Cashier or convenience store clerk

11 Taxi driver

12 Timber cutter

13 Fisherman

14 Metal worker

15 Roofer

16 Firefighter

17 Groundskeeper or gardener

18 Automobile mechanic

19 Welder

20 Electric power installer

. . . And a Few of the Safest

1 Lawyer

2 Banker

3 Insurance agent

4 Government administrator

5 Accountant

6 Legislator

Other Dangerous Jobs in the World

In addition to the jobs on the U.S. Department of Labor's and OSHA's lists, there are other very dangerous occupations that either do not attract a lot of job applicants, are highly specialized, or have a high degree of secrecy. The men and women who hold these jobs certainly risk their lives every day on the job, and they deserve to be mentioned. They are not listed in order of danger; all of these jobs are just plain dangerous.

- **Fire (or smoke) jumpers:** The huge forest fires that break out each year around the world are the workplace of fire jumpers, who parachute into these raging infernos to better fight and control them. There are only about 400 to 500 smoke jumpers in the United States, and they generally work part-time, during the busy forest fire season.

- **Vulcanologists:** These scientists stalk volcanoes and lava flow, often trekking dangerously close to gather the data and photographs they need.

- **Plague fighters:** Specialized medical staff who go into a plague-ridden region of the world in Africa, Asia, and other developing locations and attempt to identify and isolate the cause of plagues, as well as treat the victims.

- **Bike messengers in New York City:** Speed counts in this job, which involves transporting letters and packages around the city. The faster you are, the more assignments you can complete, the more money you make. Bike messengers reportedly break all traffic laws and even hold onto the backs of vehicles to speed up their trips. You can just imagine what happens when a car stops suddenly.

- **Sand hogs:** That's what they call individuals who work among the tunnels in a city's underground water system. In a city like New York, the system is incredibly intricate—and dangerous, especially when explosives need to be set off.

- **Explosives experts:** Have a bomb to disarm? Who you gonna call? Bomb busters. Explosives experts need nerves of steel (and armor of steel), steady hands, and a cool head.

- **Blowout control experts:** Remember the out-of-control oil fires that sprang up in Kuwait during the Gulf War? Someone had to put caps on those oil wells. Experts from eight different countries worked to cap 732 oil wells. Of course, these accidents occur other places as well. It's a filthy, smelly, dangerous job, but someone has to do it.

- **Bodyguards:** The purpose of a bodyguard is to "take the bullet." Need we say more? Most bodyguards work for businesspeople. In their spare time, they apparently get together with other bodyguards through an International Bodyguard Association in Brighton, Tennessee (901-837-1915).

- **Bounty hunters:** Yes, there are still bounty hunters in the United States. Today's bounty hunters usually work for bail bondsmen, rounding up people who have jumped bail. Bounty hunters typically get 10 to 30 percent of the fugitives' bail amount. Because some of the approximately 20,000 fugitives that are returned each year by bounty hunters are considered dangerous—and bounty hunters are not allowed to use guns in many states—the job has a great element of danger.

- **CIA spy:** Perhaps James Bond gets the martinis and the fancy cars, but real-life spies and secret agents don't always live so well. The real secret spy stuff is done in the Clandestine Service of the Central Intelligence Agency. Ask for it by name when applying for a job there.

- **Delta Force:** The estimated 2,500 to 8,000 men and women who do this job for the U.S. government are trained in antiterrorism tactics and then sent out to use them in fun places like Iran and Iraq. At their training headquarters at Fort Bragg, they learn to storm buildings and planes and rescue hostages. Delta Force is said to employ the world's best markspeople. The average candidate is about 31 years old, has been recruited from the Green Berets or Rangers (two high-caliber, army special operations forces), and has an above-average IQ. Candidates are trained in spy operations, shooting, air assaults, bodyguarding, and high-speed driving.

- **Mine sweepers:** There are many countries that need a good sweep, and about 20 companies that specialize in locating and removing land mines. During the five months that Iraq occupied Kuwait, a total of 7 million land mines were deployed by Iraqi forces and by U.S.-led allied forces, and it cost Kuwait about $1 billion dollars to clean them up. There was a human cost as well: 83 mine sweepers lost their lives.

- **SEALs:** These are Specialists in Naval Special Warfare (SEa, Air, Land), a job classification that was created by President Kennedy in 1962. SEALs go through 27 weeks of what can only be called torturous training, much of it in frigid water at night. SEALs perform many of the same covert activities that Delta Force personnel do, but they do it mostly in locations near the world's oceans, lakes, and rivers.

Part IV

Crucial Facts about the Human Body

Nearly 500 years ago, a Belgian professor of anatomy and surgery at the University of Padua published a book that completely changed our understanding of the human body and how it works. Although dissecting human bodies was illegal at the time, Andreas Vesalius did it anyway, and presented his revolutionary findings in the book, *The Fabric of the Human Body*. He showed the intricate structure of the brain, how nerves are connected to bone, and how bones are nourished. For his efforts, he was sentenced to death, but the sentence was later reduced.

Vesalius's work was a catalyst for things to come. Since his time, researchers have learned much about the human body, how its different parts function, and the factors that can cause disease and dysfunction.

There are so many fascinating things about the human body that it is hard to know where to start. In this section of the book, we have brought together topics that seem to interest people most. For example, how much do you actually know about your own body parts? We've included a basic inventory of the human body, and described how some of the parts work. What types of limits can your body endure? Pain, noise, cancer-causing agents, and tobacco are all challenges to the human body. Each of these issues is brought to light in ways that allow you to better protect your health.

No discussion of health would be complete without a look at high-calorie foods and how to burn them off. We introduce you to some of America's favorite fast—and fattening—foods, as well as ways to burn off those excess calories. Could eating some of those high-fat foods be a cause of some of the diseases that affect so many Americans today? You can read about that and more in the chapters on disease risk factors and common ailments by age group.

Because no one likes being sick or undergoing medical procedures, we offer a list of recovery times associated with various diseases and medical procedures, so you will have a better idea of what to expect if you face either situation.

chapter forty

151 Body Parts: What They're Called and What They Do

Sometimes it's surprising how little we really know about what we are made of. For example, how well educated are you about the many organs that are packed so efficiently under your very own skin? What are they called? What do they do? Are they replaceable?

We hope this list will help you "take stock" of yourself. It includes just a few of the many body parts, both inside and out, that you carry around with you every day. Perhaps you'll find a few things you didn't know you had on the shelves.

(Any word or phrase in **bold** within an entry means there is a separate, individual entry for that body part.)

1 **Abdomen.** The area of the body between the chest and the pelvis. The abdomen consists of the **stomach**, **large** and **small intestines**, **liver**, **gallbladder**, **pancreas**, **spleen**, and **bladder**.

2 **Adenoids.** Glands that filter out and destroy bacteria, especially those that cause respiratory infections. Adenoids usually continue to grow until a child is about 6 years old; then they gradually shrink down to nothing.

3 **Adrenal glands.** A pair of glands that are located on top of the kidneys. The adrenal glands secrete several different hormones that affect the body's response to stress, metabolic rate, growth, blood glucose (sugar) concentration, and loss and retention of minerals.

4 **Alveolus.** The singular form (alveoli is the plural) for a small air sac found in the lungs, or a milk-secreting portion of the breast.

5 **Aorta.** The largest **artery** of the body. It supplies oxygenated blood to all other arteries except the **pulmonary artery**.

6 **Appendix.** A tiny, twisted, coiled tube attached to the **cecum** in the large intestine. The appendix apparently has no function.

7 **Arm.** The portion of the upper limb from the elbow to the shoulder. No, "arm" does *not* pertain to the entire limb. See **forearm**.

8 **Arteries.** The elastic, muscular tubes that carry blood away from the heart to other parts of the body. They are the largest of the blood vessels.

9 **Atriums.** The two upper chambers of the **heart**. The left atrium receives fully oxygenated blood from the lungs and the right receives oxygen-deficient blood from the upper and lower parts of the body.

10 **Axilla.** Another name for the armpit, the small hollow under the arm where it joins the body at the shoulders.

11 **Bladder.** A muscular sac, located in the lower abdomen, that receives urine from the kidneys and stores it until it can be eliminated through the **urethra**, prompted by contractions from the bladder muscles.

12 **Blood.** A fluid **connective tissue** that has four main functions: 1) transports oxygen from the lungs to cells throughout the body and carbon dioxide from cells to the lungs; 2) clots to protect against excessive loss from the body; 3) regulates the pH of fluids in the body, body temperature, and the water content of cells; and 4) uses specific blood cells—white blood cells—to protect against disease.

13 **Brain.** Hippocrates said that "from the brain and from the brain only arise our pleasures, joys, laughter, and jests as well as our sorrows, pains, griefs, and fears." Although not a scientific explanation, Hippocrates' thoughts were on target. The brain is the center of the nervous system and of the entire body. It is the core of intellectual, emotional, and physical activity, voluntary and involuntary, as well as your conscious and unconscious self.

14 **Brain stem.** The portion of the brain that lies immediately above the spinal cord. It is composed of the **medulla oblongata**, **pons**, and **midbrain**.

15 **Buttocks.** The two fleshy masses located on the posterior portion of the back of the trunk. Sometimes referred to as the gluteus maximus (*glut* means buttock, *maximus* means largest).

16 **Calcaneal tendon.** The technical name for the Achilles tendon, which is located at the back of the heel.

17 **Capillaries.** These are the smallest blood vessels in the body and are the location for the exchange of nutrients and wastes between the blood and the tissue cells. Capillaries are so narrow that blood cells must pass through them in single file.

18 **Carpal bones.** The eight bones located in the wrist. This is the area affected in people who have carpal tunnel syndrome.

19 **Cartilage.** A tough type of connective tissue partly composed of elastic fibers and collagen. Perhaps your most "prominent" cartilage is in your nose.

20 **Cecum.** The first segment of the **large intestine**. It is where the appendix is attached.

21 **Cerebellum.** One of three regions of the **brain**. The cerebellum is located behind the **brain stem** and is a center for balance and the control of fine movement.

22 **Cerebrum.** The largest part of the brain. It is composed of two hemispheres and contains the centers for personality, the senses, voluntary movement, and thought.

23 **Cervix.** Generically, "cervix" means *neck*, so it can refer to the neck or a constricted portion of any organ. In women, it specifically refers to the neck portion of the **uterus**.

24 **Chromosome.** One of the minuscule, threadlike structures found in the nucleus of a cell that contain genetic material. Human cells normally have 46 chromosomes.

25 **Clitoris.** A highly sensitive organ in females that has specialized nerve endings. Like the **penis**, the clitoris contains tissues that become engorged with blood during sexual stimulation.

26 **Coccyx.** The fused bones at the far end of the **vertebral column**, sometimes referred to as the tailbone.

27 **Cochlea.** The coiled structure in the inner ear that transforms sound vibrations into nerve signals that are sent to the brain, where they are interpreted.

28 **Colon.** This is the longest portion of the **large intestine**. It begins at the cecum, ascends on the right side of the **abdomen** (ascending colon), turns left under the **liver** and abdomen (transverse colon), descends past the **spleen** (descending colon), and turns into the sigmoid colon near the left hip bone. It then ends at the **rectum**. The primary function of the colon is to absorb water from the contents of the bowel and to conserve it.

29 **Cones.** Specialized photoreceptor cells in the **retina** that allow us to see colors in bright light.

30 **Conjunctiva.** The fragile membrane that covers the lining of the eye and the **eyeball**.

31 **Connective tissue.** One of four types of tissue found in the human body, and the most abundant. It binds and supports other body tissues, protects organs, and is the major transportation system within the body (because **blood** is considered to be a fluid connective tissue).

32 **Cornea.** The transparent dome located at the front of the **eyeball**. The cornea is the main focusing part of the eyeball.

33 **Corpus collosum.** The "great divide" in the **brain** that separates the cerebral hemispheres—the right brain from the left brain.

34 **Cowper gland.** Tiny gland in the male reproductive system that secretes a protective and lubricating mucus that makes up part of the semen.

35 Cranium. The section of the **skull** that protects the **brain** as well as the organs of hearing, sight, and balance. It consists of eight bones: two parietal bones, two temporal bones, and the frontal, occipital, sphenoid, and ethmoid bones.

36 Deep fascia. A sheet of **connective tissue** that is wrapped around a muscle to hold it in place.

37 Dermis. The middle of three layers of **skin**. The dermis is composed of dense, irregular connective tissue.

38 Diaphragm. The muscular band that separates the chest from the **abdomen**. During inhalation, the diaphragm contracts and flattens, which creates space for the expanding **lungs**. During exhalation, it relaxes, forcing air from the lungs.

39 Disks. The cartilage pads that lie between the **vertebrae** in the spine. The disks protect the **vertebral column** by absorbing shock and concussion.

40 Diverticulum. A pouch or sac found in the wall of an organ or canal. They are most prominent in the **colon**, where they can lead to a painful inflammation known as diverticulitis.

41 Duodenum. The first 10 inches of the **small intestine**, which connects the **stomach** and the **ileum**. People who have duodenal ulcers are aware of this area of their bodies.

42 Dura mater. The membrane that covers and protects the **brain** and **spinal cord**.

43 Eardrum. The membrane that separates the outer ear from the **middle ear**. The eardrum vibrates in response to sound waves that enter the ear.

44 Endocrine glands. Glands that secrete substances called hormones directly into the **blood** without going through a channel or duct. Examples of endocrine glands are the **adrenal**, **pituitary**, and **thyroid glands**.

45 Epidermis. The top, outer layer of **skin**. It is the body's first line of protection against invasion from foreign objects and organisms.

46 **Epiglottis.** A small, valvelike piece of cartilage that seals off the windpipe when you swallow, thus preventing you from choking.

47 **Eustachian tube.** The tube that connects the back of the nose to the **middle ear**. The eustachian tube equalizes air pressure on both sides of the **eardrum** and also drains secretions from the middle ear.

48 **Exocrine glands.** Glands that secrete substances, such as saliva, perspiration, oil, earwax, and milk, through ducts into body cavities, directly onto a surface, or into the lining of an organ. Examples of exocrine glands are sweat glands and **salivary glands**.

49 **Eyeball.** A globe, one inch in diameter in adults, that is the organ of sight. The eye contains more than 50 percent of the sensory receptors in the entire human body.

50 **Eyebrow.** The ridge above the eye that protects the eye against foreign objects, direct sunlight, and perspiration.

51 **Eyelids.** The upper and lower eyelids are thin skin layers that protect the eyes from excessive light and foreign objects, shade the eyes during sleep, and spread secretions over the eyeballs by blinking.

52 **Fallopian tube.** One of a pair of tubes that runs from an **ovary** to the **uterus**. Each month in menstruating women, one of the ovaries releases an egg, which is transported to the uterus through a fallopian tube.

53 **Femur.** The femur is the thigh bone—the longest, heaviest, and strongest bone in the human body. It extends from the hip to the knee, or **patella**.

54 **Foot.** The end of the lower limb, extending from the ankle to the toes. The bones in the foot are arranged in two arches, which allow the foot to support the body's weight and provide leverage while walking.

55 **Forearm.** The portion of the upper limb that extends between the elbow and the wrist.

56 **Forebrain.** Located in the front of the **cerebrum**, the forebrain is the site of the most complex functions of human action, emotion, and thought, including memory, reasoning, speech, the formation of words, and judgment.

57 Gallbladder. The small, pear-shaped organ that is located just below the **liver**. The gallbladder stores bile, a digestive juice that is produced by the liver. Bile is used by the body to break down fatty foods.

58 Gene. A segment of a **chromosome** that contains specific hereditary information.

59 Glans penis. The slightly enlarged area at the end of the **penis**, which is rich in nerve cells.

60 Hair. A threadlike structure that develops in the **skin**. Hair emerges from a hair follicle, a tiny structure that lies in the top layer of the skin.

61 Hand. The end portion of an upper limb. The muscles that move the hand are located in the **forearm**.

62 Heart. The heart is a muscle that consists of two pumps, each of which has two chambers. The right side of the heart receives oxygen-deficient **blood**, which it pumps to the **lungs**. The left side receives oxygenated blood from the lungs and pumps it to the rest of the body. Because the right side works harder than the left, the left side of the heart is smaller than the right.

63 Hindbrain. The hindbrain's main function is to coordinate muscle activity and amplify signals that travel from the **brain** to the muscles.

64 Hippocampus. A portion of the **brain** that is a center for learning and long-term memory.

65 Hymen. A thin mucous membrane located at the vaginal opening. A torn or punctured hymen is commonly regarded as a sign that a woman has "lost" her virginity; however, it can be broken by physical activities such as horseback riding, gymnastics, and bike riding.

66 Hyoid bone. An unusual bone in that it doesn't touch any other bones in the body, but it is supported by many muscles. This U-shaped bone forms part of the **larynx** and supports the **tongue**.

67 Hypothalamus. A small part of the **brain**, located at its base, where the hormonal and nervous systems interact. The hypothalamus is responsible for body functions such as blood pressure, appetite, thirst, and body temperature.

68 **Ileum.** The final segment of the **small intestine**. The ileum is where absorption of nutrients is completed.

69 **Iris.** The colored portion of the **eyeball**. The iris contains muscles that constrict and contract to regulate the amount of light that passes through the eye's lens.

70 **Jejunum.** The midsection of the **small intestine**. It is about 3 feet long and was so named because it is empty at death (*jejunum* means "empty").

71 **Joints.** Structures that allow two or more bones to move easily in relation to each other. Joints consist of **cartilage** and **ligaments**, which hold the bones together.

72 **Kidney.** One of two bean-shaped organs that are located in back of the abdominal cavity. Each kidney filters the **blood**, removes waste materials from the blood, and regulates the body's fluid and salt content.

73 **Lacrimal glands.** Two glands, one over each eye, that secrete tears through lacrimal ducts onto the upper **eyelid**. Tears are critical for keeping the eyes healthy and lubricated.

74 **Large intestine.** This is the last part of the gastrointestinal tract, and it is responsible for completing the absorption of food, the production of some vitamins, the formation of stool, and the elimination of stool from the body. Its average diameter is 2.5 inches and its length is about 5 feet. The large intestine is composed of four main sections: **cecum**, **colon**, **rectum**, and anal canal.

75 **Larynx.** The structure in the neck at the top of the windpipe that contains the vocal cords. The larynx automatically moves up and down when you swallow.

76 **Leg.** The portion of the lower limb that extends between the knee and the ankle. Technically, the part of the lower limb above the knee is not the leg, but the **thigh**.

77 **Lens.** A transparent structure in the **eyeball** composed of layers of elastic protein fibers. It focuses light rays onto the **retina**.

78 **Ligament.** A band of tissue that is composed primarily of collagen—a fibrous, elastic protein. Ligaments support bones, mainly around the joints.

79 **Liver.** The largest organ in the human body, the liver is located in the upper right **abdomen**. The liver's main functions are to produce bile and cholesterol from the breakdown of old red blood cells and fat; make proteins; and remove toxins and waste products from the blood or convert them into safer substances such as urea, which is a component of urine.

80 **Lumbar spine.** Portion of the lower spine, extending from the lowest ribs to the bottom of the spine. The lumbar spine is the area where the diagnostic procedure known as a spinal tap (or lumbar puncture) is performed. (See Chapter 26).

81 **Lungs.** Two cone-shaped, spongelike structures located in the chest cavity and protected by the rib cage. The **lungs** are a transfer station: When air enters the lungs, the lungs filter out oxygen to the **capillaries** so it can circulate throughout the body. Carbon dioxide delivered to the lungs by the capillaries is then exhaled from the lungs.

82 **Lunula.** The semicircle-shaped white area at the base of a nail. Did you even know this had a name?

83 **Lymph nodes.** Small, oval glands that contain white blood cells, which are part of the body's barrier against infection. Lymph nodes are found in small groups along **lymphatic vessels** throughout the body, but they are most concentrated in the neck, groin, and armpits. They act as a barrier against infection and they filter out and destroy toxic substances and microorganisms.

84 **Lymphatic vessels.** Large vessels that collect lymph fluid. Lymphatic vessels are similar to **veins** but they have thinner walls and more valves. They have several functions, which include transporting cholesterol and fat-soluble vitamins (A, D, E, and K) from the gastrointestinal tract to the **blood** and helping protect the body against invading organisms.

85 **Mammary gland.** A modified sweat gland in females that produces milk. It is a type of **exocrine gland**.

86 **Marrow.** The spongy center part of bone that comes in two types. Red bone marrow produces blood cells, while yellow bone marrow consists mostly of fat tissue and does not make blood cells.

87 **Medulla oblongata.** This structure is part of the **brain stem** and is a continuation of the **spinal cord**. The medulla is like a way station, in that it contains all the sensory and motor fibers that extend between the spinal cord and the other parts of the **brain**.

88 **Meninges.** The three membrane layers that cover and protect the **brain** and the **spinal cord**.

89 **Midbrain.** Located appropriately in the middle of the brain, the midbrain controls vision and eye reflexes, involuntary muscle activities, and motor responses of the torso and head. It also connects the **forebrain** with the **hindbrain**.

90 **Middle ear.** The part of the ear that reaches from the eardrum to the skull. It contains the three bones that make it possible for people to hear.

91 **Muscles.** Tissues designed to contract, either voluntarily or involuntarily. There are approximately 700 muscles in the human body, and they are divided into three types: skeletal, which are responsible for voluntary movement of the bones; smooth, which are found in the organs and blood vessels and are associated with involuntary movement; and cardiac, which is the heart. By the way, the Latin word *musculus* means "little mouse." What does that have to do with muscles? No one knows for sure.

92 **Myocardium.** The muscular middle layer of the **heart** wall. The myocardium makes up the bulk of the heart and is the area damaged in people who experience a myocardial infarction, or heart attack.

93 **Nails.** Nails are composed of a protein called keratin and act as protective armor for fingertips and toes. Although nails have no nerves and thus cannot feel, they can act as shock absorbers when you stub your toe. It takes from three to six months for a nail to grow from its base to its top.

94 **Nipple.** A pigmented projection on the breast. The openings of the milk ducts are located here.

95 **Nose.** Everyone knows the nose is the organ of smell, but it also has other roles. The nose acts as a filter for approximately 500 cubic feet of air per day, filtering out dust, bacteria, and other microscopic particles, and warming air to the same temperature as your blood. The nose also gives your voice resonance.

96 **Optic nerve.** The bundle of nerves that runs from the back of the **eyeball** to the **brain** and transmits image signals. Excessive use of alcohol and tobacco can damage the optic nerve.

97 **Otoliths.** Minute particles of calcium carbonate that reside in the ear. These "ear rocks," as they are often referred to, help maintain equilibrium.

98 **Ovaries.** These two glands are found only in women. Located in the pelvic region, the ovaries secrete two female hormones: estrogen and progesterone.

99 **Palate.** The roof of the mouth, consisting of a bony front portion (the hard palate) and a soft back portion (soft palate).

100 **Pancreas.** The pancreas is perhaps best known as the organ that produces insulin, the all-important hormone that regulates the use of glucose (sugar) in the body. When the pancreas does not produce insulin, the result is diabetes. The pancreas also produces digestive enzymes and glucagon.

101 **Parathyroid glands.** Four glands located on the **thyroid gland**, near the base of the throat. The parathyroid glands produce a hormone that helps control calcium levels in the blood by increasing the amount of calcium absorbed in the intestines and reducing the amount eliminated from the **kidneys**.

102 **Patella.** The medical term for the knee. The word *patella* means "little dish."

103 **Pelvis.** A dish or basin-like bony structure that consists of the hip bones, the sacrum, and the **coccyx**. The pelvis provides stable support for the **vertebral column**, attaches the lower limbs to the rest of the skeleton, and protects the pelvic organs, including the reproductive organs, in both men and women.

104   **Penis.** The male sexual organ made of spongy tissue that contains many blood vessels. During sexual arousal, the penis is capable of increasing in both size and length. The **urethra**, which runs inside the penis, is the tube through which both semen and urine leave the body.

105   **Pericardium.** The membrane that surrounds (*peri-* means around) and protects the **heart** and holds it in place in the chest cavity. Inflammation of the pericardium is known as pericarditis.

106   **Phalanges.** The jointed, flexible bones in the ends of the fingers. They make it possible for the fingers to flex and bend—to play the piano, make finger puppets, or type a letter.

107   **Pharynx.** The technical name for the throat. The pharynx is approximately 5 inches long and is part of two body systems—the respiratory and the digestive—as it is a highway for both air and food.

108   **Pineal gland.** The pea-sized pineal gland is located at the base of the **brain**. Although it is active metabolically, its actual function is unknown.

109   **Pinna.** The projecting part of the external ear that is shaped like the flared end of a horn. It is made of **cartilage** and covered with **skin** and helps capture sound waves for the ear.

110   **Pituitary gland.** A pea-sized gland located near the base of the **brain**. The pituitary gland, sometimes referred to as the "master gland," controls all other major **endocrine glands** (ductless glands that produce secretions that are circulated throughout the body). It secretes several hormones that regulate many different processes, including reproduction, growth, and metabolism.

111   **Pons.** The part of the **brain stem** that forms a connection or "bridge" between the **medulla oblongata** and the **midbrain**.

112   **Prostate gland.** A part of the male reproductive system, the prostate gland is a walnut-sized structure located below the **bladder**. The prostate gland produces secretions that mix with the sperm cells. These secretions enable the sperm to swim and move freely after ejaculation.

113   **Pulmonary artery.** The artery that delivers fully oxygenated **blood** from the **lungs** to the **heart**.

114   **Pupil.** The hole in the center of the **iris**, through which light enters the **eyeball**.

115   **Rectum.** The end of the **large intestine**, located just above the anus. It is about 8 inches long and is where stool passes out of the body.

116   **Retina.** The light-sensitive portion of the eye, located at the back of the **eyeball**. When an image enters the eye in the form of light, the retina converts the image to signals that are sent to the **brain** along the **optic nerve**.

117   **Rods.** Specialized cells in the eye that allow us to see in dim light. Unlike **cones**, which allow us to see colors, rods let us see shades of gray.

118   **Salivary glands.** Three pairs of glands (parotid, sublingual, and submandibular) that secret saliva through ducts that drain into the mouth.

119   **Sciatic nerves.** The two largest nerves in the body, each one originates at the base of the spine and travels through the **buttocks** down the back side of the **thigh** and down the **leg**. Sciatica, a type of nerve pain that can be felt anywhere along the course of either sciatic nerve, is caused by compression of or damage to the nerve.

120   **Scrotum.** The part of the male reproductive system that contains and protects the **testes**. The scrotum is divided into two compartments, each of which contains one testis.

121   **Sebaceous glands.** You could call these sweat glands the goosebump glands. They are located all over the body except on the soles of the feet and the palms of the hands. Sebaceous glands are connected to hair follicles and secrete an oil called sebum, which keeps the **skin** soft and prevents the **hair** from becoming brittle. When you are cold or frightened, a muscle attached to the hair follicles pulls the hair erect, which releases sebum onto the skin. When the glands are pushed up, goosebumps are the result.

122   **Semicircular canals.** Three bony channels located in the ear. They contain the receptors that are responsible for equilibrium.

123   **Sinuses.** The nasal sinuses are eight air spaces in the **skull**. One pair is located just above the **eyebrows**; another is on either side of the bridge of the nose. A third pair is deep behind the **nose**, and the last pair is in the cheekbones. The size of the sinuses has an impact on the resonance of your voice. When the nose doesn't produce enough mucus, the sinuses produce the difference.

124   **Skin.** This is the largest organ, and it makes up about 5 percent of the body's weight. The skin is the body's first defense against invading organisms; it also helps regulate body temperature and is an important indicator of the body's physical and emotional health, based on changes in its appearance.

125   **Skull.** The skull is a bony protective covering for the **brain** and is composed of two main parts—the **cranium** and the facial bones. The base of the skull is thicker and stronger than the sides and top.

126   **Small intestine.** A coiled, 16-foot-long tube that is composed of three parts: **duodenum**, **jejunum**, and **ileum**. When partially processed food from the **stomach** enters the small intestine, it is completely broken down by bile—juice from the **pancreas**—and intestinal secretions so the body can use the nutrients.

127   **Spinal cord.** The mass of nerve tissue that is located in the vertebral canal (spinal column). It is from 16 to 18 inches long and is the origination point for 31 pairs of nerves. The spinal cord is the highway for nerve impulses to travel from the **brain** to the periphery of the body, and it is the coordinator of spinal cord reflexes (automatic responses to sensory signals that enter the spinal cord).

128   **Spleen.** A soft, spongy organ that sits behind the **stomach**. It performs many essential functions, including production of blood cells, destruction of old blood cells, and maintaining a reserve blood supply. Despite performing these important tasks, the spleen can be removed without the body missing it.

129   **Stomach.** A hollow, J-shaped organ located just below the **diaphragm**. In the stomach, food is mixed thoroughly with digestive juices secreted by the stomach lining. The stomach then gradually releases the processed food into the **small intestine**.

130   **Subcutaneous layer**. The bottom of three layers of the skin. This layer is composed of fat.

131   **Teeth.** Hard, **connective tissue** structures, composed of calcium, which are embedded in the jaw. Technically, they are known as *dentes*, which explains why you go to a *dentist* for your teeth.

132   **Tendons.** Tough cords of tissue found at the ends of **muscles** that attach to bones. Tendons are responsible for transmitting the force of muscle contractions to cause movement.

133   **Testes.** The two male reproductive glands that are contained in and protected by the **scrotum**. The testes make the male sex hormone called testosterone, as well as sperm cells, which fertilize the female egg or ovum.

134   **Thalamus.** A portion of the **brain** consisting of two masses, located in the **midbrain**. It is the primary relay station for sensory signals from the **spinal cord**, **brain stem**, **cerebellum**, and other parts of the brain. It is responsible for the crude perception of some sensations, such as pressure, temperature, and pain. It also has a role in awareness.

135   **Thigh.** The portion of the lower limb that extends between the hip and the knee.

136   **Thumb.** *Pollex*, Latin for "strong," is the technical name for the thumb. The thumb is opposed to the other fingers, which makes it useful for picking up objects.

137   **Thymus gland.** Composed of two oval lobes, the thymus gland is located behind the breastbone. It is responsible for the development of the immune system. During infancy and childhood, the thymus is large, but it shrinks to the size of a grape by adulthood.

138   **Thyroid gland.** Located on either side of the **trachea**, the thyroid gland has two lobes that secrete iodine-based hormones. These hormones are responsible for regulating mental and physical growth, oxidation, blood pressure, heart rate, body temperature, and the absorption and utilization of glucose (sugar), which is critical for energy use and production.

139   **Tongue.** Composed primarily of **muscles**, the tongue is a very versatile organ. It plays critical roles in eating, tasting, and speaking, and registers pain if something is too hot or rejection if something is foul. The top of the tongue is covered with a thick mucous membrane that houses the taste buds and nerves.

140   **Tonsils.** Located at the entrance of the throat, these lymphatic tissues help fight infections. Tonsils frequently become chronically infected in children, and so they are often removed.

141   **Trachea.** The tubular passageway for air to enter the **lungs**. Also known as the windpipe, it is lined with mucous membrane and supported by **cartilage**. This is the structure into which doctors make an incision to create an emergency air passageway (a procedure called a tracheostomy) if there is a breathing obstruction above the chest level.

142   **Trunk.** The main part of the body to which the upper and lower limbs are attached.

143   **Umbilical cord.** The ropelike structure that connects a mother with her fetus. The cord contains umbilical arteries, through which pass wastes from the fetus, and an umbilical vein, through which nutrients and oxygen are passed to the fetus.

144   **Urethra.** In men, it is a narrow, S-shaped tube that runs from the **bladder**, inside the **penis**, to the outside of the body. It performs two main functions in men: It carries urine from the bladder to the exterior of the body; and it is the passageway through which semen travels from the **prostate gland** to the penis. In women, the urethra runs from the bladder to the outside of the body and carries urine only.

145   **Uterus.** An organ of the female reproductive system, on whose walls a fertilized egg attaches itself and eventually develops into a fetus.

146   **Uvula.** The fleshy piece of muscular tissue and mucous membrane that hangs down from the soft **palate** at the back of the throat. The uvula, which is Latin for "little grape," helps close off the nasal passages when you swallow. But it's real claim to fame is the fact that it vibrates when breath goes across it. The result: snoring.

147 **Vagina.** A narrow, 4- to 6-inch-long canal or tube in females that leads from the **uterus** to the external opening. The vagina is composed of **muscle** and fibroelastic **connective tissue** and has an amazing ability to expand enough to allow the passage of an infant.

148 **Veins.** The small blood vessels responsible for transporting oxygen-depleted blood.

149 **Ventricles.** The lower chambers of the **heart**, which are responsible for pumping oxygen-depleted blood through the **pulmonary artery** to the **lungs** (right ventricle) and oxygen-rich blood to the aorta and the rest of the body (left ventricle).

150 **Vertebral column.** Also known as the spine or the backbone, the vertebral column is composed of 26 spinal bones, or vertebrae, in adults, and 33 vertebrae in children. The column encloses and protects the **spinal cord** and is where the ribs and back muscles attach.

151 **Vulva.** An external reproductive organ in females that is made up of several components: the mons pubis (a pad of fatty tissue that covers the pubic bone), the labia majora and labia minora (folds of fatty tissue that protect the genitals within), and the **clitoris**.

Replacement Body Parts: Now and in the Future

Currently there are four main types of replacement body parts: human donor parts, animal parts, artificial or prosthetic parts, and human regeneration. When it comes to human donors, there are never enough to meet the demand. As of May 2000, there was a waiting list for 69,728 organs in the United States. The majority of the people waiting for replacement organs need a kidney (45,273), with liver (15,359) and heart (4,143) coming in second and third. Unfortunately, fewer than 6,000 organs are donated each year.

The use of animal parts raises questions of incompatibility and ethics. The use of artificial parts has been limited, although it is somewhat successful in the case of limbs. The regeneration of human tissue is rather new technology that appears to be promising, especially in the case of regenerated cartilage.

Here is where medical technology stands today, and the direction many see it going in.

- **Heart valves:** *Now:* Plastic and metal valves, as well as those taken from pigs, lambs, and other animals. *Future:* We may have heart valves grown from a patient's own cells.

- **Limbs:** *Now:* Artificial (prosthetic) limbs that are attached to the nervous system, which allows the limbs to move. *Future:* Prosthetic limbs will be able to feel sensations.

- **Bone and cartilage:** *Now:* Hormones can be injected into fractured bones to help them regenerate. *Future:* The body will create its own new bone and cartilage by building on plastic mesh, which surgeons will implant in the body.

- **Nerves:** *Now:* Nerves can be reconstructed using cultivated pig nerve cells. *Future:* Scientists will make synthetic nerves from a material called polymer.

- **Organs:** *Now:* Organs are transplanted from donors, and researchers can grow small pieces of human liver tissue. *Future:* By 2020, scientists foresee the ability to grow human organs from human tissue in the laboratory.

- **Eyes:** *Now:* Laser surgery, contact lenses, and glasses are the techniques to correct vision. *Future:* Surgically implanted permanent lenses will eliminate the need for glasses and contact lenses.

- **Skin:** *Now:* Artificial skin is available, made from human cells and synthetic materials. *Future:* Researchers will take stem cells (immature cells that have not yet become specialized) and stimulate them with growth hormones to grow skin.

- **Hair:** *Now:* Hair transplants are available, but they can take years to complete and then are not always successful. *Future:* Scientists hope to use growth proteins to stimulate hair to regenerate.

- **Blood vessels:** *Now:* Synthetic and animal cells are used to create new arteries and veins. The body rejects many of these foreign blood vessels, so the recipients must take antirejection drugs. *Future:* Scientists will grow new arteries and veins from a patient's own cells.

chapter forty-one

Body Inventory:
Trillions of Cells, Millions of
Capillaries, and More

If your insurance company asked you to take an inventory of your home, you could do it in one of several ways. You could do it room by room, listing all the items in each one. Or you could do it by category—say, furniture, small appliances, large appliances, jewelry, and so on. In both cases, you would be listing items you can easily visualize and touch.

What if you had to make an inventory of your body? Easy, right? Two arms, two legs, ten toes . . . sure, that's the obvious stuff. But what about the stuff that's not so obvious? For example, how many miles of "highway" does your blood travel throughout your body each day? How many bones do you have? How about the number of cells, body systems, or neurons?

Here are some inventory numbers taken from the human body. We think you'll find them fascinating.

Note: The figures given here refer to adults, unless otherwise noted.

- 100 trillion: Approximate number of cells in the human body. This encompasses all types of cells, including but not limited to blood, nerve, muscle, sperm, skin, and so on.

- 25 trillion: Approximate number of red blood cells. Red blood cells are so small, a pile of 500 measure only four one-hundredths of an inch high. Each red blood cell lives about four months.

- 1 trillion-plus: Number of platelets (the smallest of the blood cells) in the bloodstream. Platelets are responsible for making blood clot. Each platelet lives for only 10 days, and 200 billion new ones enter circulation each day.

- 100 billion: Approximate number of neurons—nerve cells—in the body. Nerve cells develop thin strands up to 3 feet long that transmit signals to and from the brain.

- 220 million: Number of quarts of blood the heart pumps through itself over a 70-year average lifetime.

- 100 million: The approximate number of rods (cells that discern light and dark, shape, and movement) in the eye.

- 6 to 7 million: Average number of eggs (ova) human females are born with in their ovaries. The number of eggs gradually declines as a woman ages, until menopause (around age 50), when the supply is depleted.

- 6 million: Number of olfactory receptor cells (neurons) in each nostril. These specialized cells can detect between 4,000 and 10,000 different smells.

- 3 million: Number of red blood cells that die every second. At the same time, another 3 million are being produced in the bone marrow.

- 3 million: Approximate number of cones (cells that discern color) in the eye.

- 2 to 3 million: Number of eccrine sweat glands in the body. The highest concentration are found in the soles of the feet, palms of the hands, and armpits. Eccrine sweat glands help regulate body temperature.

- 1 million-plus: Number of sperm cells one testis produces each day. As many as 500 million sperm may be found in one ejaculation, but fewer than 500 actually reach the upper part of the fallopian tube in a woman, where fertilization takes place.

- 1 million: Estimated number of surface skin cells (epidermis) that are shed every 40 minutes.

- 250,000: Number of sweat glands in your feet. Feet tend to sweat more than other parts of the body. In fact, there are more sweat glands per square inch in your feet than in any other body part.

- 90,000 miles: Approximate length of the blood vessel system (arteries, veins, and capillaries) if placed end to end. That's enough "roadway" to circle the globe nearly four times.

- 60,000: Approximate number of melanocytes per square inch of skin. Melanocytes are spider-shaped cells that produce the skin pigment melanin.

- 50,000: Estimated number of lobules in the liver. Lobules are tiny compartments that help the liver process about 1 quart of blood per minute.

- 9,000: Average number of taste buds on the tongue. There are four kinds of taste buds: sour, sweet, salty, and bitter. Everyone has a different number of each kind and different patterns of distribution on the tongue.

- 1,000: Average number of hairs per square inch on a human head. The average area of a head is 120 square inches. Not everyone has the same number of hairs on their heads, however. Generally, blondes have a total of 140,000; brunettes, 110,000; those with black hair have 108,000, while redheads have 90,000.

- 650: Approximate number of sweat glands in one square inch of skin.

- 600-plus: Number of skeletal muscles in the body

- 574: Number of amino acids in a hemoglobin molecule. It takes about 90 seconds for a hemoglobin molecule to form. The number of amino acids in any given protein molecule and the time it takes to complete formation of the molecule depend on the type of protein being created.

- 425: Gallons of blood the kidneys process each day. This is remarkable, considering that each kidney weighs a mere 5 ounces.

- 350: Number of bones in a newborn.

- 206: Average number of bones in an adult. The number is "average" because some people have an extra rib or one less, and some have one or two fewer vertebrae.

- 50: Approximate number of taste cells in each taste bud. Each taste cell lives about 7 to 10 days, so if you burn your tongue, new taste cells will be coming soon to replace those you lost.

- 46: Number of chromosomes (structures that carry the body's genetic information) in the nucleus of every human cell.

- 33: Number of vertebrae in the spinal column. They are divided into five categories: cervical (7 vertebrae), thoracic (12), lumbar (5), sacrum (5), and coccyx (4). In adults, the 5 sacral vertebrae fuse to form the sacrum, and the 4 coccygeal vertebrae fuse to form the coccyx; so while there are 33 vertebrae in children, there are 26 in adults.

- 32: Number of permanent teeth, including the wisdom teeth, which typically appear by the time a person is in the late teens or early twenties.

- 31: Pairs of nerves that travel through the gaps between the vertebrae in the spinal cord and disperse out to body organs and tissues.

- 26: Number of bones in each foot. The number of bones in both feet combined comprise 25 percent of the bones in the body.

- 22: Number of bones that make up the skull.

- 21: Length in feet of the small intestine. The designation "small" refers to the diameter of the intestine and not its length. The large intestine is much shorter than the small one.

- 17: Length (average) in inches of the spinal cord, which descends from the neck to the lumbar (lower) part of the back. The spinal cord is up to 3/4 of an inch thick.

- 15 to 20: Number of sections, called lobes, in the human female breast. Each lobe ends in many smaller lobules, which further end in tiny bulbs that produce milk during lactation.

- 12: Number of body systems. They are: cardiovascular (or circulatory), digestive, endocrine (specific glands), immune, integumentary (skin and related components), lymphatic, muscular, nervous, respiratory, reproductive, skeletal, and urinary.

- 12: Pairs of ribs found in 95 percent of people. About 5 percent are born with one or more extra ribs, while individuals with Down's syndrome have one pair less.

- 12: Pairs of cranial nerves that branch out from the underside of the brain to relay signals primarily to the face, head, shoulders, and throat.

- 6 to 10: Average weight (in pounds) of the skin. If stretched out, the adult skin would cover an area of about 3 feet by 7 feet.

- 5 feet: Length of the large intestine.

- 5 liters: Amount of blood in the body. All that blood travels along an estimated 90,000 miles of blood vessel highway.

- 5 senses: Smell, taste, hearing, touch, and sight. Many would argue that some people are gifted with a sixth sense, which has been referred to as intuition or extrasensory perception.

- 3: Number of parts to the brain. They are: cerebrum, cerebellum, and cerebral cortex.

- 3: Number of ounces the brain loses from age 20 to age 80. Even though the brain shrinks from its peak of 3 pounds at age 20 years, the shrinkage isn't necessarily associated with a decline in mental capacity. It is true that the ability to process information rapidly and to make quick decisions declines with age, but intellectual performance often does not follow suit.

chapter forty-two

Pain, Pain, Go Away:

7 Types of Pain and How to Treat Them

Pain. It's been called a gift, a blessing, and a friend; not because we look forward to experiencing it, but because it can literally save our lives. When we're in the throes of pain—a burn from a spilled pot of boiling water, a broken bone, a finger smashed in a car door—we aren't thinking, "Gee, I'm so glad I feel this way." But if we didn't feel the burning, pounding, stabbing, or piercing sensations, we wouldn't know that something serious is wrong and that we need to take action.

What Is Pain?

According to the International Association for the Study of Pain, this phenomenon is "an unpleasant sensory and emotional experience associated with actual or potential tissue damage, or described in terms of such damage." Do you truly understand what pain is after reading that definition? If not, don't feel bad; even scientists and researchers have a hard time describing, measuring, and categorizing pain. That's because pain is a very complicated physical and psychological experience. That said, here's a brief explanation of the very complicated pain cycle.

1. Throughout the body there are pain receptors, which some sort of stimulus, such as hitting your finger with a hammer or stepping on a tack, can

prompt into action. The receptors then send the message of pain as electrical impulses along the nerves to the spinal cord.

2. The spinal cord transmits the message to the brain. At the same time, depending on the stimulus, other messages may trigger a response. If you stepped on a tack, for example, you would quickly pull your foot up and away from it. This is a reflex response, but at this point, you are not yet consciously aware of the pain.

3. The brain receives the pain signal and processes it, and now you are aware that you hurt. Because all of this happens so quickly, it seems to you that you both reacted and felt the pain at the same time, but there was really a split second of time between the two events.

Types of Pain

Before we even tackle categorizing pain, here are the two main types of pain with which most people are familiar.

- **Acute pain** is short-lived and usually can be identified, observed, or described easily. A smashed finger, broken leg, migraine, or sore throat are typical examples of acute pain. This type of pain usually disappears within a few hours to a few days, but may last up to three months. Acute pain that lasts longer than a few weeks and up to three months is sometimes referred to as subacute pain.

- **Chronic pain** is long-term; that is, any pain that lasts for more than three months. This type of pain often adversely affects a person's quality of life. Chronic back pain associated with a dislocated disk or pinched nerve and cancer pain are examples of chronic pain.

Categories of Pain

When it comes to categorizing pain, you will find the types organized according to the source of the pain, how it originated, how it manifests itself, or whether it is associated with a medical condition. This list is an incorporation of the categories used by the U.S. Department of Health and Human Services and several institutions dedicated to the study and treatment of pain. Remember that within any category, pain can be either acute or chronic. To read more about treatments, see Chapters 3 (herbal remediess), 4 (vitamins), 5 (minerals), 6 (alternative supplements), 29 (prescription drugs), 30 (homeopathic remedies), and 67 (acupuncture and acupressure).

1 ARTHRITIS PAIN

Symptoms of the more than 100 different types of arthritis usually include pain and inflammation. Although inflammation is a healthy response to tissue injury (because it means that body fluids are bringing cells to the injured area to destroy toxins at the damaged site), it also causes increased pressure against the surrounding tissues and causes pain.

Common types of arthritis include osteoarthritis, rheumatoid arthritis, systemic lupus erythematosus, gout, and fibromyalgia.

Conventional treatment:

- Nonsteroidal anti-inflammatory drugs (NSAIDS) such as ibuprofen.
- The newer COX-2 inhibitors, celecoxib and relecoxib.
- Corticosteroid injections for more advanced cases.
- Exercise to build mobility and strength and thus help reduce pain.
- Application of deep heat and ultrasound to relieve painful joints.

Alternative approaches:

- Acupressure and acupuncture done by a professional.
- Chiropractic manipulation of the spine and joints.
- Dietary approaches. Some people benefit by identifying which foods they are allergic to and eliminating them from their diet. Common allergens include grains, meat, eggs, and dairy products. Some people are allergic to the nightshade vegetables, which include tomatoes, eggplant, potatoes, and green peppers. Others get pain relief by following a low-fat, low-protein, vegetarian diet.
- Herbs such as boswellia, bromelein, cayenne, ginger, and willow bark.
- Homeopathic remedies, including arnica, bryonia, and rhus toxicodendron.
- Nutritional supplements: Glucosamine and chondroitan are helpful for many people; vitamins C, B6, and E may also be useful.

2 GYNECOLOGICAL PAIN

This category encompasses any pain related to a woman's reproductive system. The most frequently occurring conditions of this type include painful menstruation, endometriosis, and premenstrual syndrome (PMS). Pelvic inflammatory disease (PID) is also common. Unlike the three other very common conditions in this category, PID results from an infection, which must be treated to bring about pain relief.

Conventional treatment:

- Analgesics, such as naproxen and ibuprofen.
- Antibiotics (for pelvic inflammatory disease).
- Hormones, in the form of birth control pills or as individual hormone therapy (estrogen, progesterone, or male hormones).

Alternative approaches:

- Acupressure can relieve cramping pain.
- Herbs such as black cohosh, valerian, and skullcap; for PID, try oregon grape or echinacea.
- Nutritional supplements, such as vitamin B complex, calcium, magnesium, and essential fatty acids.
- Yoga can relieve cramping and back pain associated with many gynecological conditions.

3 HEAD PAIN

Nearly everyone experiences at least one headache during his or her lifetime. Tension headache is the most prevalent type; others include sinus headache, migraine, and cluster headache.

Conventional treatment:

- Analgesics such as acetaminophen, aspirin, or ibuprofen for tension headache; antihistamines and decongestants for sinus headache.
- Prescription medications such as sumatriptan and zolmitriptan for migraines; for cluster headache, corticosteroids, methysergide maleate, and lithium carbonate may be helpful.

Alternative approaches:

- Acupuncture and acupressure to help relieve all types of head pain.
- Aromatherapy to relieve the pain of tension, sinus, and migraine headaches. Lavender, eucalyptus, peppermint, and rosemary oils have proven useful.
- Biofeedback to help calm migraine and tension headache.
- Chiropractic for tension headache to remove stress in the muscles; sometimes helpful for migraine.
- Herbs for tension headache include valerian and passionflower; for cluster headache, cayenne; and for migraine, feverfew.
- Homeopathic remedies for tension headache include belladonna, bryonia, and rhus toxicodendron.
- Meditation to relieve tension headache.
- Nutritional supplements, especially magnesium, to help reduce the pain of both migraines and cluster headache.
- Progressive relaxation exercises to relieve tension headache.

4 MUSCLE AND OVERUSE PAIN

Sprains and strains, torn muscles and ligaments, bursitis, tendonitis, bruises, fractures, and carpal tunnel syndrome fall into this category. And let's not forget the most common of muscle-related pain—back pain.

Conventional treatment:

- Analgesics, such as aspirin and ibuprofen.
- Corticosteroids; injections in some cases of carpal tunnel syndrome or tennis elbow.
- RICE: rest, ice, compression, and elevation.
- Surgery in severe cases of carpal tunnel syndrome.

Alternative approaches:

- Acupuncture for bursitis and carpal tunnel syndrome.
- Homeopathic remedies such as arnica cream applied to painful sites or oral rhus toxicodendron for pain.

- Nutritional supplements, including vitamin E to improve blood circulation and promote healing of damaged tissues; vitamin B6 to improve nerve inflammation; and vitamins C and A to promote tissue-building and repair of injured tendons.

5 Neurological and Neuropathic Pain

Neuropathic pain is caused by a disturbance in the path of pain signals as they are transmitted to the spinal cord, which then causes the brain to misinterpret the message. The cause of neuropathic pain is usually unknown, but in some cases it can be due to a growth that compresses nerves of the spinal cord, damage caused by surgery or other trauma, or chemical damage related to cancer treatment.

Inflamed nerve cells, such as occur with an infected tooth or with shingles, are examples of neurological pain. A broad term used to describe severe, sharp nerve pain is *neuralgia*. Sciatica and trigeminal neuralgia are two common neuralgias. Diabetic neuropathy is also associated with neurological pain.

Neuropathic pain is the most difficult pain to treat.

Conventional treatment:

- Prescription analgesics for mild cases and opioid drugs for severe cases.
- Anticonvulsants such as carbamazepine and phenytoin can relieve the pain of trigeminal neuralgia.
- Surgery to destroy the offending nerve is reserved for severe cases that don't respond to any medical treatment. A treatment called thermocoagulation uses heat from an electrical current to destroy nerve cells.
- TENS—transcutaneous electrical nerve stimulator—is a battery-powered device that is attached to painful areas using electrodes. TENS stimulates the nerves, which then may block the transmission of the painful impulses to the brain.

Alternative approaches:

- Acupuncture and deep tissue massage may relieve the pain of trigeminal neuralgia.
- Chiropractic may help sciatica.
- Homeopathic remedies: bryonia for the shooting pain of sciatica.
- Hypnotherapy and visualization can help people cope with chronic neuropathic pain.

- Nutritional supplements: Taking high doses of vitamin E (500 IU three times daily under a doctor's supervision) relieves the pain for some people with shingles. High doses of calcium and magnesium (1,000 and 400 mg, respectively) taken at bedtime may help sciatica.

6 PEDIATRIC PAIN

Infants and children experience special types of painful medical conditions, including teething, colic, ear infections, and growing pains.

Conventional treatment:

- Acetaminophen (do not give aspirin to children).

Alternative approaches:

- Acupressure can relieve pain associated with teething, ear infections, and colic.
- Herbs: For ear pain, a few drops of garlic or mullein oil in the ear can ease pain; use chamomile or peppermint tea for colic.
- Homeopathic remedies include belladonna and calcarea carbonica for ear infections, teething, and growing pains; and bryonia and colocynthis for colic.

7 POSTSURGICAL PAIN

Surgery—either oral or regular surgery—places a great deal of stress on the nervous and circulatory systems and compromises the immune system. The pain that follows the trauma of surgery can be quite severe, and proper management is necessary not only for comfort but to aid the healing process.

Conventional treatment:

- Analgesics, such as aspirin, acetaminophen, ibuprofen, and the COX-2 inhibitor relecoxib.
- Opioid analgesics, such as codeine, hydromorphone morphine, oxymorphone, oxycodone, and pentazocine.

Alternative approaches:

- Herbs, including bromelain and cayenne.
- Homeopathic remedies, including arnica and hypericum.

- Guided imagery and visualization.
- Meditation.

Other Categories of Pain

Other medical conditions that cause pain do not fit neatly into any of the previous categories. Although these conditions are diverse, conventional practicioners often treat these kinds of pain in similar ways, either with an over-the-counter or prescription analgesic, or with surgery. There is much more diversity, however, among the alternative treatments. The options are:

Burns

- *Conventional:* aspirin, acetaminophen.
- *Alternatives:* the herbs calendula or aloe; vitamin E liquid on the affected area.

Hemorrhoids

- *Conventional:* acetaminophen, an injection of phenol, cauterization (burning the end of the hemorrhoid), or surgery.
- *Alternatives:* acupuncture; herbal ointment of pilewort; homeopathic remedies of hamamelis, aesculus, or sulfur; nutritional supplements of psyllium; yoga.

TMJ (temporomandibular joint syndrome)

- *Conventional:* an over-the-counter analgesic or a muscle relaxant such as diazepam.
- *Alternatives:* biofeedback, acupressure or acupuncture, massage, chiropractic, relaxation exercises, guided imagery and visualization.

Ulcers

- *Conventional:* antacids, histamine H2 blockers (cimetidine, ranitidine, famotidine), and antibiotics.
- *Alternatives:* the herb licorice; stress-reducing strategies including biofeedback, meditation, massage, and yoga.

chapter forty-three

49 Ways
to Burn Calories

In the December 30, 1999 issue of the *New England Journal of Medicine*, researchers James Levine of the Mayo Clinic in Rochester, Minnesota, and Ioannis Pavlidis of the Honeywell Technology Center in Minneapolis, Minnesota, suggested that chewing gum regularly could lead to a loss of 10 pounds over a one-year period. If you're like me, you're prepared to lay in a year's supply of sugar-free gum tomorrow. Did you know that you burn 17 calories when you drink a 16-ounce glass of ice water? That's because your body needs to raise the temperature of the water, and that takes more energy than drinking room-temperature water.

Everything you do burns calories. If you simply lie in bed all day and don't move, you burn calories. That's because every function of the body—breathing, digestion, blinking—requires energy, and calories are energy.

How many calories an individual burns depends on many factors. Statements like "You burn X number of calories when you do Y" are not as simple as they first appear. The amount of calories you burn during an activity depends on, among other things:

- Your body size: If you weigh 90 pounds, 1 hour of vigorous tennis will burn about 350 calories. But if you weigh 200 pounds, you could burn about 700 calories.

- How much effort you put into the activity: If you jog a 14-minute mile, you will burn fewer calories than if you jog a 10-minute mile.

- The percentage of body fat and muscle: Exercise burns fat as well as calories. When you replace fat with muscle, you get a bonus as well. That's because pound for pound, muscle uses more calories to maintain itself than fat does. So the more muscle and the less fat you have, the more calories you can consume without gaining weight.

- Environmental factors: Jogging into a strong wind burns more calories than jogging on a windless day. Swimmers burn more calories in cold water and when swimming against a current than in warmer, tranquil water.

Exercise does more than just burn calories while you're doing it. Vigorous exercise can raise your metabolism (the rate at which your body burns calories) so that your body continues to burn fat for many hours after you stop exercising. For example, let's say you normally burn 100 calories an hour just sitting in a chair and 400 calories an hour running. If you were to sit in a chair for several hours after you ran for one hour, you would burn more than 100 calories per hour, about 20 to 30 percent more.

Are you ready to start burning? Here are some common activities and exercises, and approximately how many calories each will burn in an hour. The calorie cost is based on a 154-pound person. If you weigh less or more, the amount you burn will likely be less or more, respectively. By the way: If you have a chubby cow, let her chew her cud. Researchers Levine and Pavlidis also noted in their study that cows that chew their cud expend 20 percent more calories than their non-cud-chewing peers.

Activity	Calories Burned per Hour
1 Sitting	60–85
2 Talking on the telephone	60–85
3 Sleeping	60–85
4 Reading	60–85
5 Standing	120–150
6 Driving	120–150
7 Slow walking, 1 mph	120–150

Activity	Calories Burned per Hour
8 Walking on flat surface, 2 mph	150–240
9 Cycling, 5 mph	150–240
10 Horseback riding (walk)	150–240
11 Mopping the floor	240–300
12 Bowling	240–300
13 Cycling, 6 mph	240–300
14 Golfing, pulling a cart	240–300
15 Lawn mowing (power)	240–300
16 Walking, 3 mph	240–300
17 Badminton (singles)	300–360
18 Walking, 3.5 mph	300–360
19 Ping-Pong	300–360
20 Cycling, 8 mph	300–360
21 Golfing, carrying clubs	300–360
22 Tennis (doubles)	300–360
23 Raking leaves	300–360
24 Walking, 4 mph	360–420
25 Cycling, 10 mph	360–420
26 Roller-skating	360–420
27 Horseback riding (trot)	360–420
28 Canoeing, 4 mph	360–420

Activity	Calories Burned per Hour
29 Walking, 5 mph	420–480
30 Cycling, 11 mph	420–480
31 Tennis (singles)	420–480
32 Downhill skiing (easy)	420–480
33 Waterskiing	420–480
34 Cross-country skiing, 2.5 mph	420–480
35 Shoveling snow	420–480
36 Jogging, 5 mph	480–600
37 Cycling, 12 mph	480–600
38 Downhill skiing (vigorous)	480–600
39 Horseback (gallop)	480–600
40 Basketball	480–600
41 Ice hockey	480–600
42 Running, 5.5 mph	600–660
43 Cycling, 13 mph	600–660
44 Fencing	600–660
45 Basketball (vigorous)	600–660
46 Handball (social)	600–660
47 Cross-country skiing, 4 mph	600–660
48 Running, 6 to 10 mph	More than 660
49 Handball (competitive)	More than 660

25 High-Calorie Fast Foods (or How to Pack on the Pounds...Fast) and 40 Lower-Calorie Alternatives

Most of us identify high-calorie foods as having a lot of fat. We know that butter, oil, lard, and nuts are fattening, while cucumbers, carrots, and oranges are not. Simple enough.

Or at least it would be simple enough if most of us didn't live in denial about much of the other food we consume. You know about denial: It's that place in our heads where we believe we can eat more double-fudge and butterscotch chip cookies because the package says they're "low-fat."

The facts, as you probably know deep in your heart, are that "low-fat" and "no-fat" don't necessarily translate into significantly fewer calories. For example, the full-fat version of Skippy peanut butter contains 190 calories per 32 grams (5.9 calories per gram). Low-fat Skippy contains 180 calories per 35 grams (5.1 calories per gram). Another example is Oreo cookies. The full-fat version: 160 calories per 32 grams (5 calories per gram); the low-fat variety, 140 in 33 grams (4.24 calories per gram). Not much of a difference. But if you're in denial, you're thinking, "These are low-fat, so I'll have two instead of one." Net result: You've eaten more calories than if you had stuck with the full-fat version.

Quicker Isn't Better

Americans love fast food. It's convenient, there are no dishes to wash, and much of it, although laced with preservatives and other chemicals, just plain tastes good. Unfortunately, that's because it's loaded with tasty fat grams.

This list includes some of the highest-calorie foods on the fast-food market. Along with the number of calories for each serving, we've included the number of fat grams, just to make it interesting.

Bon appetit!

HIGH-CALORIE FAST FOODS

Food Item	Calories	Grams of Fat
1 Schlotzsky's Deluxe Original Sandwich	2,638	152
2 Schlotzsky's Turkey Original	2,083	104
3 Schlotzsky's Large Original	1,917	102
4 Schlotzsky's Cheese Original	1,857	98
5 Schlotzsky's Roast Beef & Cheese (large)	1,749	70
6 Denny's Appetizer Sampler	1,405	80
7 Denny's Double Decker Burger	1,247	80
8 Denny's Meat Lover's Skillet	1,147	93
9 Denny's Cinnamon Swirl Slam	1,105	78
10 Hardee's Monster Burger	1,060	79
11 Denny's Cinnamon Swirl French Toast	1,030	49
12 Jack in the Box Bacon Ultimate Cheeseburger	1,020	71
13 Burger King Double Whopper with Cheese	1,010	67
14 Schlotzsky's Chicken Breast (large)	1,008	15
15 Denny's Country Slam	1,000	66

Food Item	Calories	Grams of Fat
16 Schlotzsky's Albacore Tuna (large)	1,000	26
17 Denny's T-Bone and Eggs	991	77
18 Dairy Queen Chocolate Chip Cookie Dough Blizzard	950	36
19 Denny's Buffalo Wings	940	68
20 Carl's Jr. Double Western Bacon Cheese	900	49
21 Dairy Queen Chocolate Malt (regular)	880	22
22 Arby's Chicken Finger Meal	880	47
23 Boston Market Meat Loaf Sandwich with Cheese	860	33
24 Taco Bell Taco Salad with Salsa	850	52
25 McDonald's Big Xtra with Cheese	810	55

LOWER-CALORIE FAST-FOOD ALTERNATIVES

If you still wish to frequent fast-food restaurants, here are some lower-calorie alternatives to the gut-busters in the previous list. But remember: no dressing or sauce on the salads or sandwiches.

Food Item	Calories	Grams of Fat
1 Long John Silver's Side Salad	20	0
2 Schlotzsky's Small Garden Salad	25	1
3 Jack in the Box Salad	50	3
4 Carl's Jr. Garden Salad To Go	50	2.5
5 Wendy's Caesar Side Salad	100	4
6 Subway Turkey Breast Salad	101	2
7 Wendy's Deluxe Garden Salad	110	6

Food Item	Calories	Grams of Fat
8 Subway Club Salad	123	3
9 Denny's Grilled Chicken Breast	130	4
10 White Castle Hamburger	135	7
11 White Castle Fish Sandwich	160	6
12 Denny's Sr. Menu Pot Roast	160	6
13 Panda Express Chicken with Mushrooms	170	9
14 Taco Bell Taco	170	10
15 Jack in the Box Taco	170	10
16 Panda Express Broccoli and Beef	180	11
17 Long John Silver's Country Style Breaded Fish (1)	200	10
18 Taco Bell Taco Supreme	210	14
19 Subway Ham Deli Sandwich	224	3
20 Subway Veggie Delite 6" Sub	232	3
21 Subway Turkey Deli Sandwich	227	4
22 Taco Bell Tostada	250	12
23 Arby's Light Roast Chicken Deluxe Sandwich	260	5
24 Hardee's Hamburger	270	11
25 Taco Bell Country Breakfast Burrito	270	14
26 Wendy's Jr. Hamburger	270	10
27 KFC Tender Roast Chicken Sandwich without Sauce	270	5
28 McDonald's Hamburger	270	9
29 Whataburger Justaburger	276	11

Food Item	Calories	Grams of Fat
30 Jack in the Box Hamburger	280	12
31 Jack in the Box Breakfast Jack	280	12
32 Carl's Jr. BBQ Chicken Sandwich	280	3
33 Chick-fil-a Chargrilled Chicken Sandwich	280	3
34 Dairy Queen Chili Dog	280	16
35 Denny's Kid's Meal Burgerlucious	296	17
36 Blimpie Turkey Sub (6-inch)	320	4.5
37 Burger King Whopper Jr., no cheese	320	15
38 Scholtzsky's Dijon Chicken (small)	330	4
39 Long John Silver's Chicken Sandwich	340	14
40 Boston Market Turkey, no cheese or sauce	400	3.5

chapter forty-five

Your Risk for *78* Diseases, Factored by Family, Age, Gender, and Environment

What is your risk for developing heart disease? Diabetes? Gallstones? Would you be surprised to learn that only 6 to 10 percent of breast cancer cases are caused by genetics, and that a woman has a fourfold increase in her risk of getting breast cancer if her brother has had prostate cancer?

Sometimes the risk factors for a disease are readily apparent. Older age, for example, is a risk for Alzheimer's disease. It would be very rare to see someone in the thirties with the disease. And it is well known that smoking is a risk factor for lung cancer.

But not all risk factors are so obvious. The prostate and breast cancer connection is a good example. Many other little-known risk factors for common diseases and ailments are important for you to know. If nothing else, they can be a call to action.

The 78 diseases and medical conditions listed here cover all age groups. The "Family" category refers to the likelihood that the condition is passed along genetically; that is, that it runs in families. "Environment" refers to lifestyle habits or situations that are risk factors for or aggravate the disease. An "N/S" entry means the factor is Not Significant for that particular disease.

1 *Acute Leukemia* A blood cancer in which a large number of abnormal or immature white blood cells are produced by the bone marrow. There are two main types: acute lymphoblastic leukemia (ALL; abnormal lymphocyte cells) and acute myeloid leukemia (AML; abnormal myeloblast cells).

- *Family:* ALL and AML—N/S
- *Age:* ALL—Most common cancer in children. AML—More common in people older than 60.
- *Gender:* ALL—More common in boys. AML—Occurs in men and women equally.
- *Environment:* Most cases have no identifiable cause. Prior exposure to radiation or toxic chemicals is a risk factor.

2 *AIDS*

- *Family:* N/S
- *Age:* Leading cause of death in Hispanics and Blacks in the U.S. between the ages of 25 and 44, not because of age but because of less access to advanced medical therapies.
- *Gender:* N/S
- *Environment:* Unprotected sex with multiple partners; intravenous drug use.

3 *Alzheimer's Disease*

- *Family:* Sometimes runs in families.
- *Age:* Primarily strikes people 65 years and older.
- *Gender:* Women twice as susceptible as men.
- *Environment:* There is much debate over possible lifestyle or environmental risk factors for Alzheimer's disease. Some say exposure to toxic chemicals, such as aluminum, is a risk factor.

4 *Aortic Aneurysm* Enlargement of a portion of the aorta because of a weakness in the artery wall.

- *Family:* Sometimes runs in families.
- *Age:* Most common after age 65.
- *Gender:* More common in males.
- *Environment:* High-fat diet, lack of exercise, obesity, and smoking.

5 *Asthma*   Narrowing of the airways that results in shortness of breath and wheezing.

- *Family:* Sometimes runs in families.
- *Age:* About 50 percent of new cases appear in children younger than 10 years, but it can occur in people of any age.
- *Gender:* More common in males.
- *Environment:* Frequent exposure to tobacco smoke.

6 *Atherosclerosis*   The accumulation of fatty substances on the walls of the arteries.

- *Family:* Family history increases the risk of developing heart problems.
- *Age:* Tends to affect people older than 35.
- *Gender:* Premenopausal women are less likely than men of the same age to have atherosclerosis; but after menopause, the risk for men and women is about equal.
- *Environment:* High-fat diet, lack of exercise, obesity, smoking.

7 *Bladder Cancer*   Cancerous growths that develop in the lining of the bladder.

- *Family:* Heredity may play a role.
- *Age:* More common among people older than 50.
- *Gender:* Three times more common in males.
- *Environment:* Smoking, working in the rubber manufacturing or industrial dye or solvent industries; possibly nitrates in smoked meats, caffeine.

8 *Bone Metastases (Cancer)*   Secondary bone cancer, also known as bone metastases, are tumors that have spread to the bone from another area of the body. Bone metastases most often appear in the ribs, pelvis, skull, or spine, and are much more common than primary bone cancer.

- *Family:* Depends on the type of primary cancer that has spread.
- *Age:* More common in elderly people.
- *Gender:* N/S
- *Environment:* N/S

9 *Breast Cancer*

- *Family:* Family history increases risk: A woman who has a sister who developed breast cancer has a 2.5 times greater risk of getting the disease; her risk increases twofold if her mother had breast cancer before age 40; and her risk increases fourfold if her brother has had prostate cancer.

- *Age:* Postmenopausal women who are 50 or older are more likely to get breast cancer than premenopausal women.

- *Gender:* Fewer than 1 percent of cases occur in men.

- *Environment:* Exposure to hormones, especially estrogen, either naturally or through oral contraceptive or hormone treatment; obesity, high-fat diet, radiation, alcohol consumption.

10 *Carpal Tunnel Syndrome*   Pain and tingling that occur in the hand and forearm, caused by compression of a nerve in the wrist.

- *Family:* N/S

- *Age:* Most common between the ages of 40 and 60.

- *Gender:* More common in females.

- *Environment:* Work or leisure activity that involves repetitive hand and wrist movement.

11 *Cataracts*   Clouding of the lens of the eye, which results in loss of vision.

- *Family:* Sometimes caused by an abnormal chromosome.

- *Age:* Most common in people older than 75, but occasionally it is present at birth.

- *Gender:* N/S

- *Environment:* Exposure to the sun, contact sports, vitamin deficiencies, excessive alcohol consumption, cigarette smoke, air pollution.

12 *Celiac Disease*   Malabsorption of food due to the lining of the small intestine being damaged by a negative reaction to the protein gluten.

- *Family:* Sometimes runs in families.

- *Age:* Usually occurs in the first year of life.

- *Gender:* More common in females.
- *Environment:* N/S

13 *Cerebral Palsy*   A group of disorders that includes abnormalities of movement and postures caused by damage to the developing brain.

- *Family:* N/S
- *Age:* Damage can occur before or during birth, or during a child's early years.
- *Gender:* N/S
- *Environment:* N/S

14 *Cervical Cancer*   Cancerous tumor found in the lower end of the cervix.

- *Family:* N/S
- *Age:* Most common between the ages of 45 and 65.
- *Gender:* Women only.
- *Environment:* Unprotected sex at an early age, sex with multiple partners, smoking.

15 *Chlamydia Cervicitis*   The most common sexually transmitted disease, it is an infection of the genital tract in women.

- *Family:* N/S
- *Age:* Can affect sexually active women of any age.
- *Gender:* Women only.
- *Environment:* Unprotected sexual activity and sex with multiple partners.

16 *Cholecystitis*   Inflammation of the gallbladder.

- *Family:* Sometimes runs in families.
- *Age:* More common in people older than 40.
- *Gender:* Twice as common in females.
- *Environment:* High-fat diet, obesity.

17 *Chronic Fatigue Syndrome*   Prolonged fatigue (of at least 6 months' duration) accompanied by many other symptoms, such as headache, sore throat, tender lymph nodes, muscle and joint pain.

- *Family:* N/S
- *Age:* Most common between the ages of 25 and 45.
- *Gender:* More common in females.
- *Environment:* N/S

18 *Chronic Obstructive Pulmonary Disease*   Progressive damage to the lungs, usually caused by smoking.

- *Family:* In very rare cases, it can be caused by an abnormal gene inherited from both parents.
- *Age:* More common in people older than 40.
- *Gender:* Twice as common in males.
- *Environment:* Smoking; air pollution; airborne pollutants from a work environment, such as dust, noxious gases, or chemicals.

19 *Cirrhosis*   Irreversible scarring of the liver that occurs in the late stages of various liver disorders.

- *Family:* Most cases are not related to family history.
- *Age:* More common in people older than 40.
- *Gender:* More common in males.
- *Environment:* Long-term, excessive alcohol use.

20 *Colorectal Cancer*   Cancerous tumor of the lining of the rectum or colon.

- *Family:* It is inherited in some cases.
- *Age:* Becomes more common in people older than 40.
- *Gender:* Rectal cancer is more common in males; colon cancer is more common in females.
- *Environment:* Low-fiber, high-fat diet, alcohol abuse, obesity.

21 *Conjunctivitis*   Inflammation of the membrane that covers the white of the eye (conjunctiva) and the inside of the eyelids.

- *Family:* N/S
- *Age:* N/S
- *Gender:* N/S
- *Environment:* Wearing contact lenses; using cosmetics or eyedrops that cause an allergic reaction; exposure to ultraviolet light, smoke, or air pollution.

22 *Coronary Artery Disease*   A narrowing of the coronary arteries (which supply the heart with blood) that leads to heart damage.

- *Family:* Sometimes runs in families.
- *Age:* Likelihood increases with age.
- *Gender:* More common among men until age 60, then found equally in men and women.
- *Environment:* Obesity, high-fat diet, lack of exercise, smoking.

23 *Crohn's Disease*   Chronic inflammatory disease that can affect any part of the digestive tract.

- *Family:* Sometimes runs in families, and is more common among people of Jewish origin.
- *Age:* Most commonly occurs in people between ages of 15 and 30.
- *Gender:* N/S
- *Environment:* Smoking.

24 *Cystic Fibrosis*   An inherited condition in which the fluid- and mucus-producing glands have abnormally thick secretions.

- *Family:* Most common, severe, inherited disease among people of European and North American origin. Caused by an abnormal gene inherited from both parents.
- *Age:* Present at birth.
- *Gender:* N/S
- *Environment:* N/S

25 *Cystitis*   Inflammation of the lining of the bladder, resulting in painful, frequent urination.

- *Family:* N/S
- *Age:* More common in adolescent girls.
- *Gender:* Much more common in females.
- *Environment:* Sexual intercourse may trigger the condition in some women.

26 *Deep Vein Thrombosis*   Presence of a blood clot in a deep-lying vein.

- *Family:* Sometimes runs in families.
- *Age:* More common in people older than 40.
- *Gender:* Slightly more common in females.
- *Environment:* Obesity and prolonged inactivity (for example, being bedridden, lengthy automobile or plane travel).

27 *Diabetes Mellitus*   A chronic disease in which the body either cannot produce insulin, which allows the body to use sugar (glucose) for energy (type I diabetes); or the body produces an inadequate amount of insulin or cannot properly use the insulin it does produce (type II diabetes).

- *Family:* Sometimes runs in families.
- *Age:* Type I—Childhood or adolescence. Type II—Usually people older than 40.
- *Gender:* N/S
- *Environment:* Type I—Cause unknown. Type II—Obesity.

28 *Diverticulosis*   Presence of tiny pouches in the colon.

- *Family:* N/S
- *Age:* More common in people older than 50.
- *Gender:* N/S
- *Environment:* Low-fiber diet is a risk factor.

29 *Down's Syndrome*   A chromosome disorder that affects physical appearance and mental development.

- *Family:* Caused by an extra chromosome; more likely to occur in infants born to older women. Risk is 1 in 1,500 in women who conceive at age 20 and 1 in 100 in women who conceive at 37.
- *Age:* Present at birth.
- *Gender:* N/S
- *Environment:* N/S

30 *Eczema*   Patches of itchy, red, blistering skin; also called dermatitis. There are several types of eczema, including atopic, contact, seborrheic, and nummular.

- *Family:* Atopic—People with an inherited tendency to allergies and asthma are more susceptible to this form of eczema. Contact, Seborrheic, and Nummular—N/S
- *Age:* Atopic—Appears first in infancy and can recur throughout life. Contact—Can occur at any age. Seborrheic—Affects infants and adults. Nummular—Affects adults.
- *Gender:* Atopic, Contact, and Seborrheic—N/S. Nummular—More common in men than women.
- *Environment:* Atopic—May be aggravated by stress, extreme temperatures, or certain foods. Contact—Exposure to or contact with an irritating substance. Seborrheic—N/S. Nummular—N/S.

31 *Endometriosis*   A condition in which pieces of endometrial tissue (from the lining of the uterus) attach themselves to other organs in the abdomen.

- *Family:* Sometimes runs in families.
- *Age:* Most common between ages 30 and 45.
- *Gender:* Women only.
- *Environment:* Never having children, delaying pregnancy until later in life.

32 *Epilepsy*   A brain disorder in which seizures recur.
- *Family:* Some types run in families.
- *Age:* Most often develops in children and young adults.

- *Gender:* N/S
- *Environment:* N/S

33 *Gallstones* Stones, usually composed of cholesterol, pigments, and salts, that form in the gallbladder.

- *Family:* Sometimes runs in families; more common among Hispanic and Native American people.
- *Age:* More common in people older than 40.
- *Gender:* Twice as common in males.
- *Environment:* High-fat diet, obesity.

34 *Gastritis* An acute or chronic condition in which the lining of the stomach is inflamed.

- *Family:* Sometimes runs in families.
- *Age:* More common in people older than 50.
- *Gender:* N/S
- *Environment:* Smoking, alcohol abuse.

35 *Gastroenteritis* Inflammation of the lining of the stomach and intestines, usually caused by a bacterial or viral infection.

- *Family:* N/S
- *Age:* Most common in infants and children, but can occur at any age.
- *Gender:* N/S
- *Environment:* Unsanitary conditions, contaminated food or water.

36 *Genital Herpes* Painful recurring blisters on and around the genitals, caused by a viral infection.

- *Family:* N/S
- *Age:* Sexually active people of any age.
- *Gender:* N/S
- *Environment:* Unprotected sex with multiple partners.

37 *Glaucoma*   Abnormally high pressure of the fluid inside the eye. Two types: acute and chronic.

- *Family:* Acute—Sometimes runs in families; more common in Blacks and Asians. Chronic—Sometimes runs in families; more common in Blacks.
- *Age:* Most common in people older than age 60.
- *Gender:* N/S
- *Environment:* N/S

38 *Gout*   A type of arthritis in which deposits of uric acid crystals are deposited in the joints, especially in the big toe.

- *Family:* Often runs in families.
- *Age:* Most common between the ages of 30 and 50.
- *Gender:* Twenty times more common in males.
- *Environment:* Obesity, excessive alcohol use.

39 *Hemochromatosis*   An inherited disorder in which there is an excess amount of iron deposited in the body's tissues.

- *Family:* Caused by an abnormal gene that is inherited from both parents.
- *Age:* Present at birth but usually doesn't become apparent until after age 40.
- *Gender:* Much more common among males.
- *Environment:* Excessive alcohol intake aggravates the condition.

40 *Hemorrhoids*   Swellings around the anus and inside the rectum.

- *Family:* N/S
- *Age:* More common in adults.
- *Gender:* More common in females during pregnancy and childbirth.
- *Environment:* Obesity, low-fiber diet.

41 *Herpes Zoster (Shingles)*   A painful, blistering rash along the path of a nerve; it is caused by the chickenpox virus.

- *Family:* N/S
- *Age:* Most common in people between the ages of 50 and 70.

- *Gender:* N/S
- *Environment:* May be brought on by stress.

42 *Hypertension* Chronic high blood pressure that may damage the arteries and heart.

- *Family:* Sometimes runs in families; is more common among Blacks.
- *Age:* More common as people age.
- *Gender:* More common in males.
- *Environment:* Alcohol abuse, smoking, stress, high-salt diet, obesity.

43 *Hyperthyroidism* An overproduction of thyroid hormones, which leads to overstimulation of some bodily functions, such as metabolism, heart beat, anxiety, and bowel movements.

- *Family:* Sometimes runs in families.
- *Age:* Most common in people between the ages of 20 and 50.
- *Gender:* Seven to ten times more common in females.
- *Environment:* N/S

44 *Hypothyroidism* The underproduction of thyroid hormones, which causes many body functions to slow down.

- *Family:* Sometimes runs in families.
- *Age:* Most common in people older than 40.
- *Gender:* More common in females.
- *Environment:* An iodine deficiency is a risk factor.

45 *Irritable Bowel Syndrome* Intermittent abdominal pain, diarrhea, and/or constipation.

- *Family:* Sometimes runs in families.
- *Age:* Most common among people 20 to 30.
- *Gender:* Twice as common in females.
- *Environment:* Stress, some foods (for example, fatty foods, fruit, sorbitol) may aggravate the condition.

46 *Kidney Stones*   Deposits of crystallized stones in the kidney.

- *Family:* Inherited in some cases.
- *Age:* Most common between the ages of 30 and 50.
- *Gender:* More common in males.
- *Environment:* Dehydration, high intake of calcium.

47 *Liver Cancer*   Cancerous tumor that originates in the liver.

- *Family:* N/S
- *Age:* More common with increasing age.
- *Gender:* About four times more common among males.
- *Environment:* Alcohol abuse, intravenous drug abuse.

48 *Lung Cancer*   Cancerous tumor that develops in the lung tissue.

- *Family:* N/S
- *Age:* Usually seen in people between the ages of 50 and 70.
- *Gender:* More common in males.
- *Environment:* Smoking, occupational risk from exposure to asbestos, radioactive materials, nickel, and chromium.

49 *Macular Degeneration*   Progressive damage to the macula, the area near the center of the retina, where sharp vision occurs.

- *Family:* Sometimes runs in families.
- *Age:* Most common with advancing age, usually after age 70.
- *Gender:* More common in females.
- *Environment:* Excessive exposure to sunlight, smoking.

50 *Migraine*   A severe headache that is often accompanied by nausea, vomiting, and visual disturbances.

- *Family:* Sometimes runs in families.
- *Age:* Usually first occurs by age 30.
- *Gender:* More common in females.
- *Environment:* Stress, food allergies, lack of sleep, missed meals, menstruation.

51 *Multiple Sclerosis* A progressive disease of the nerves in the brain and spinal cord, which results in weakness, loss of sensation, movement problems, and vision damage.

- *Family:* Sometimes runs in families.
- *Age:* Usually develops between the ages of 20 and 40.
- *Gender:* More common in females.
- *Environment:* Stress and heat may aggravate symptoms.

52 *Muscular Dystrophy*   An umbrella term for various genetic conditions in which the muscles become wasted and weak.

- *Family:* Caused by an abnormal gene on the X chromosome.
- *Age:* Present at birth.
- *Gender:* Nearly all cases affect males.
- *Environment:* N/S

53 *Osteoarthritis*   Gradual deterioration of the protective cartilage that covers the ends of the bones in the joints.

- *Family:* Runs in some families.
- *Age:* Common among people older than 60; rare in those younger than 45.
- *Gender:* Twice as likely to occur in women than men.
- *Environment:* Obesity and repetitive, strenuous activity.

54 *Osteoporosis* Loss of bone density, which causes the bones to become brittle and susceptible to fracture.

- *Family:* Sometimes runs in families.
- *Age:* Common in people older than 50.
- *Gender:* Much more common in women.
- *Environment:* Poor diet, insufficient exercise, tobacco and alcohol use.

55 *Ovarian Cancer*   Cancerous tumor that develops in one or both ovaries.

- *Family:* Sometimes runs in families.

- *Age:* Most common between the ages of 50 and 70.
- *Gender:* Women only.
- *Environment:* Not having had children, late menopause.

56 *Ovarian Cysts*   Fluid-filled sacs that grow in or on one or both ovaries.

- *Family:* N/S
- *Age:* Most common between the ages of 30 and 45.
- *Gender:* Women only.
- *Environment:* N/S

57 *Pancreatic Cancer*   Cancerous tumor of the pancreas.

- *Family:* Slightly more common among Blacks and Polynesians.
- *Age:* More common in people older than 50.
- *Gender:* Almost twice as common in males.
- *Environment:* High-fat diet, smoking, alcohol abuse.

58 *Pancreatitis (Acute, Chronic)*   Sudden (acute) or long-term (chronic) inflammation of the pancreas.

- *Family:* Acute and Chronic—N/S
- *Age:* Acute—Most cases affect adults. Chronic—Most common in people 35 to 45 years of age.
- *Gender:* N/S
- *Environment:* Excessive alcohol use.

59 *Parkinson's Disease*   A progressive disorder of the brain that results in problems with movement.

- *Family:* Sometimes runs in families.
- *Age:* More common in people older than 60.
- *Gender:* Slightly more common in males.
- *Environment:* N/S

60 *Pelvic Inflammatory Disease* Inflammation of the female reproduction organs.

- *Family:* N/S
- *Age:* Most common in females between the ages of 15 and 24.
- *Gender:* Females only.
- *Environment:* Unprotected sexual activity.

61 *Peptic Ulcer* A damaged area of the lining of the stomach or the start of the small intestine (the duodenum).

- *Family:* Sometimes runs in families.
- *Age:* Stomach ulcers are more common in people older than 50; duodenal ulcers are most common in people 20 to 45.
- *Gender:* Duodenal ulcers are more common in males.
- *Environment:* Stress, smoking, unsanitary conditions, excessive alcohol use.

62 *Pneumonia* Inflammation of the air sacs in the lungs, usually caused by an infection.

- *Family:* N/S
- *Age:* Most common in infants, children, and the elderly.
- *Gender:* N/S
- *Environment:* Smoking, alcohol abuse, malnutrition.

63 *Polycystic Ovary Syndrome* Multiple, small, fluid-filled cysts in the ovaries that are usually caused by an imbalance in the sex hormones.

- *Family:* Sometimes runs in families.
- *Age:* Women of childbearing age.
- *Gender:* Women only.
- *Environment:* N/S

64 *Prostate Cancer* Cancerous tumor located in the glandular tissue of the prostate gland.

- *Family:* Sometimes runs in families; more common in Blacks.

- *Age:* Increasingly common in men older than 65.
- *Gender:* Men only.
- *Environment:* N/S

65 *Prostatitis*   Inflammation of the prostate gland, sometimes caused by a bacterial infection.

- *Family:* N/S
- *Age:* Most common between the ages of 30 and 50.
- *Gender:* Men only.
- *Environment:* Unprotected sexual activity with multiple partners is a risk factor.

66 *Psoriasis*

- *Family:* Often runs in families.
- *Age:* Depends on the type. Plaque psoriasis affects any age; guttate affects children and adolescents; pustular affects mainly adults; and inverse affects the elderly.
- *Gender:* N/S
- *Environment:* Stress can trigger an attack; use of some drugs, such as antidepressants, antihypertensives, beta blockers, and antimalarial medications.

67 *Pyelonephritis*   Inflammation of one or both kidneys, usually caused by a bacterial infection.

- *Family:* N/S
- *Age:* Most common between the ages of 16 and 45.
- *Gender:* Much more common in females.
- *Environment:* Possibly associated with sexual activity in females.

68 *Raynaud's Phenomenon*   Intermittent and sudden narrowing of the arteries in the hands, and sometimes the feet.

- *Family:* Sometimes runs in families.
- *Age:* Usually between the ages of 15 and 45.

- *Gender:* More common in females.
- *Environment:* Exposure to cold and smoking can trigger attacks.

69 *Rheumatoid Arthritis*   Chronic swelling, pain, and stiffness of the joints that often leads to deformity.

- *Family:* May run in some families.
- *Age:* Generally people older than 40.
- *Gender:* Affects three times more women than men.
- *Environment:* N/S

70 *Rosacea*   Long-term, sometimes chronic pimples and redness on the forehead and cheeks.

- *Family:* Often runs in families.
- *Age:* Most common between the ages of 30 and 55.
- *Gender:* More common among women.
- *Environment:* Use of alcohol, spicy foods, and coffee may prompt an attack.

71 *Schizophrenia*   A serious mental disorder in which people have an inability to function socially, loss of a sense of reality, and hallucinations, including hearing voices.

- *Family:* Sometimes runs in families.
- *Age:* Usually develops in males aged 18 to 25 and in females aged 26 to 45.
- *Gender:* N/S
- *Environment:* Stressful life situations can be a risk factor.

72 *Sickle-Cell Anemia*   An inherited type of anemia in which the red blood cells are distorted into a sickle shape.

- *Family:* An inherited condition caused by an abnormal gene inherited from both parents. Most cases occur in Blacks.
- *Age:* First symptoms appear within 6 months of birth.
- *Gender:* N/S
- *Environment:* Symptoms can be triggered by strenuous exercise and high altitudes.

73 *Stomach Cancer*   Cancerous tumor in the stomach lining.

- *Family:* More common in people with type A blood. Sometimes runs in families.
- *Age:* Most common in people older than 50.
- *Gender:* Twice as common in males.
- *Environment:* Smoking, certain foods (salty, smoked), high alcohol use.

74 *Systemic Lupus Erythematosus*   Inflammation of the body's connective tissues, which then damages the joints, internal organs, and skin.

- *Family:* Sometimes runs in families.
- *Age:* Usually occurs between ages 16 and 55.
- *Gender:* Much more common in females.
- *Environment:* Exposure to sunlight and stress appear to be risk factors.

75 *Testicular Cancer*   Cancerous tumor that develops within a testis.

- *Family:* Sometimes runs in families.
- *Age:* Most common between the ages of 20 and 40.
- *Gender:* Males only.
- *Environment:* N/S

76 *Ulcerative Colitis*   Chronic, intermittent inflammation and ulceration of the colon and rectum.

- *Family:* Sometimes runs in families; more common in Caucasians.
- *Age:* Onset usually occurs between the ages of 15 and 35.
- *Gender:* N/S
- *Environment:* More common among nonsmokers and ex-smokers.

77 *Uterine Cancer*   Cancerous tumor found in the lining of the uterus.

- *Family:* N/S
- *Age:* Most common between the ages of 55 and 65.

- *Gender:* Women only.
- *Environment:* Obesity, not having had children.

78 *Varicose Veins* Presence of swollen, distorted veins just under the skin's surface, usually appearing on the legs.

- *Family:* Often runs in families.
- *Age:* Most common in elderly people.
- *Gender:* More common in females.
- *Environment:* Pregnancy, prolonged standing, excess weight.

chapter forty-six

Recovery Time for *99* Diseases, Procedures, and Operations

In today's busy world, we're always concerned about time. How much time will it take for the mechanic to repair the car? How much time will you have to wait in line at the bank? Will you have time to run all your errands before your kids get home from school? Likewise, when an illness, medical procedure, or operation upsets our normal schedule and disrupts our sense of time, we typically want to know how much time it will take for our lives to get back to normal.

This list gives you the average amount of time it takes to recover from various illnesses, medical procedures, and surgeries. Your actual recovery time may differ, depending on your overall physical, emotional, and mental condition.

Illnesses

1 **Altitude Sickness:** Adverse reactions to high altitude, marked by headache, nausea, vomiting, stupor, shortness of breath, visual disturbances, and other symptoms, depending on the height people reach and how long they stay at that altitude. *Recovery:* 1 to 3 days.

2 **Athlete's Foot:** Contagious fungal infection of the skin on the feet. *Recovery:* Usually 3 weeks, but it commonly recurs.

3 **Bronchitis (acute):** Inflammation of the air passages of the lungs. *Recovery:* 2 weeks.

4 **Canker Sores:** Painful sores that form inside the mouth. *Recovery:* Most heal without scarring within 2 weeks, but they often recur.

5 **Chickenpox:** Contagious mild disease caused by the herpes zoster virus. *Recovery:* 7 to 10 days for children; typically longer for adults.

6 **Common Cold:** Contagious viral infection usually characterized by sneezing, sore throat, fever, runny nose, and headache. *Recovery:* Spontaneously within 7 to 14 days.

7 **Conjunctivitis:** Inflammation of the membrane (conjunctiva) that covers the white of the eye and the inside of the eyelids. *Recovery:* Bacterial conjunctivitis usually resolves within 48 hours with antibiotic treatment, but treatment should continue for up to 10 days. Viral conjunctivitis usually clears up within 2 to 3 weeks with treatment.

8 **Diphtheria:** Highly contagious throat infection. *Recovery:* Curable within 1 week, but recovery may take several weeks.

9 **Fifth Disease:** Mild, infectious viral disease characterized by a "slapped cheek" rash on the face. *Recovery:* 10 days to 2 weeks.

10 **Gastroenteritis:** Inflammation of the lining of the stomach and intestines, usually caused by a bacterial or viral infection. *Recovery:* Most people recover within a few days. In infants, diarrhea may persist for days or weeks.

11 **Gonorrhea:** Sexually transmitted disease that affects the reproductive organs and occasionally the eyes. *Recovery:* 1 to 2 weeks with treatment.

12 **Heat Stroke or Heat Exhaustion:** Illness caused by prolonged exposure to high temperatures, limited intake of fluids, or dysfunction of the temperature control mechanisms in the brain. *Recovery:* With prompt treatment, 1 to 2 days.

13 **Hepatitis (viral):** Inflammation of the liver caused by a hepatitis virus, most commonly hepatitis A or B. *Recovery:* People in otherwise good health, 1 to 4 months; a small percentage develop chronic hepatitis.

14 **Herpes Zoster (shingles):** Painful rash that is the reemergence of the chickenpox virus in adults. *Recovery:* Most recover within 2 to 6 weeks, but up to 50 percent of people older than 50 develop posttherapeutic neuralgia, prolonged pain that continues for months after the rash disappears.

15 **Impetigo:** Common, contagious bacterial skin disease. *Recovery:* 7 to 10 days with treatment.

16 **Influenza:** Common, contagious, respiratory viral infection. *Recovery:* Spontaneous within 7 to 14 days without complications; 3 to 6 weeks if complications occur.

17 **Kidney Infection (acute):** Noncontagious, bacterial infection of the kidneys. *Recovery:* 10 to 14 days with treatment.

18 **Laryngitis:** Inflammation of the larynx (voice box) and the surrounding tissue, resulting in hoarseness. *Recovery:* For viral laryngitis, spontaneous within 10 to 14 days; for bacterial laryngitis, with treatment, 7 to 10 days.

19 **Measles:** Highly contagious viral infection that affects the respiratory tract and skin. *Recovery:* Symptoms usually subside in 3 days.

20 **Migraine:** A severe headache that is often accompanied by nausea and visual disturbances. *Recovery:* A few hours to a few days.

21 **Mononucleosis:** Viral infection that affects the respiratory tract, liver, and lymph system. *Recovery:* Spontaneous in 10 days to 6 months. Fatigue frequently lasts for 3 to 6 weeks after other symptoms disappear.

22 **Mumps:** Viral disease that causes painful inflammation of the salivary glands. *Recovery:* Spontaneous within 10 days.

23 **Otitis Media (middle ear infection):** Inflammation of the middle ear, usually due to an infection. *Recovery:* The pain usually resolves within a few days with antibiotic treatment and analgesics. Mild hearing loss may linger for a few weeks.

24 **Pelvic Inflammatory Disease:** Infection of the internal reproductive organs of the female. If it was transmitted by sexual activity it is contagious. *Recovery:* With early treatment, 1 to 6 weeks, depending on severity.

25 **Pericarditis (acute):** Inflammation of the pericardium (thin membrane around the heart). *Recovery:* Curable within 6 months unless caused by cancer.

26 **Pertussis (whooping cough):** A bacterial infection that inflames the windpipe and the airways in the lungs, resulting in a violent cough that often ends in a high-pitched "whoop" in children. Adults don't usually have the accompanying sound. *Recovery:* Symptoms improve within 4 to 10 weeks, but a dry cough may persist for several more months.

27 **Pleurisy:** Inflammation and irritation of the thin membrane (pleura) that lines the lung and chest cavity. *Recovery:* Spontaneously in 2 weeks, if there are no complications.

28 **Pneumonia:** Inflammation of the air sacs in the lungs, usually caused by an infection. *Recovery:* Young individuals who are in otherwise good health usually recover within 2 to 3 weeks. In people with immune system disorders, the disease can be fatal.

29 **Pyelonephritis:** A very common kidney disorder in which one or both kidneys are inflamed due to a bacterial infection. *Recovery:* Oral antibiotic treatment can result in symptom improvement within 2 days. Recurrent pyelonephritis may need to be treated over 6 months to 2 years to help reduce the frequency of attacks.

30 **Respiratory Syncytial Virus:** Contagious respiratory viral infection that occurs in epidemics. *Recovery:* 7 to 12 days in mild cases.

31 **Rheumatic Fever:** An inflammatory complication of streptococcal infections that affects many parts of the body, especially the skin, joints, and heart. *Recovery:* Treatable but not curable.

32 **Rubella:** Mild, contagious viral illness that results in rash and other symptoms. *Recovery:* Spontaneously in 1 week.

33 **Scarlet Fever:** A contagious childhood disorder with a rash. *Recovery:* In 10 days with antibiotic treatment.

34 **Sinusitis:** Inflammation of the sinus cavities. It can be acute (usually caused by an allergy or virus) or chronic (often from a bacterial infection). *Recovery:* 3 weeks with treatment.

35 **Strep Throat:** An infection and inflammation of the pharynx by streptococcal bacteria. *Recovery:* Usually curable within 10 to 12 days with antibiotic treatment.

36 **Sty:** A pus-filled, painful swelling located at the root of an eyelash. *Recovery:* Usually resolves within a few days without treatment. If it does not, antibiotic treatment is usually needed, and the sty should then clear up within 2 to 3 days.

37 **Syphilis:** Sexually transmitted disease that causes widespread tissue destruction. *Recovery:* Curable in 3 months with treatment.

38 **Thrush:** Common fungal infection of the mouth. *Recovery:* 3 days with treatment, but it often recurs.

39 **Tonsillitis:** Inflammation of the tonsils, lymph tissue located at the back of the throat. *Recovery:* Improvement occurs within 2 to 3 days.

40 **Urethritis:** Inflammation of the urethra. *Recovery:* With prompt diagnosis and treatment, symptoms usually resolve within 24 hours.

41 **Vaginitis:** A yeast infection caused by *Monilia* or *Candida albicans*. *Recovery:* Usually curable within 2 weeks but often recurs.

42 **Valley Fever:** A pulmonary infection caused by inhalation of fungi in the soil. The disease sometimes spreads to the bone, skin, and brain. *Recovery:* If it doesn't spread, spontaneous healing within 3 to 6 weeks.

Procedures and Operations

43 **Aneurysm Removal:** Surgical removal of an aneurysm (a ballooning in the wall of an artery) and insertion of a synthetic graft to replace it. *Recovery:* 6 weeks.

44 **Appendectomy:** Removal of the appendix. *Recovery:* 3 weeks.

45 **Arthroplasty (hip):** Surgery to alter or reform the hip. *Recovery:* 6 weeks.

46 **Bone Marrow Aspiration and Biopsy:** Procedure to diagnose blood disorders such as leukemia and severe anemias. Both a fine-needle syringe and a large needle are used to obtain the aspiration and marrow, respectively. *Recovery:* Soreness at the collection site for a few days.

47 **Breast Augmentation:** Surgery to increase the size of the breasts. *Recovery:* 2 weeks.

48 **Breast Reduction:** Surgery to reduce the size of the breasts. *Recovery:* 4 weeks.

49 **Bunion Surgery:** Surgery to remove a bunion—an inflamed, thickened bony growth at the base of the big toe that can cause a foot deformity. *Recovery:* About 6 weeks before normal activity can resume.

50 **Carotid Endarterectomy:** Surgical removal of an obstruction in the carotid artery, usually caused by a buildup of cholesterol. *Recovery:* 2 weeks.

51 **Carpal Tunnel Repair:** Surgery to relieve pressure on the nerve and to remove any scar tissue in the wrist area. *Recovery:* 4 weeks.

52 **Cataract Surgery:** Removal of a diseased lens of the eye and implantation of an artificial lens. *Recovery:* 3 to 4 days.

53 **Cervical Biopsy:** A minor procedure that involves collecting a tissue sample from the cervix. *Recovery:* 2 to 4 days.

54 **Cesarean Section:** Delivery of one or more infants through an incision rather than through the birth canal. *Recovery:* 4 weeks.

55 **Circumcision:** Removal of the foreskin from the penis. *Recovery:* 3 weeks.

56 **Colonoscopy:** A diagnostic procedure that involves inserting a fiber-optic endoscope into the colon to view possible abnormalities. *Recovery:* 4 days.

57 **Colostomy:** Creation of an opening in the abdomen where the colon can be redirected to the outside of the body. *Recovery:* 6 weeks.

58 **Cornea Transplant:** Removal of a diseased cornea and implantation of a donor cornea. *Recovery:* 3 to 4 weeks.

59 **Coronary Artery Bypass:** Removal of a blood vessel from the leg or chest to be used to bypass one or more blocked arteries in the heart. *Recovery:* 6 weeks.

60 **Culdocentesis:** The use of a needle and syringe to collect a fluid sample from deep in the vagina, behind and under the cervix. *Recovery:* 1 week.

61 **Disk Removal (ruptured):** Removal of a damaged disk from the spine. *Recovery:* 5 weeks.

62 **Endometrial Biopsy:** Procedure to remove a tissue sample from the endometrium. *Recovery:* 1 week.

63 **Episiotomy:** An incision made at the exterior of the vaginal opening to create a larger opening for delivery of an infant. *Recovery:* 6 weeks.

64 **Face Lift:** Cosmetic surgery that involves removal of excess skin, fat, and tissue from the face to eliminate wrinkles, tighten the skin, and remove a double chin. *Recovery:* 6 weeks.

65 **Fractured Bone:** A broken bone. *Recovery:* Varies depending on the type of fracture and extent of tissue damage. Children heal faster; bones in the elderly often never heal completely.

66 **Hair Transplant:** Relocation of segments of hair-bearing skin to bare areas. *Recovery:* It may take several months to know if the procedure has worked, so recovery can take months.

67 **Heart Transplant:** Removal of a diseased heart and implantation of a functioning one. *Recovery:* 6 weeks.

68 **Heart Valve Replacement:** Removal of a damaged heart valve and replacement with a donor or artificial valve. *Recovery:* 4 weeks.

69 **Hemorroidectomy:** Removal of hemorrhoids. *Recovery:* 3 weeks.

70 **Hernia Repair (incisional):** When the intestine protrudes through a weakened area in the abdomen. *Recovery:* 2 weeks.

71 **Hernia Repair (inguinal):** When the intestine extends through an internal weakness or defect. *Recovery:* 6 weeks.

72 **Hysterectomy:** Surgical removal of the cervix and uterus; may also include removal of the fallopian tubes and ovaries. *Recovery:* 6 weeks.

73 **Kidney Removal:** Surgical removal of a damaged kidney. *Recovery:* 4 weeks.

74 **Kidney Stone Removal:** Removal of kidney stone(s). *Recovery:* 2 weeks.

75 **Laparoscopy:** Procedure that allows visual examination and some treatment of the pelvic and abdominal organs. *Recovery:* 6 days.

76 **Laryngectomy:** Removal of the voice box (larynx), usually because of cancer. *Recovery:* 4 weeks.

77 **Liposuction:** Use of suction equipment to permanently remove deposits of fat through an incision. *Recovery:* Depends on the extent of the procedure.

78 **Liver Transplant:** Removal of a diseased liver and implantation of a functioning one. *Recovery:* 6 months.

79 **Lumbar Puncture:** A lumbar puncture involves drawing a sample of cerebrospinal fluid from the spine as a test for meningitis or other nervous system conditions. *Recovery:* You should remain lying down for at least 1 hour after the procedure to avoid getting a severe headache.

80 **Mastectomy (complete):** Removal of one or both breasts and nearby lymph nodes. *Recovery:* 6 weeks.

81 **Mastectomy (lumpectomy):** Removal of a lump in the breast. *Recovery:* 2 weeks.

82 **Meniscectomy:** Removal of a damaged knee. *Recovery:* 6 weeks.

83 **Orchiectomy:** Removal of a testicle because of gangrene or cancer. *Recovery:* 3 weeks.

84 **Ovarian Cyst Removal:** Removal of a cyst from one or both ovaries. *Recovery:* 4 weeks.

85 **Pacemaker Implantation:** Implantation of a pacemaker into the chest. *Recovery:* 2 weeks.

86 **Penile Implant:** Device implanted in the penis to help it become erect. *Recovery:* 4 weeks.

87 **Polypectomy:** Removal of a polyp from the colon. *Recovery:* 12 days.

88 **Prostatectomy (through lower abdomen):** Removal of part or all of an enlarged prostate gland through an incision in the lower abdomen. *Recovery:* 6 weeks.

89 **Prostatectomy (transurethral):** Removal of part or all of an enlarged prostate gland using a cystoscope, a thin instrument that is inserted through the urethra. *Recovery:* 3 weeks.

90 **Rhinoplasty:** Cosmetic reconstruction of the nose. *Recovery:* 3 weeks.

91 **Splenectomy:** Removal of the spleen. *Recovery:* 4 weeks.

92 **Sterilization (female):** Tubal ligation, in which the fallopian tubes are cut and tied. *Recovery:* 2 weeks.

93 **Strabismus Surgery:** Correction of cross-eye. *Recovery:* 2 weeks.

94 **Thyroidectomy:** Removal of the thyroid gland. *Recovery:* 6 weeks.

95 **Tonsillectomy:** Removal of the tonsils. *Recovery:* 3 weeks.

96 **Tracheostomy:** An incision made into the trachea to create an airway. *Recovery:* 2 weeks.

97 **Tummy Tuck (abdominoplasty):** Removal of excess fat and skin from the abdominal area. *Recovery:* 10 weeks.

98 **Varicose Vein Removal:** Removal of swollen veins, usually in the legs. *Recovery:* 11 weeks.

99 **Vasectomy:** Male sterilization, in which a small section of each sperm duct is removed through the scrotum. *Recovery:* 6 days.

chapter forty-seven

Health Risks for Infants:
21 Typical Ailments
and What to Do about Them

The first 12 months in the life of a child are full of wonder, discovery, and learning for both child and parents. It is also a time when medical problems can be frightening, because during the first 4 to 6 months of life, the immune system is not developed enough to fight disease and infection effectively.

Most illnesses in infants are minor and usually disappear within a few days. Occasionally, symptoms such as fever, diarrhea, or vomiting are associated with more worrisome problems, however, or a child acquires a more serious disease. Below is a list of common symptoms and medical conditions an infant might typically experience, along with some tips on what to do about them.

1 **Atopic dermatitis**, also known as eczema, is a red, scaly, dry, itchy rash that may or may not be accompanied by blisters. It most often appears on the face, neck, backs of the knees, and the insides of the elbows. About 50 percent of all cases among infants resolve by age 18 months.

Cause: The cause is unknown, although it tends to occur in children who have a family history of asthma or allergies.

Treatment: To help prevent the infant from rubbing the itchy spots and causing them to bleed (which increases the risk of infection), keep the affected areas moist by giving the child lukewarm baths daily or by applying moisturizing lotions several times a day. Use small amounts of moisturizing soap and apply lotion to the baby's damp skin after the bath to seal in moisture. Dress the child in long-sleeved clothing and keep the nails short. Your doctor may recommend an over-the-counter corticosteroid cream or an antihistamine, but do not use these products without first consulting your pediatrician.

2 Blisters (sucking) can develop on the lips of infants. They are usually harmless and don't normally interfere with feeding.

Cause: The blisters can form as infants suck either on the breast or a bottle's nipple.

Treatment: Do not pop the blisters. Blisters generally heal themselves. If the blisters spread to other parts of the baby's body, contact your doctor.

3 Bronchiolitis is an infection of the bronchioles, the tiny breathing passages in the lungs. Six months is the most common age for this condition. Symptoms include sneezing, mild cough, runny nose, high fever, and wheezing. The skin around the nails and mouth may turn blue because the child cannot get enough oxygen.

Cause: The most common virus that causes this condition is called respiratory syncytial virus (RSV).

Treatment: Bring the child to a doctor, who can collect nasal samples to determine if the cause of the illness is RSV. Because antibiotics don't work against viruses, the doctor may prescribe a bronchodilator. A cool-mist vaporizer in the child's room aids breathing.

4 Colic is the term for unexplained, prolonged periods of crying. It affects about 20 percent of all infants. The condition generally disappears by age 3 months.

Cause: The cause of colic is unknown.

Treatment: Having a colicky baby can be stressful to parents. Motion seems to soothe many crying infants. Walking or rocking them or going for a ride in the car may help. White noise can also be calming. Run a hair dryer or vacuum cleaner where the infant can hear it. Natural remedies include herbal teas that contain ingredients to reduce gas. Cooled peppermint, chamomile, or lemon balm teas may help.

5 Common cold is the most frequent infection for people of all ages, and infants are not exempt. Symptoms include runny nose, chest congestion, sneezing, dry cough, irritability, and watery eyes. A cold in a newborn (2 months old or less) can be dangerous, so contact your doctor if your new infant gets a cold.

Cause: A cold can be caused by any one of many viruses.

Treatment: Acetaminophen can relieve discomfort, but give it only on the advice of your doctor. Prevent dehydration by giving your infant plenty of fluids.

6 Conjunctivitis, or pinkeye, is inflammation of the lining of the inside of the eyelids (conjuctiva). Symptoms include pain, a thick, crusty discharge from the eyes, and eyelids that are stuck shut, especially during sleep. The eyes may tear a lot, and the eyelids may swell.

Cause: Although conjunctivitis is often caused by bacteria, it can also be caused by allergies, viruses, or an irritating chemical or other pollutant.

Treatment: To remove discharge from the eyes, wipe the eyes with a clean cotton ball soaked in cool water several times a day. Wipe in a direction away from the infant's nose, and wash your hands before and after touching your baby's face, as conjunctivitis is contagious. Your doctor will determine if the condition is caused by a bacterial or viral infection. For bacterial infections, antibiotic eyedrops are usually prescribed; for a viral infection, over-the-counter eyedrops can be used to relieve the irritation until the condition clears up on its own, usually within 8 to 10 days. Natural treatments for conjunctivitis include an eyewash made from the herb eyebright or from chamomile in a cool solution, or the homeopathic remedies apis, argentum nitricum, or pulsatilla. See a knowledgeable professional for dosage instructions.

7 Constipation is the presence of hard, infrequent stools.

Cause: Among infants, constipation commonly occurs when they are first fed solid foods.

Treatment: Infant foods such as prunes, apricots, beans, and plums and a decrease in foods such as bananas, applesauce, and rice often corrects the problem. Changing the formula may also help, but consult your doctor before making a change.

8 Cradle cap is a common type of skin irritation that can occur in infants up to 6 months of age. Cradle cap is a harmless form of dermatitis that usually clears up on its own.

Cause: Cradle cap is caused by a buildup of scaly skin and oil on the scalp.

Treatment: Run unscented baby oil into the infant's scalp and leave it on overnight. The next day, wash the scalp and hair with a gentle shampoo and use a fine-tooth comb to comb out the dead skin. Keep the scalp clean and dry between treatments. The condition often returns, and the treatment remains the same.

9 **Croup** is an infection of the upper airway that is characterized by fever and a dry, barking cough that is worse at night. Other symptoms include loss of appetite, irritability, and fatigue. It is most common in children ages 6 months to 3 years. It commonly occurs in late fall and early spring.

Cause: Croup is caused by a viral infection.

Treatment: Most cases of croup can be treated successfully at home. Place a humidifier in your child's room to help make breathing easier. To prevent dehydration, give the child plenty of fluids. If the symptoms don't improve within 3 to 5 days, contact the doctor. He may give your child a breathing treatment. Natural treatments for croup include the homeopathic remedies aconite, spongia, and hepar sulphuris. See a homeopath for dosage instructions.

10 **Diaper rash** is a condition in which skin covered by diapers—on the genitals, thighs, and buttocks—becomes red and inflamed. Most cases of diaper rash last only a few days, but it can recur.

Cause: Moisture, not the type of diaper, is the culprit in diaper rash. Keeping your infant dry and clean is the prevention.

Treatment: An over-the-counter ointment that contains zinc oxide protects the skin. If your infant has developed an infection, your doctor may prescribe a topical antibiotic. A natural remedy for diaper rash includes a combination of sandalwood, peppermint, and lavender oils (2 drops of each) mixed with 4 tablespoons of a neutral oil such as almond or safflower and gently applied to the affected area.

11 **Diarrhea** is the passing of frequent, watery stools.

Cause: In infants, diarrhea can result from many different factors. These include prescription medication, especially those that contain sugar; starting solid foods too early; reaction to cow's milk; introduction of sugar into the diet; and infection of the stomach or intestines. A doctor should be consulted whenever an infant has diarrhea, especially if it is accompanied by fever, vomiting, or reduced urination, as the condition can become serious.

Treatment: Treatment will depend on the cause. Your doctor will guide you.

12 **Ear infection** (otitis media) is the most frequently occurring illness among infants and young children, after the common cold. They happen most often between the ages of 6 and 12 months. Symptoms include pain, which the infant usually indicates by pulling on his or her ear and by being irritable and fussy; fever, which usually ranges from 101 to 104 degrees F; and a yellow or white fluid that drains from the ear.

Cause: Ear infections are often associated with a throat or nose infection, a cold, or an allergy. Any of these conditions can cause the eustachian tube—a channel that connects the middle ear to the back of the throat and nose—to become blocked. This blockage allows fluid to collect in the middle ear, where it becomes infected, causing the eardrum to swell. Other risk factors for ear infections include exposure to secondhand smoke, having a weakened immune system, and having a family history of the problem.

Treatment: Doctors usually prescribe antibiotics, which can kill the bacteria that cause the infection, while acetaminophen or ibuprofen can relieve pain and discomfort. Follow the doctor's instructions carefully. Natural remedies include a few drops of warm garlic oil in the ear to reduce pain.

13 **Failure to thrive** is diagnosed for infants who do not steadily and progressively grow according to predetermined growth charts.

Cause: The major cause is inadequate nutrition, usually because of a feeding problem. Malabsorption, in which the infant does not digest food properly, is also common. An undetected problem with the kidneys, thyroid, lungs, adrenal glands, nervous system, intestines, or heart may also be the cause.

Treatment: Treatment depends on the cause, which, once corrected, results in normal growth.

14 **Fever** is not a disease but a symptom, usually indicating an infection. The body's normal temperature fluctuates from about 97.6 degrees F in the morning to about 99.5 degrees F in the late afternoon.

Cause: Fever is usually caused by a bacterial or viral infection. If an infant who is less than 3 months of age has a fever of 100.4 degrees F (rectal) or higher, contact your doctor immediately. A fever this high may indicate a bacterial infection that could affect various organs and cause serious disease, such as meningitis and pneumonia.

Treatment: In infants older than 2 months of age, acetaminophen can be given if the fever is higher than 102 degrees F, which usually reduces the temperature by 1 or 2 degrees within 2 hours. Ibuprofen can be used in children older than 6 months.

15 **Jaundice** is a yellow-green discoloration of the skin and the whites of the eyes. In the majority of cases, jaundice in infants is harmless.

Cause: Jaundice is common in newborn infants because their livers cannot keep up with the amount of bilirubin, a pigment formed naturally in the body. The excess bilirubin is dumped into the bloodstream and causes the skin and eyes to change color.

Treatment: Most cases clear up on their own. If the jaundice is more serious, a doctor may prescribe phototherapy, which involves placing the infant under white or blue ultraviolet B light. The light changes the bilirubin so that it can pass into the bloodstream and out with the urine.

16 **Respiratory Distress Syndrome (RDS)** is the most common lung disease in premature infants and can be deadly.

Cause: RDS is caused by a deficiency of a chemical called surfactant, which protects the air sacs in the lungs. Some premature infants don't have an adequate amount of this protection, and their lungs can collapse.

Treatment: Infants born with RDS go into an intensive care unit for oxygen treatment and may also receive a surfactant replacement. With treatment, most infants recover within 1 to 2 weeks.

17 **Roseola** is a common infection that develops in about one-third of all children between the ages of 6 months and 3 years. Symptoms include a rapidly rising fever that disappears and is followed in one to two days by a rash that looks like small red blotches all over the body.

Cause: Roseola is caused by a virus, but it is not especially contagious.

Treatment: This is a relatively harmless illness that can be treated with acetaminophen or ibuprofen to bring down the fever. The child should be given plenty of fluids and rest. Recovery is usually complete within a week.

18 **Sudden Infant Death Syndrome (SIDS)** is the sudden, unexplained death of an infant younger than 12 months of age. It is the main cause of death among infants between the ages of 1 month and 1 year.

Cause: The cause is unknown, although some risk factors seem to include premature birth; a mother who abused alcohol, tobacco, or other drugs during pregnancy; low birthweight; and inadequate prenatal care.

Treatment: Prevention, not treatment, is recommended for all parents, because there is no way to predict who will fall victim to SIDS. Infants should be placed on their backs for sleeping, and items that could cause suffocation (blankets, toys) should be kept away from their faces.

19   **Thrush** is an infection that often occurs in the mouth of both breast- and bottle-fed infants. Signs of thrush include creamy yellow or white spots throughout the inside of the infant's mouth and throat. They are painful when rubbed.

Cause: A fungus called *Candida albicans* is the cause of thrush. Some infants get thrush if their mothers had a vaginal yeast infection at the time of birth.

Treatment: Your doctor will prescribe an antifungal medication, which should resolve thrush within a few days. However, thrush can recur. If you bottle-feed your child, boil the nipples for 20 minutes before using them. If you are breast-feeding, always wash your breasts after your infant feeds.

20   **Vomiting**, unlike spitting up, can be a sign of medical problems. It is common for infants to spit up while they are being fed or immediately afterward. However, if the child is vomiting after two or more consecutive feedings, if his or her vomit is tinged with blood or colored brown or green, or if the child is vomiting and not gaining weight, consult a doctor immediately.

Cause: Vomiting can result from a virus that affects the ears, respiratory system, urinary tract, or central nervous system.

Treatment: Treatment depends on the cause. Contact your doctor immediately if your infant is younger than 1 month and has vomited more than once. You should also call your doctor if your infant has bloody, green, or dark brown vomit; is very irritable; has convulsions; has difficulty swallowing; or has not urinated in 8 hours or more.

21   **Whooping cough**, also known as pertussis, is a contagious infection that affects the lungs. It most often affects infants. A vaccine for whooping cough is given to most children, but it is only 70 to 90 percent effective. Initial symptoms include runny nose, low-grade fever, sneezing, and a mild cough. The cough progresses to severe bouts that can last up to a minute and deprive the child of oxygen. Some children make the characteristic "whoop" sound as they gasp for breath.

Cause: Whooping cough is caused by the bacteria pertussis. The disease is spread by inhaling the viral particles released during sneezing, coughing, and talking.

Treatment: Doctors usually prescribe antibiotics and recommend lots of liquids. Infants sometimes need to be hospitalized.

chapter forty-eight

25 Medical Conditions That Typically Appear between the Ages of 1 and 12

The toddler years—ages 1 to 3 years—is a time when children are learning to explore their environment and learning how to socialize. It is also a time when they are exposed to a vast number of germs and other nasty microbes. A couple of years later, they are off to school, where their exposure increases even more. But if children have been taught basic hygiene habits—washing their hands often, especially after using the bathroom and before eating, and covering their mouths and noses when sneezing or coughing—eat a healthy diet, and get adequate exercise, they will likely weather any infection that comes their way.

The list of symptoms and diseases presented here includes ailments that typically first appear in children between their toddler years and their teen years. Many of the conditions may also strike adults, but are not as common in that age group. Childhood diseases that were once common, including measles, chickenpox, mumps, and German measles (rubella), are now seldom seen because of vaccinations; but because outbreaks can occur, they are included as well.

1 **Asthma** is a chronic respiratory disease that affects the airways connecting the lungs to the windpipe. In people with asthma, these airways swell and become blocked with mucus, making breathing difficult. Asthma is the most common chronic disease among children: Approximately 5 million children and adolescents in the United States have asthma. Although it can happen at any age, most children develop asthma before age 5. It tends to run in families and affects boys more than girls.

Causes: Asthma attacks may be triggered by a respiratory infection, environmental irritants (e.g., tobacco smoke, pollen), emotional stress, certain drugs (e.g., aspirin, ibuprofen), certain foods (e.g., milk, beef, eggs, and nuts are common triggers), and exercise.

Treatment: Medications include bronchodilators (which relax the muscles in the airways), corticosteroids (fight inflammation), and cromolyn sodium (prevents release of chemicals that trigger an attack). Yoga has been shown to reduce stress-induced asthma attacks, and acupressure and reflexology can be used to help relieve symptoms.

2   Attention Deficit Disorder (ADD) and Attention Deficit Hyperactivity Disorder (ADHD) are the two main types of attention disorders. Children with either ADD or ADHD are easily distracted, have difficulty paying attention, and act impulsively. Many of them also lack motivation, are depressed, and have sleep disorders and learning disabilities. Children with ADHD are hyperactive as well. Although these behaviors can be found in many children, boys and girls diagnosed with attention disorders have these problems consistently for 6 months or longer. It is estimated that 3 to 5 percent of children have an attention disorder, although some experts believe the number is higher. Attention disorders tend to affect boys more than girls and also run in families. These disorders cannot be diagnosed until a child is 3 years old, because a certain level of development is needed to conduct the tests.

Causes: The exact causes are unknown. Possible causes include brain injury, abnormally slow brain development, effects from a mother who used drugs during pregnancy, or a nervous system abnormality. Some experts believe diet—especially the chemicals and other additives found in foods—can disrupt a child's chemical balance and cause the disorder.

Treatment: Options include drugs (e.g., Ritalin), dietary changes (elimination of sugars and food additives), behavior modification therapy, and family therapy.

3   Chickenpox is a highly contagious disease that can be prevented by a vaccine. Before the introduction of the vaccine in the early 1990s, most children got chickenpox by the time they were 10 years old. Today, there are far fewer cases. Symptoms include a mild fever and a rash characterized by fluid-filled blisters. Headache, chills, and irritability may also be present. After 5 to 7 days the blisters usually dry up and turn into scabs.

Causes: Chickenpox is caused by the varicella virus and is spread by direct contact with an affected person or by a virus that becomes airborne by an infected person's sneezing, coughing, or talking.

Treatment: Calamine lotion or oatmeal baths can help relieve the itching. Acetaminophen or ibuprofen can help reduce the fever and ease aches and pains.

4 **Constipation** is the passing of a dry, hard stool that may require straining and cause pain. The bowel habits of children vary widely; whether a child goes two or three times a day or once every two days may be fine for that child if the stool is of normal consistency.

Causes: Constipation can have many different causes. Among toddlers who are in toilet training, some become constipated when they withhold stool. It may also occur if the child is not getting enough fiber or fluids. If your child has prolonged constipation, hard stools with blood streaks, or a distended abdomen, contact your doctor.

Treatment: Depends on the cause. If your toddler becomes constipated during toilet training, you may need to stop the training until the constipation resolves. For constipation that results from poor eating habits, adding fiber or more fluids to the diet can often resolve constipation within a day or two.

5 **Diarrhea** is a common childhood symptom that can have many causes. Diagnosis depends on what other symptoms may be occurring along with the diarrhea, such as stomach pain or fever.

Causes: Diarrhea that is accompanied by a fever of 101 degrees F or higher may be a sign of gastroenteritis (an infection of the stomach and intestines), while bloody diarrhea may signal an ulcer or intestinal disorder. Excitement and nervousness, especially about going to school or making new friends, is a common cause of diarrhea. Other causes include use of antibiotics, failing to chew food properly, or drinking too much fruit juice. If diarrhea persists for several days, call your doctor.

Treatment: Treatment depends on the cause. Your doctor can recommend the appropriate remedy. To prevent dehydration, make sure you give your child enough liquids.

6 **Ear infections** often occur until a child is about 5 years old. In fact, by age 3, 80 percent of children have had at least one ear infection. Some children develop chronic ear infections that lead to hearing loss. Prolonged hearing loss during these early years can cause problems with language development and speech.

Causes: Ear infections are often associated with a throat or nose infection, a cold, or an allergy. Any of these conditions can cause the eustachian tube—a channel that connects the middle ear to the back of the child's throat and nose—to become blocked. This blockage allows fluid to collect in the middle ear, where it becomes infected, causing the eardrum to swell. This is called middle ear infection, or otitis media, the most common type of ear infection. Other risk factors for ear infections include exposure to secondhand smoke, having a weakened immune system, and having a family history of the problem.

Treatment: Antibiotics are usually prescribed, and acetaminophen or ibuprofen can be given for pain relief. Follow the doctor's instructions carefully for dosing of these drugs. Natural remedies include a few drops of warm garlic oil in the ear to reduce pain.

7 **Erythema multiforme** is a severe rash that most often occurs in children older than 3 years of age. Although most cases resolve without any problems, serious complications can result in some children. Symptoms include an itchy, red rash with some spots that look like a bull's eye. The rash usually appears mostly on the arms and legs, and sometimes it is raised, like hives. Other symptoms that may occur include headache, fever, diarrhea, sore throat, and muscle aches. In severe cases, the rash spreads to the eyes, digestive tract, mouth, and genitals and develops into open sores.

Causes: Some cases of erythema multiforme are a reaction to medication, such as penicillin or sulfa; others accompany viral or bacterial infections, such as strep throat, or to a vaccination. About 50 percent of cases have no known cause.

Treatment: If the case is caused by a medication, the drug should be stopped immediately. A doctor can prescribe corticosteroids to help reduce inflammation and antihistamines to relieve itching. The rash usually disappears in 2 to 4 weeks, but it can recur.

8 **Febrile seizures** are convulsions and loss of consciousness resulting from a rapidly rising fever. They occur in up to 5 percent of children, usually between the ages of 6 months and 5 years. About one-third of children who experience one febrile seizure will have at least one more. Signs of febrile seizure include a fever that rises quickly, usually associated with an infection. The child then loses consciousness and begins to have sudden, uncontrolled body movements. Some children also lose bowel and urinary functioning. A seizure can last up to 15 minutes, after which the child regains consciousness. In most cases, the child suffers no harm from the seizure.

Cause: Febrile seizures tend to run in families. They are apparently brought on by the sudden rise in body temperature, but no one knows why some children develop seizures while others do not.

Treatment: To help prevent a child from harm, parents should ease the child onto the ground and remove any objects in the immediate area. Once the seizure has stopped, first make sure the child is breathing, then call your doctor. Acetaminophen or ibuprofen can be given to help reduce the fever.

9   **Fifth disease**, also known as erythema infectiosum, is a viral infection that causes a rash on the arms, cheeks, and legs. It appears most often among children 5 to 11 years old and during the winter and spring. Symptoms may include mild fever, body aches, mild cold symptoms, and irritability, followed by an itchy rash.

Cause: The viral infection is spread in the air through coughing and sneezing.

Treatment: Fifth disease is harmless for most children and no treatment is needed. Children with a compromised immune system (e.g., sickle-cell anemia or cancer) should be treated by a doctor. Oatmeal baths or topical corticosteroid cream can be used to reduce the itching.

10   **German measles**, also known as rubella, is a contagious infection against which children are vaccinated usually at 12 to 15 months of age and again at 4 to 6 years. Symptoms include a mild fever, body rash, and swollen glands in the neck and behind the ears.

Cause: German measles is caused by a virus that is spread when an infected individual sneezes, coughs, or speaks.

Treatment: Most cases don't require any treatment except plenty of fluids and rest. Acetaminophen can be given to help reduce fever, and oatmeal baths or calamine lotion can relieve itching.

11   **Hand-foot-and-mouth disease** is a viral infection that causes painful sores in the throat and mouth and a rash on the feet and hands. It most commonly affects children who are in day care or nursery school and rarely is seen in children older than 10. The first signs of the disease are a sudden fever from 100 degrees to 103 degrees F, a runny nose, and sore throat. These are followed by blisters in the mouth and throat, which make eating painful. Sometimes the rash spreads. Symptoms are generally mild and disappear within 10 days.

Causes: The virus spreads by coughing or sneezing, when children fail to wash their hands after going to the bathroom, or by touching the open blisters of an infected person.

Treatment: Acetaminophen can be given to reduce fever. Cold foods and liquids can help ease mouth pain.

12 **Intussusception** is an intestinal disorder in which the intestine folds in on itself, partly or completely blocking the digestion of food or the absorption of nutrients. It occurs most often in children 6 months to 2 years old, but is seen in older children as well. Signs of intussusception include sudden abdominal pain, vomiting, irritability, and diarrhea followed by stool that has a jelly consistency.

Cause: The cause is unknown. Some experts believe it may be caused by a viral infection.

Treatment: A barium enema is usually used to treat this disorder. The pressure from the enema usually eliminates the fold. If this is unsuccessful, surgery is usually required.

13 **Juvenile rheumatoid arthritis (JRA)** is the persistent inflammation of a child's joints and internal organs that lasts for months. The disease typically begins between the ages of 2 and 5 years or 9 and 12 years and affects the elbows, ankles, and knees most often. Other symptoms of the disease are chronic fever and anemia. More than 20,000 children in the United States have JRA. There are three types of JRA: pauciarticular (meaning affecting "few joints") is the most common; polyarticular (meaning "affecting many joints") is the next most common; and systemic (meaning "throughout the body"), which affects joints and internal organs.

Cause: The cause is unknown, although experts do know that it is the result of an abnormal response by the immune system. It tends to run in families.

Treatment: Doctors can prescribe ibuprofen, aspirin, or other anti-inflammatory drugs for mild to moderate cases, or corticosteroids for severe cases. Physical therapy and a regular exercise program are often recommended to help retain flexibility in the joints. JRA resolves in most children by the time they are young adults.

14 **Lactose intolerance** is an inability to digest a sugar known as lactose, which is found in milk and milk products, because of an inadequate amount of an enzyme called lactase.

Cause: This condition can be inherited or acquired, and usually develops in children at 5 years and older. Symptoms include bloating, watery diarrhea, vomiting, and stomach cramps after eating dairy products.

Treatment: The best treatment is to avoid milk and its products and to substitute similar soy products, such as soy milk, soy yogurt, and soy-based frozen desserts. Lactose-free baby formulas are available, as are lactase enzyme supplements that can help children digest lactose in milk.

15 **Measles**, also know as rubeola, is a highly contagious, viral disease that is spread by coughing and sneezing. The first symptoms of measles include runny nose, hacking cough, red eyes, and low-grade fever, followed by the appearance of small red spots that first appear in the mouth and then spread to the body. Fortunately, since the development of a vaccine, measles has become a rarity these days.

Cause: Measles is caused by a virus that is spread through coughing, sneezing, and talking.

Treatment: To treat the fever, give the child acetaminophen and lots of fluids. A humidifier in the child's room can help relieve the coughing. The disease usually clears up in 7 to 10 days.

16 **Meningitis** is a contagious disease that affects the meninges, the lining that covers the brain and spinal cord. Although it is more common among children younger than 5, it can affect children of any age. Meningitis may develop after a cold, throat infection, flu, or other illness that compromises the immune system. Signs and symptoms include nausea, fever, irritability, vomiting, severe headache, stiff neck, back and shoulder pain, and sensitivity to light. Some children develop a rash.

Causes: Meningitis can be caused by the bacterium *Haemophilus influenzae* type b, most often seen in children ages 3 months to 3 years; or *Neisseria meningitidis* and *Streptococcus pneumoniae*, which is seen in older children. Meningitis can also be caused by a group of viruses called enteroviruses.

Treatment: Intravenous antibiotics are given for bacterial meningitis, along with plenty of fluids and rest. Viral meningitis is mostly treated with fluids and rest.

17 **Molluscum contagiosum** is a skin infection that is common among young children. It is characterized by small, round, raised bumps that are smooth and pearly white. The bumps are filled with a cheesy substance, which contains the infection. Scratching or breaking open the bumps will spread the infection to other parts of the body or to other people.

Cause: Molluscum contagiosum is caused by a virus and can be spread by direct contact or by sharing towels or swimming in a pool with an infected person.

Treatment: A doctor can remove the bumps by applying chemicals that kill the virus or by cutting each bump open and removing the center. These treatments will need to be repeated every few weeks. The bumps usually disappear by themselves within several months to 2 years.

18   **Mumps** is a contagious viral infection that causes the salivary glands in the back of the cheeks to swell. It most often affects children between the ages of 2 and 12 years. Although most children are vaccinated against this disease, those who are not immunized are susceptible to the disease, as are the approximately 5 percent of children for whom the vaccine does not work. In addition to swollen salivary glands, other symptoms may include fever, loss of appetite, and headache. Infrequently, mumps infection spreads to the ovaries, testes, brain, or pancreas.

Causes: The virus is spread by sneezing, talking, and coughing, or by direct contact with the saliva of an infected person.

Treatment: There is no treatment for mumps. An ice or heat pack can be placed on the swollen area to help relieve any pain. Acetaminophen also can be given for pain.

19   **Obesity** among children is defined as weighing 20 percent or more over ideal body weight for the child's height and sex. Up to 10 percent of children younger than age 12 are obese in the United States. These children risk developing high blood pressure, heart disease, diabetes, gallbladder disease, arthritis, kidney disease, and cancer at a younger age than other adults.

Causes: Eating too many fatty and sugary foods and lack of sufficient exercise are the two main causes of childhood obesity.

Treatment: The best treatment is attention to a healthy diet and regular exercise. Diet drugs are not recommended for use in children.

20   **Pica** is an abnormal eating behavior in which children eat things that are not food, including dirt, plaster, wood, animal feces, paint, hair, or clay. Up to 20 percent of children younger than 6 years old practice this behavior. Most children outgrow it, but some carry the behavior into adulthood.

Causes: Pica is more common among children who lack sufficient emotional and intellectual stimulation. Anemia and lead poisoning often result from pica.

Treatment: Counseling is needed to help these children change their behavior. Unsafe substances need to be hidden or stored away from where the children can reach them.

21   **Pigeon toe** is a minor deformity in which the feet and toes point inward. It is extremely common among children 2 to 4 years old, and usually resolves by the time they are 8.

Cause and Treatment: Once a doctor has ruled out any bone problems, treatment is usually not needed. Children can do specific exercises to help strength the leg muscles. Special orthopedic shoes may be required in severe cases.

22   **Pinworms** are minute worms that take up residence in the intestines. The anus of a child with pinworms is red and irritated, and the child may be restless and scratch the area, especially during sleep. In girls, pinworms may invade the vagina or urethra and cause itching, irritation, and a vaginal discharge.

Causes: Pinworm eggs can enter the body on contaminated fingers, toys, or toilet seats, or be inhaled from the air.

Treatment: The goal is to break the cycle of reinfection, which takes up to 3 weeks. Children should avoid putting their hands or fingers into their mouths and their nails should be cut short. Contaminated bedding, clothing, and towels should be washed in hot, soapy water. If this attempt does not work, medication can be taken by the child and all members of the family to avoid infestation.

23   **Scarlet fever** is a contagious bacterial infection that most often affects children between the ages of 2 and 10 years. Symptoms include a bright red rash that begins on the neck, groin, and armpits, and then spreads to the back, chest, and extremities. It is accompanied by a bright red tongue, high fever, sore throat, swollen glands, vomiting, and coughing.

Cause: Scarlet fever usually develops after a bout of streptococcal throat infection.

Treatment: Antibiotics are the usual treatment. Acetaminophen or ibuprofen for the fever and plenty of liquids to prevent dehydration are recommended.

24   **Strep infection** is a contagious infection that is most common among school-age children. It affects the throat most often, but it can also infect the skin. Strep is spread by sneezing, coughing, and talking or, in the case of skin strep infection, through a wound or cut. Symptoms of strep throat include sore throat, fever, and tender, swollen glands in the neck. Skin strep causes red, swollen, tender areas that drain pus.

Cause: The streptococcus bacteria cause strep infections.

Treatment: Your doctor will prescribe antibiotics, plenty of fluids, and acetaminophen for fever and pain. Gargling with salt water helps relieve the sore throat.

25 **Tonsillitis** is inflammation of the two small masses of tissue on both sides of the back of the throat. Tonsillitis affects most children at least once, and it is most common in children between the ages of 5 and 10 years. Symptoms include red, sore, swollen tonsils and difficulty swallowing. Fever, chills, headache, and bad breath may also occur. Ear pain and difficulty breathing often accompany severe tonsillitis.

Cause: Tonsillitis occurs when the tonsils cannot handle the bacteria and viruses that invade the body.

Treatment: Your doctor will do a culture to determine the cause of the tonsillitis. If the cause is bacteria, he or she will prescribe antibiotics. Children who have tonsillitis caused by a virus should not take antibiotics. Acetaminophen to relieve the pain, plenty of fluids, and rest are prescribed for all cases.

chapter forty-nine

10 Common Health Problems for Kids between 12 and 20

Between the ages of 12 and 20, the adolescent years, children rapidly go through a tremendous number of intense physical, social, and psychological changes. The big event of the adolescent years is the onset of puberty (from the Latin *puber* for "adult"), which is the stage of maturation during which girls and boys become physically capable of reproduction. Although this fact is enough to frighten some parents into wanting to lock their teenagers up until adulthood, puberty does have purposes other than driving parents crazy.

What we call puberty is actually a host of effects that result from the so-called "raging hormones" secreted by the endocrine glands. Not all the changes that happen to kids at this age are related to the reproductive system, however. The growth hormone, for example, causes more dramatic increases in height and weight than in earlier years, and the percentage of body fat tends to increase in girls and decrease in boys.

Health concerns that affect adolescents are, for the most part, associated with hormonal changes and tend to present themselves in the form of mind–body conditions. This isn't surprising. After all, the teen years are difficult. Seeking acceptance from others while struggling to understand oneself; dealing with physical changes that may be upsetting or baffling; and coping with huge emotional swings that seem to come and go of their own accord would be a tall order for anyone.

Here are 10 typical health concerns that face adolescents. Most can be handled easily with medical intervention, but remember—a dose of our understanding, patience, and guidance doesn't hurt either.

1 **Acne.** Approximately 80 percent of teenagers experience some degree of acne. Girls tend to get acne earlier than do boys, but boys generally get more severe cases. Most of the pimples, pustules, and cysts of acne appear on the face, chest, upper back, and shoulders.

Cause: The surge in hormone production during puberty stimulates the production of an oily substance called sebum, which is found in sebaceous glands in the skin. These glands are more numerous in the areas where acne most often appears. Although sebum normally reaches the skin surface without a problem, it can result in a pimple or blackhead if the channels leading from the glands to the skin become blocked by dead cells. It's not known why some teens suffer with severe acne while others have little or no problem. It is not believed to be caused by diet or dirt on the skin.

Treatment: Medications commonly used to treat acne include benzoyl peroxide, which kills skin bacteria; tretinoin, which helps unclog pores and eliminates blackheads; and antibiotics, which can reduce bacteria on the skin. The prescription drug isotretinoin (Accutane) is very potent and can cause significant side effects such as liver problems and birth defects if taken during pregnancy. Azelaic acid (Azelex) is a grain-based topical drug that inhibits skin bacteria and decreases the sebum that plugs the pores. Among herbal remedies, tea tree oil (as a topical) and calendula or goldenseal infusions (strong teas) may be helpful.

2 **Chlamydia.** The sexually transmitted disease chlamydia is a bacterial disease that is very common among young adults and teenagers. The Centers for Disease Control and Prevention report that 50 percent of cases of chlamydia reported in 1995 were among teenagers. The typical case of chlamydia, says the CDC, is female and between the ages of 12 and 19. It's been estimated that 4 million people in the United States have the disease, yet many people don't know they are infected: About 75 percent of infected women and half of infected men are symptom-free. Too often, women discover they had chlamydia years earlier when they try to get pregnant and learn they are infertile from the disease.

Cause: Chlamydia is transmitted through sexual contact and is caused by the bacterium *Chlamydia trachomatis.*

Treatment: Chlamydia can easily be treated and cured with antibiotics. An individual's sex partner or partners need to be treated as well.

3 Depression. It's been estimated that at least 5 percent of adolescents have a major depressive problem—not just a case of feeling sad or blue, but a chronic, deeply disturbed mood that lasts for months. Depression is often difficult to detect in teenagers because their depressive behaviors are often taken as "normal" adolescent defiance or acting out. But depression among teens can be very serious. Suicide is the third leading cause of death among people 15 to 24. A study conducted by the Centers for Disease Control and Prevention found that 27 percent of high school students questioned had considered suicide, 16 percent had made a plan, and 8 percent had already attempted it.

Depression appears in twice as many girls as boys. Signs of the illness in an adolescent can include long-term sadness, loss of enthusiasm in once-enjoyed activities, angry outbursts, and acting out by using drugs, engaging in sexual activity, fighting, and criminal activities. Physical complaints may include fatigue, insomnia, wanting to sleep all the time, loss of appetite, or uncontrollable hunger.

Cause: May include social pressures, high parental expectations, significant losses (death of someone close, or move to a new area and loss of friends), family crisis (divorce, remarriage, introduction of stepchildren), or heredity.

Treatment: Antidepressants, cognitive behavioral therapy, or often both are recommended, depending on the severity of the depression.

4 Dysmenorrhea (painful menstruation). When a young woman's menstrual cycle first begins, she is likely to experience few if any problems except for minor cramping and a headache. For some, however, cramps can be severe and may be accompanied by nausea, diarrhea, headache, and difficulty with concentration.

Cause: Chemicals called prostaglandins, which are released into the bloodstream during menstruation, cause adverse effects in some women. Among the most common effects are muscle contractions of the uterus, which translate into painful cramps. Prostaglandins are also responsible for the other symptoms associated with menstruation.

Treatment: Over-the-counter medications such as ibuprofen, naproxen, and ketoprofen reduce inflammation and inhibit the activity of the prostaglandins. Other pain relievers without prostaglandin-hindering actions may also be helpful, including acetaminophen (Tylenol and others) and combination products such as Midol and Pamprin. Herbal remedies include dong quai, valerian, feverfew, and cramp bark. A heating pad on the lower abdomen can provide some relief.

5 **Eating disorders.** The eating disorders anorexia nervosa and bulimia are all too common among teenagers—an estimated 10 percent of teenage girls have one or both of these disorders. Boys are less affected, but it is more common among them than once thought. Anorexia nervosa is a condition in which self-imposed starvation leads to a body weight that is at least 15 percent lower than the norm for a person's age and height. Adolescents with anorexia nervosa are typically high-achievers and perfectionists, constantly trying to please family and friends but always feeling as if they are failing. In an attempt to have control over something in their lives, they say "no" to food and relentlessly starve themselves. They suffer from low self-esteem and have a severely distorted body image, believing they are fat when they are in fact often dangerously thin. A small percentage of these kids die of the disease, and most have residual effects such as poor bone density, heart damage, and among girls, menstrual problems in later years once they recover from the weight loss.

Teens with bulimia binge on large quantities of food and then purge their bodies by vomiting and using laxatives. Many bulimics appear to be of normal weight, but some alternate their binges with very low-calorie diets and experience weight fluctuations. Bulimia can cause serious health problems, including hormonal imbalance; damage to the heart, liver, and other organs; dehydration; and a deficiency of important nutrients.

Causes: Factors that contribute to these eating disorders include social and cultural pressures to be thin, especially for women, as a way to be successful and desirable; a perfectionist personality; and an imbalance of neurotransmitters in the brain.

Treatment: A team approach is usually needed to treat these disorders, including individual therapy, family counseling, and the medical help of a family physician, nutritionist, and sometimes medication. Many of these young people also suffer from depression, substance abuse, and anxiety.

6 **Mononucleosis.** Often referred to as mono, this disease is an acute viral infection that occurs most commonly during adolescence. Symptoms include headache, fatigue, and a low-grade fever, all of which last a few days. These symptoms are followed by a sore throat, a higher fever, and swollen lymph nodes, and occasionally swollen tonsils, nausea, and vomiting. These symptoms usually last for several weeks, then slowly resolve. Fatigue and an enlarged spleen, which causes some abdominal tenderness, may linger for several weeks longer.

Cause: The Epstein-Barr virus is the culprit, a virus that infects nearly everyone by the time they reach adulthood. In most people, however, the infection occurs during early childhood and causes mild symptoms or none at all.

Treatment: There are no effective drugs against the Epstein-Barr virus, so the best treatment is rest, ibuprofen or acetaminophen for pain relief or fever, and liquids.

7   Plantar warts. These benign tumors, which appear on the bottoms of the feet, affect teenagers more often than adults or children. They can be quite painful, and if not treated, they can grow to more than an inch in circumference and spread into clusters. Infections are most common in moist environments, such as gym locker rooms and showers, which explains their prevalence among teenage boys, especially those involved in team sports.

Cause: Plantar warts are caused by a virus that invades the skin through a small cut or crack. They are usually contracted by walking barefoot on infected surfaces where the virus lurks. They can be spread by touching, scratching, or shedding.

Treatment: The warts can disappear spontaneously and then recur in the same location. Self-treatment using over-the-counter remedies is not recommended. A procedure called carbon dioxide laser cautery can be performed in a doctor's office to remove the wart.

8   Premenstrual Syndrome (PMS). Teenage girls are not too young to experience PMS, and many of them do. Symptoms include bloating, fluid retention, breast tenderness, backache, fatigue, dizziness, headache, irritability, anxiety, depression, insomnia, and food cravings. These symptoms appear between ovulation and menstruation.

Cause: No specific cause has been identified for PMS.

Treatment: Birth control pills can relieve symptoms, but if these are not parentally acceptable, the herbs chaste berry, dandelion, dong quai, and skullcap can be helpful, as can nutritional supplements of magnesium, calcium, and vitamin B6. It is best to avoid or reduce the intake of white flour, sugar, caffeine, and dairy products during times of PMS.

9 **Scoliosis.** People with scoliosis have an abnormal sideways curvature of the spine. Most cases occur in girls and become apparent during the rapid growth years of early adolescence. It is such a concern that screening for scoliosis is now done in junior high and middle schools. Scoliosis becomes apparent when one shoulder appears higher than the other.

Causes: The causes are not well understood. The most common form of the disorder may be genetically inherited. Less common cases occur following trauma or accompany diseases such as cerebral palsy or muscle diseases.

Treatment: The extent of the curvature determines how it will be treated. If the curvature is less than 30 degrees, routine exercises to strengthen the torso are usually prescribed to prevent further progression of the condition. More severe cases may require a back brace and extensive physical therapy. Emotional support is also very important for these teenagers, as the limitations imposed by the treatment can be very upsetting.

10 **Social phobia.** People with social phobia are terrified of social contact and interaction because they fear others are scrutinizing them. Social phobia and depression often occur together, and both of them appear more often in teenage girls than in boys. Studies show that symptoms of social phobia begin to appear in late adolescence, but Dr. Una McCann, chief of anxiety disorders at the National Institute of Mental Health, believes that it occurs by early adolescence or even childhood.

Cause: Many teens who were simply shy as children develop symptoms of social phobia when they are confronted with the social and emotional pressures of adolescence. For some the symptoms come on suddenly after an especially stressful or emotional event, such as being humiliated in front of peers. Others become phobic when they are called upon to speak in public or accept an honor before an audience.

Treatment: Recommended treatment is cognitive behavioral therapy, with antidepressants if needed.

chapter fifty

23 Common Ailments of People between 20 and 90

Unlike the ubiquitous common cold, many diseases and medical conditions first appear within a predictable time range. You won't see a 40-year-old man with croup or an infant with Alzheimer's disease. You're also not likely to encounter a 5-year-old girl with breast cancer or a 52-year-old woman with mumps. There's a time and place for everything, and so it seems to be with illness.

A line also seems to exist between infant, child, or adolescent illnesses and adult medical problems. In those rare cases when medical conditions cross that line, they seem to affect people on either side of the line differently, as if they "know" they don't belong in that age category. For example, chickenpox is a relatively mild disease when it strikes children. A few days of itching, a low-grade fever, a week of feeling tired, and then the kids bounce back. Not so for adults. When adults get this "childhood" disease, the consequences can be serious. A pregnant woman who gets chickenpox risks having a child with birth defects, and pneumonia is a common complication of chickenpox in all adults.

Here are 23 adult illnesses and diseases that tend to manifest after adolescence. They have been placed into three broad age groups: 20 to 40; 40 to 65; and 65-plus. These categories reflect when the diseases are typically first apparent.

Ages 20 to 40

1 **Cervical cancer.** The early stages of cervical cancer, which affects the narrow neck of the uterus (the cervix), cause no symptoms. More advanced stages can cause a watery or bloody vaginal discharge, vaginal bleeding after intercourse or between menstrual periods, and abnormally heavy menstrual periods.

Age: Abnormal cervical cells usually appear in women between the ages of 25 and 35, with detectable cancer showing between 30 and 40. Invasive cancer usually is apparent between 40 and 60.

Causes: About 80 percent of cervical cancer cases are related to sexually transmitted viral infections. Other risk factors include having sexual intercourse before age 18, having multiple sex partners, or a history of sexually transmitted disease.

Treatment: Most cases are cured using a combination of surgery to remove the cancer, followed by radiation or chemotherapy.

2 **Crohn's disease.** This chronic inflammatory condition of the intestines makes digestion difficult and causes cramps and pain after eating. Crohn's disease is also characterized by low-grade fever, loss of appetite, fatigue, and weight loss. It is more common in women than in men and rare among blacks or Asians.

Age: Crohn's disease is usually diagnosed in people in their twenties and thirties.

Cause: The actual cause of Crohn's disease is unknown, but it is believed to be an autoimmune disease. Possible triggers include a virus, irritation from food additives, and smoking. Stress aggravates the symptoms.

Treatment: Because this disease is not curable, treatment must be lifelong. An anti-inflammatory drug called sulfasalazine is prescribed most often, along with short-term prednisone, to reduce inflammation. Natural remedies that provide some relief include the herbs slippery elm, chamomile, and marsh mallow. Stress reduction techniques, including yoga, tai chi, and meditation, are also recommended.

3 **Systemic lupus erythematosus (SLE).** SLE is a chronic, autoimmune, inflammatory condition. Patients with lupus have unusual antibodies in their blood that target their own body tissues. The disease is characterized by a rash, extreme sensitivity to the sun, severe fatigue, low-grade fever, enlarged lymph nodes, poor circulation in the toes and fingers, muscle aches, and joint pain. Women make up 90 percent of all SLE cases, and it strikes blacks three times more often than whites.

Age: Most people with SLE are between the ages of 20 and 45.

Causes: Although no single cause has been identified, some experts believe SLE is caused by a combination of genetic, immunologic, and hormonal factors.

Treatment: Because there are so many symptoms, treatment can be difficult. Nonsteroidal anti-inflammatory drugs such as ibuprofen can be taken to relieve joint pain, and chronic rash may respond to antimalarial medications. People with SLE often have food allergies. If they are identified and the foods are avoided, symptoms often improve.

4 Testicular cancer. This form of cancer affects the testes in men and is characterized by a change in size or shape of a testicle, swelling of the testicles, a feeling of heaviness in the testicles, and a firm, initially painless lump in a testicle. This disease affects more whites than blacks.

Age: Testicular cancer is the most common type of cancer in men between the ages of 15 and 35.

Cause: The cause is unknown. About 10 percent of testicular cancer cases occur in men who were born with an undescended testicle, and it has been shown to run in families. Other risk factors include a sedentary lifestyle, having had mumps, injury to the testicles, overexposure to radiation or pesticides, and early puberty.

Treatment: Removal of the testicle is done in the majority of cases, followed by radiation and chemotherapy.

Ages 40 to 65

5 Amyotrophic lateral sclerosis (ALS). Also known as Lou Gehrig's disease, ALS is a motor neuron disease. This means that it affects the nerves that leave the spinal cord. These nerves are responsible for supplying electrical stimulation to the muscles. When the signals fail, so does the ability to move the muscles.

Age: ALS occurs most often in people in the fifth through seventh decades of life.

Cause: The cause is unknown.

Treatment: There is no cure for ALS. Treatment is to relieve symptoms of the disease. Only one drug has been approved by the Food and Drug Administration (riluzole, trade name Rilutek), which can prolong life in some ALS patients. The usual causes of death are infections that develop because the body is so weak. Once a person contracts ALS, death typically occurs within 2 to 7 years.

6   Benign prostatic hyperplasia. Enlargement of the prostate gland, accompanied by difficulties in urination, dribbling, an inability to empty the bladder, and having to get up frequently during the night to urinate are symptoms of benign prostatic hyperplasia.

Age: Enlargement of the prostate usually appears after age 45.

Cause: The exact cause is not known, although it seems to be associated with age-related hormone changes, specifically a decline in testosterone and a rise in other hormones.

Treatment: Several medications can ease urination (terazosin, prazosin) or reduce prostate size (finasteride). Helpful herbs include saw palmetto, nettle, and Asian ginseng. In severe cases or when cancer is present, surgery is often recommended.

7   Bladder cancer. This fairly common form of cancer accounts for about 5 percent of all cancers in the United States, which is about 50,000 cases per year. Men are two to three times more likely than women to get the disease, and whites contract bladder cancer twice as often as blacks.

Age: Most bladder cancers occur after the age of 55, and the average age is 68.

Causes: Chronic irritation of the bladder appears to cause this form of cancer. People who have a history of chronic bladder infections or inflammation of the bladder are at higher risk. There is also a very strong association between exposure to cancer-causing chemicals and bladder cancer. People who work with toxins—such as painters, truckers, metalworkers, and anyone who handles industrial dyes—and people who have received radiation or certain chemotherapy agents are also at higher risk.

Treatment: Superficial tumors that are detected very early can be removed surgically or burned out with a laser. This, combined with chemotherapy, can be protective against spread (metastasis) of the disease. More advanced disease may require removal of the bladder followed by radiation and chemotherapy.

8   Breast cancer. More than 99 percent of breast cancer occurs in women. This form of cancer typically begins with the formation of a small tumor which, left undetected, can shed cells and spread to other parts of the body. Breast cancer is the most common type of cancer in women.

Age: About two-thirds of all breast cancer cases are in women older than 50.

Causes: Although the exact cause is not known, experts have devised a list of risk factors. However, most women who have these factors don't get the disease, while many others without the risk factors do. Some of those risk factors are: mother, sister, or daughter with breast cancer; postmenopausal; started menstruation before age 12, stopped menstruating after 55; took hormone therapy or birth control pills; had first child after age 30; a high-fat diet; and obesity.

Treatment: Various surgical procedures to remove the cancer can be performed, including lumpectomy, modified radical mastectomy, or radical mastectomy (see Chapter 31), followed by radiation or chemotherapy as needed.

9   **Colon (colorectal) cancer.** The large intestine, which includes the colon and rectum, is a tube that plays a major role in processing and eliminating food and waste from the body. Colorectal cancer is the second most common cause of cancer death in the United States (lung cancer is first). About 40 percent of the approximately 150,000 people who get colorectal cancer die of the disease each year. Early diagnosis and treatment are the keys to surviving colorectal cancer.

Age: Risk for the disease increases significantly after age 50 and continues to increase with age.

Causes: A family history of polyps (small tumors that grow in the colon), or various colon diseases such as colitis or Crohn's disease are risk factors for colorectal cancer. A diet low in fiber, fruits, and vegetables and high in fat also appears to be a risk factor. Some studies suggest that eating charred meats, which contain carcinogens, plays a role.

Treatment: Surgery to remove the diseased portions of the colon is the usual treatment, followed by radiation and chemotherapy. Some studies suggest that taking folic acid, calcium, and antioxidants helps protect against developing colorectal cancer.

10   **Coronary heart disease.** Coronary heart disease affects more than 7 million Americans and is the most common form of heart disease. It is the number one cause of death for both women and men in the United States, and kills more than 500,000 people every year.

Age: Coronary heart disease typically affects men beginning around age 45 and women after age 55. This difference is believed to be at least partly associated with the hormone estrogen, which decreases significantly in women after menopause.

Causes: Most of the risk factors for heart disease are controllable: high blood pressure, smoking, obesity, high cholesterol, sedentary lifestyle, stress, and diabetes. Those that are not controllable include family history of heart disease, age (risk increases with age), or, in rare cases, a congenital heart abnormality.

Treatment: Conventional treatment may include drugs to calm the heart (e.g., beta-blockers), increase blood flow (e.g., nitrates), or prevent clotting (e.g., heparin, aspirin). Lifestyle changes, such as maintaining a low-fat, high-fiber diet, exercising, stopping smoking, losing weight, and moderate intake of alcohol, are typically recommended.

11 Diabetes (type II). About 90 percent of people with diabetes have the type II (non-insulin-dependent) form. It is the result of the body's inability to process insulin properly or effectively.

Age: Adult-onset diabetes usually appears after age 40.

Cause: Obesity and the development of type II diabetes appear to go hand-in-hand. Excessive intake of food raises the level of glucose (sugar) in the blood, and the pancreas cannot produce enough insulin to convert the extra sugar into energy, which leaves the excess to circulate in the bloodstream.

Treatment: Diet and exercise can control the disease in a great number of people; however, many take drugs to manage their glucose levels. Natural remedies such as chromium, fenugreek, and garlic have proven to be helpful in controlling glucose; however, they should be used only under supervision of a doctor.

12 Gallstones. Crystal-like deposits of cholesterol that develop in the gallbladder may lie dormant for years before they decide to make their presence known. In fact, about 10 percent of people in the United States have gallstones, but many don't know it. It can take 25 years or more for gallstones to become lodged in the duct that leads from the small, pear-shaped organ to the liver. When they finally do, however, the pain is severe and sudden and can cause fever, shivering, nausea, vomiting, and jaundice (yellowing of the skin).

Age: The risk of a gallbladder attack such as this increases significantly after age 40.

Causes: Several risk factors have been identified for cholesterol gallstone formation, including being female, multiple pregnancies, use of birth control pills, high-fat and low-fiber diets, obesity, rapid weight loss, some medications, intestinal diseases such as Crohn's disease, and heredity.

Treatment: Nonsurgical treatment includes drugs that dissolve the stones and the use of high-frequency sound waves to break the stones up. In many cases, the gallbladder is removed.

13 Glaucoma. Nearly 3 million people have glaucoma, a leading cause of blindness in the United States. In more than 90 percent of cases, glaucoma comes on slowly and is characterized by blurred vision, headache, teary, achy eyes, and progressive loss of peripheral vision. This type of glaucoma is called *chronic glaucoma.* Less than 10 percent of the time, glaucoma comes on suddenly and requires immediate medical attention. Symptoms of *acute glaucoma* include severe throbbing pain, blurred vision, rainbow halos around lights, dilated pupils, and occasionally nausea and vomiting.

Age: Glaucoma most commonly affects Blacks over the age of 40 and anyone older than 60.

Causes: In chronic glaucoma, there is an imbalance between the rate that fluid is produced by the cells inside the eye and the rate that the fluid drains out. In people who develop acute glaucoma, there seems to be an inherited tendency for a blockage to develop in the drainage channels in the eye. In both cases, glaucoma is the result of damage to the optic nerve when pressure from the excess fluid increases.

Treatment: Chronic glaucoma can be treated with eye drops that contain epinephrine, pilocarpine, or beta-blockers, all of which help increase the drainage of fluid from the eye. Unfortunately, these drugs can cause significant side effects, such as blurred vision, stomach upset, and headache, and they may aggravate heart problems. Natural remedies include the herb bilberry and vitamin C, chromium, and zinc.

14 Osteoarthritis. Pain and progressive stiffness and inflammation of the joints are symptoms of osteoarthritis. These symptoms are the result of a gradual loss of bone tissue in the joints. It is the most common form of arthritis, especially in the elderly.

Age: It most often appears in people older than 40.

Cause: The exact mechanism of the disease is not known, although some people seem to have a genetic tendency toward bone degeneration. Osteoarthritis is a part of the aging process, in which the cartilage and bone cannot repair themselves fast enough to keep up with the damage.

Treatment: Nonsteroidal anti-inflammatory drugs such as ibuprofen and the newer COX-2 inhibitors are often prescribed. Among natural remedies, acupressure and acupuncture, the herbs black cohosh and nettle for pain, and the supplements glucosamine and chondroitan have been effective.

15 **Osteoporosis.** Osteoporosis, which means "porous bones," is a condition in which bones lose density and gradually become thin and weakened. Of the estimated 24 million Americans with osteoporosis, 90 percent are women.

Age: Most cases of osteoporosis are discovered in women only after they experience a fracture, beginning in their mid-fifties. The disease is believed to start much earlier, however, as bone loss begins in earnest after age 35 in men and women, and accelerates in women during and for several years after menopause.

Cause: The exact cause of osteoporosis is not completely understood, but researchers understand the process of bone loss. Although bone loss is a natural part of aging, women at higher risk of bone loss are those who are thin, small-boned, fair-haired, sedentary, white or Asian, and who smoke. The decline in estrogen during and after menopause is the primary factor in osteoporosis in women.

Treatment: Hormone replacement therapy is one approach, although drugs such as raloxifine, alendronate, and calcitonin don't carry the increased risk of breast and uterine cancer associated with estrogen. Nutritional supplements, including calcium, vitamin D, and magnesium, as well as reducing the amount of protein in the diet and routine exercise, are effective approaches to slowing, stopping, or even reversing bone density loss.

16 **Parkinson's disease.** A progressive weakness and slight tremor of the hands or head, along with a shuffling gait and stooped posture, are symptoms of Parkinson's disease. Depression and other emotional problems often accompany this disease. Parkinson's disease is slightly more common in men than in women.

Age: Parkinson's disease usually first appears between the ages of 50 and 65.

Cause: The gradual degeneration of the nerve cells in the midbrain, where bodily movements are controlled, is the source of Parkinson's disease. The degeneration occurs when there is an imbalance of two substances, dopamine and acetylcholine, which are involved in nerve transmission. Why dopamine and acetylcholine are thrown off balance may be related to genetics, environmental toxins, or a viral infection, but the exact cause is unknown.

Treatment: Symptoms can be controlled for years using drugs, such as levodopa and dopamine-like drugs. A new approach called stem cell therapy, which involves implanting stem cells into the brain, may be on the horizon. Natural remedies such as acupuncture, massage, and reflexology can relieve symptoms.

17 **Rheumatoid arthritis.** This common form of arthritis affects more than 2 million Americans. It is three times more common in women than in men and affects people of all races equally. The joint inflammation characteristic of rheumatoid arthritis causes swelling, pain, stiffness, and redness in the joints. Some patients with this disease develop chronic inflammation, which leads to destruction and deformity of the joints.

Age: It most often begins after age 40 and before 60.

Cause: The cause of rheumatoid arthritis is unknown, although many experts classify the disorder as an autoimmune disease, which means the body attacks itself. In this case, an attack on the body's tissues results in inflammation. Viral, bacterial, or fungal infections, as well as certain environmental factors, could trigger the disease. A genetic cause is also possible. Smoking tobacco increases the risk of developing rheumatoid arthritis.

Treatment: Nonsteroidal anti-inflammatory drugs, corticosteroid injections, and applications of heat and ultrasound can help relieve symptoms. Natural remedies include acupuncture, acupressure, a low-fat, low-protein vegetarian diet, the supplements glucosamine and chondroitan, and identification of foods that may cause an allergic (inflammatory) reaction.

18 **Shingles.** Blisters, slight fever, chills, and deep burning, searing, aching, or stabbing pain are characteristics of shingles. The blisters typically appear along the chest, abdomen, back, or face and last about 2 weeks before they heal and scab.

Age: Shingles typically affects people 50 and older.

Cause: The herpes zoster virus, the same virus that causes chickenpox, is the culprit. In people who had chickenpox as children, this virus lies dormant for decades. In some people, physical or emotional stress, trauma, or a serious illness may prompt the virus to re-erupt as shingles.

Treatment: Although there is no known way to prevent shingles, the condition can be managed with oral or topical acyclovir, an antiviral drug. Acetaminophen can relieve pain, and corticosteroids can reduce inflammation. Herbal remedies include a cream made from cayenne to relieve pain, and topical calendula and lemon balm to reduce inflammation.

Ages 65-Plus

19 **Alzheimer's disease.** Intellectual and mental decline, along with moodiness, confusion, agitation, loss of memory for recent events, an inability to remember new information, and dizziness are all symptoms of Alzheimer's disease. This insidious illness can take a slow, moderate, or rapid course. It is the fourth leading cause of death among American adults. Women are twice as susceptible as men, and whites are four times more at risk than blacks.

Age: It usually affects people 65 and older, and by age 80, about one in three people have the disease.

Causes: Alzheimer's disease is not a normal part of aging. For reasons unknown, nerve fibers in the brain become tangled, and protein deposits form on them, causing neural damage. Some evidence points to a protein called ApoE, which transports fatty substances in the body, as a factor. Researchers are almost certain that genetics plays a role, as a person with a parent who had Alzheimer's is at higher risk.

Treatment: There is no known cure, and so far no drugs have significantly slowed progression of the disease, although several (for example donepezil, acetylcarnitine) can provide temporary improvement. The herb ginkgo biloba reportedly can relieve early symptoms.

20 **Macular degeneration.** More than 1.3 million Americans have this degenerative eye disease, which is the leading cause of vision loss in the United States. It is characterized by the gradual and painless loss of precise central vision.

Age: It rarely appears in people younger than 60.

Causes: In the majority of cases, the macula—a spot about 1/16 inch in diameter at the center of the retina—becomes scarred as deposits accumulate beneath it. This is called the *dry* form of the disease. A smaller number of cases involve the formation of abnormal blood vessels under the macula; this is referred to as the *wet* form. When these vessels leak, they cause retinal cells to die and vision becomes blurred or destroyed. Older age and the presence of diabetes, heart disease, high blood pressure, and atherosclerosis are risk factors for macular degeneration.

Treatment: Although macular degeneration cannot be cured, its progression can be slowed or stopped. A drug called verteporfin slows damage to the retina in the dry form. Laser surgery can destroy the leaking blood vessels in the wet form.

21 **Prostate cancer.** Cancer of the prostate gland, a walnut-sized gland located under a man's bladder, is diagnosed in more than 180,000 men a year and is the cause of death in about 32,000 men annually. It is the second most common cancer in men, after skin malignancies.

Age: Eighty percent of cases of prostate cancer are diagnosed in men older than 65 years.

Causes: It appears that diet plays a significant role in causing prostate cancer. Men who eat large amounts of fat, especially animal fats, are most likely to develop the disease. It is believed that high levels of the hormone testosterone, which stimulates prostate cancer, are an underlying factor in prostate cancer; fat stimulates production of testosterone.

Treatment: Many treatments can be considered, including a conventional approach—removal of the prostate, external radiation, implant radiation, chemotherapy, hormone therapy, and watchful waiting—and complementary measures, such as a Chinese herbal remedy called PC-SPES, antioxidants such as vitamins E and C and the mineral selenium, and supplements such as lycopene, curcumin, and genestein.

22 **Stroke.** When blood circulation to the brain is disrupted, the result is often stroke. Stroke can be of two main types: clot stroke, triggered by a clot in a blood vessel; or bleeding stroke, which results when an inflamed or weak blood vessel in the brain begins to leak.

Age: The majority of strokes occur in people older than age 60. Men experience stroke more often than do women, and blacks more often than whites.

Causes: The main controllable risk factors for stroke include obesity, stress, high cholesterol (usually related to a high-fat diet), smoking, lack of sufficient exercise, high blood pressure, and use of stimulant drugs such as amphetamines.

Treatment: Clot strokes are typically treated with drugs that help prevent further clotting (anticoagulants) or with thrombolytic drugs (which dissolve clots). People with bleeding stroke need to lower their blood pressure, usually with a combination of lifestyle changes and medication. Some studies suggest that ginkgo helps increase blood flow in the brain and thus may help ease the memory loss associated with stroke.

23 **Urinary incontinence.** An inability to control the flow of urine falls into three common categories:

- stress incontinence, when the bladder can't handle the increased compression during coughing, sneezing, or exercise;

- urge incontinence, caused by a sudden, involuntary contraction of the bladder; and

- mixed incontinence, a combination of the first two types.

Age: Stress incontinence usually occurs in women younger than 60, while mixed incontinence is seen in women older than 60. Urge incontinence is commonly seen in people older than 70.

Causes: Women often develop incontinence during pregnancy and childbirth or after menopause, because of weakened pelvic muscles. Older men may become incontinent after prostate surgery. Other contributors include caffeine, diet drugs, pelvic trauma, and spinal cord damage. People with multiple sclerosis often have urinary incontinence, as do elderly individuals whose thinking is impaired either by senility, drugs, or a combination of both.

Treatment: Kegel exercises, which strengthen the muscles that support the bladder and uterus, are prescribed by both conventional and alternative practitioners. Biofeedback and bladder retraining are other common approaches. Drugs such as pseudoephedrine and ephedrine may be prescribed for stress incontinence.

chapter fifty-one

21 Noisemakers: How Loud Is Your Life?

"Could you repeat that?"

"What did you say?"

"Did you say something?"

"Huh?"

If you're having trouble hearing or distinguishing certain sounds, or if you are experiencing ringing in your ears (a condition known as tinnitus), you're not alone. Hearing problems affect tens of millions of Americans, and not just older people. According to the Hearing Alliance of America, of the more than 24 million Americans who have some form of hearing loss, 40 percent of them are younger than 65, and 2 million are younger than 18. In the U.S., hearing loss is the third leading disability, behind arthritis and hypertension.

How Is Sound Measured?

Sound intensity, or loudness, is measured in decibels (dB). The decibel scale is from 0 dB to 120 dB, which is the threshold of pain, and beyond. Every increase of 10 decibels is a doubling of intensity. Therefore, 40 dB is twice as loud as 30 dB.

The Sound of Music

Every day, more than 20 million Americans are regularly exposed to hazardous sound levels, either on the job or, quite often, when listening to music. Consider this: According to an article in the March 30, 2000 issue of the *Bay Area Reporter* in San Francisco, the sound level in one popular nightclub, Sound Factory, measured 115 dB, which is louder than sandblasting. According to the Occupational Health and Safety Administration (OSHA), a mere 4 minutes and 43 seconds in the Sound Factory can leave you with permanent hearing damage.

As many rock musicians have learned, hearing loss caused by years of exposure to loud music is irreversible. Some of these hard-of-hearing rock stars got together to form a nonprofit organization called H.E.A.R. (Hearing Education and Awareness for Rockers). And it's not just hard rock that's contributing to hearing loss. A 1991 study of the members of the Chicago Symphony found that more than 50 percent of the players had significant hearing loss.

You can reduce your exposure to sound by wearing earplugs or earmuffs. Earplugs can reduce loudness by 10 to 15 decibels, while a good pair of earmuffs (like those worn by people who work around airplanes or with jackhammers) can reduce loudness by 20 to 30 decibels.

Just how loud is your life? Look at the chart and see how different sounds rate. Keep in mind that OSHA reports that 90 dB for 8 hours is the maximum safe level of noise exposure.

Noisemaker	dB Level (Average or Range)
1 Jet take-off at 25 meters	150 (Eardrum rupture)
2 Jet take-off at 50 meters	130
3 Shotgun	130
4 Disco/boom box	120
5 Thunderclap, chain saw	120

Noisemaker	dB Level (Average or Range)
6 Rock concert	110–140 (110 dB is the human pain threshold)
7 Symphony	110
8 Car horn at 1 meter	110
9 Jackhammer, garbage truck, motorcycle, outboard motor	100 (Serious damage at 8 hours)
10 Newspaper printing press	97
11 Busy city street, food blender	90
12 Subway	88
13 Dishwasher, average factory, freight train at 15 meters	80 (Possible damage)
14 Vacuum cleaner, hair dryer	70
15 Laughter	60–65
16 Conversation in office, restaurant	60
17 Quiet suburb, talking at home	50
18 Library, refrigerator humming	40
19 Quiet rural area	30
20 Rustling leaves, whisper	20
21 Breathing	10

chapter fifty-two

14 Reasons You Can't Sleep

Having trouble sleeping? You're not alone. Nearly 50 percent of Americans suffer from insomnia or some other sleep disorder. Insomnia can be transient (lasting only one or several nights and often triggered by increased stress or excitement); short-term (lasting one to three weeks, often the result of emotional stress); or long-term and chronic (lasting more than several weeks with poor sleep nearly every night).

Not everyone needs eight hours of sleep to function at their best; some people thrive on five or six. But nearly half of Americans are not reaching even that goal. Insufficient sleep can lead to mood changes, a decline in mental functioning, decreased motor skills, impaired immune system, and weight gain.

Thirty percent of high school and college students fall asleep during class at least once a week. More than 30 percent of American drivers admit they have fallen asleep at the wheel at least once during their life, and every year at least 100,000 auto accidents and 1,500 deaths are attributed to falling asleep while driving, according to the National Sleep Foundation.

For these reasons, insomnia is considered a serious problem and should be addressed aggressively. To correct it, you must be able to recognize the causes. Here are 14 causes of insomnia. How many of them apply to you?

1 Emotional distress. Anger, fear, anxiety—these emotions are the cause of transient or short-term insomnia in about 35 percent of U.S. adults.

This type of insomnia is sometimes called adjustment sleep disorder; it is a reaction to change or stress. Stress management (e.g., meditation, yoga, relaxation therapy, deep breathing) or counseling can help.

2 Depression. It can be the cause or a result of insomnia. See a professional to get an accurate diagnosis of depression and treatment options.

3 Caffeine. Avoid caffeinated beverages, chocolate, and drugs that contain caffeine (e.g., Midol, Excedrin). If you feel you must have any of these products, consume them before noon.

4 Alcohol. Avoid drinking alcohol before bedtime. It may make you fall asleep faster, but for many people it disturbs the quality of sleep.

5 Smoking. Heart rate, blood pressure, and brain wave activity all increase when you smoke. Do not smoke.

6 Night shift work. The body has a natural, circadian rhythm that is finely tuned with other body functions. Alternating day and night shifts contributes to insomnia. Many young workers in their twenties and thirties can do well under these conditions, but older individuals can develop shift-work insomnia. Switching to day shift is the best solution. If you can't switch, sleeping in a completely blacked-out room and keeping the same schedule on days off can eliminate insomnia.

7 Medications. Drugs that stimulate the body should be avoided, especially later in the day. These include those containing caffeine (see number 3), amphetamines, appetite suppressants, and corticosteroids.

8 Medical conditions. Insomnia is associated with allergies, Alzheimer's disease, arthritis, attention deficit disorder, heart disease, hypertension, hyperthyroid, and Parkinson's disease. Relaxation techniques may help, and a review of any medications you are taking should be done with your physician.

9 Artificial and natural light. The body's biological clock is triggered by sunlight. If you are not exposed to natural, well-timed cycles of sunlight and darkness that follow the body's natural rhythms, you may experience insomnia.

10 **Menstruation.** About 50 percent of women report bloating that disturbs their sleep for two to three nights per menstrual cycle. One reason is that progesterone levels fall during menstruation, and progesterone promotes sleep. Drugs should be avoided; stress management approaches may help, or discuss natural progesterone therapy with your gynecologist.

11 **Noise.** It can be environmental noise (especially if you work nights and must sleep during the day) or snoring from the person lying next to you. Earplugs can help block out noise.

12 **Jet lag.** Crossing time zones can contribute to insomnia. Take precautions when you travel: Get enough sleep before you travel, and avoid dehydration, alcohol, and caffeine before and during the flight.

13 **Excessive napping.** If you feel sleepy during the day and nap too often or for too long, you may experience insomnia. To ward off the tendency to nap, try light exercise, such as walking, yoga, or stretching, to give you energy. Avoid using stimulants such as caffeine to prevent napping, as this approach can backfire.

14 **Exercise.** Although exercise is an excellent stress and tension reducer and is recommended for everyone, do not exercise within three hours of bedtime. Exercise increases alertness and stimulates the muscles, making it harder to fall asleep.

chapter fifty-three

10 Carcinogens and What They Do to the Body

Ⅰf you want to list "the most dangerous cancer-causing substances in the environment," you can approach the project in two ways. One is to list the most dangerous and deadly substances known to humankind, even if the chances of anyone being exposed to them is extremely small. Plutonium is an example. Most experts agree that plutonium is one of the most dangerous substances, if not *the* most dangerous, on earth. But unless you work with nuclear weapons, you probably won't find yourself around any significant amount of the stuff.

The second way is to list the substances that are known to cause cancer that are the most common in our environment. They may not be as poisonous as plutonium, but they cause a lot more mischief, simply because people are constantly exposed to them.

The list presented here is based on the second approach. All of the following substances are known carcinogens, according to the National Toxicology Program (which is part of the National Institutes of Health); the National Cancer Institute; the National Center for Chronic Disease Prevention and Health Promotion; the Environmental Protection Agency; or the U.S. Department of Health and Human Services. In particular, every two years the National Toxicology Program publishes a list of known, potential, and probable toxic substances to which many Americans are exposed. As of May 2000, the list had 218 entries.

1 **Sunlight.** According to the National Center for Chronic Disease Prevention and Health Promotion, 20 percent of Americans will develop skin cancer during their lifetimes. If you're wondering how many new cases of skin cancer develop each year, the American Academy of Dermatology estimates the figure to be 1 million. The most common cause of skin cancer is sunlight exposure, specifically to ultraviolet rays. Most children get up to 80 percent of their lifetime exposure to sunlight before they reach the age of 18. One serious sunburn can double a child's risk of developing skin cancer later in life. One of the best ways to help prevent skin cancer is to use sunscreen with an SPF (sun protective factor) of at least 15 and to start using it early. That means if your infant is going to be out in the sun (and it is recommended that very young children not be exposed to direct sunlight, at least during the first 6 months of life), sunscreen should be applied. The same applies to children out playing in the park or riding their bikes. Don't be fooled into thinking that a burn is bad, but a tan is healthy. The Cancer Information Service at MD Anderson Hospital in Texas notes that "A tan is nothing more than visible evidence that skin damage has occurred."

2 **Tobacco smoke.** Tobacco smoke contains a creative mixture of more than 40 chemicals known to cause cancer, as well as many more probable carcinogens. Researchers are not entirely certain how these chemicals interact to cause disease, including cancers of the lung, throat, larynx, and mouth. Substances called nitrosamines are believed by many experts to be the most dangerous and common carcinogens in tobacco, but they are not alone. Tar, formaldehyde, nickel, nicotine, benzene, and hydrogen cyanide are just a few of the other carcinogens in tobacco smoke.

3 **Secondhand smoke.** In 1992, the Environmental Protection Agency (EPA) confirmed that secondhand smoke causes lung cancer and is linked with thousands of deaths each year. Secondhand smoke contains a mixture of exhaled mainstream smoke from nearby smokers, sidestream smoke emitted from the smoldering tobacco, and contaminants from the cigarette paper. Scientists have identified more than 4,000 substances in secondhand smoke, and more than 42 of them are known to cause cancer in people and animals.

4 **Vinyl chloride.** Do you like the smell of a new car's interior? Don't breathe too deeply; if any or all of the interior is plastic, that's vinyl chloride you're inhaling. The emission of vinyl chloride from plastic, whether it's in the interior of a car, in plastic furniture, or in other items made of plastic, is called "off-gassing." People who work in the industries that make plastics or who work in or around hazardous waste sites and landfills are also exposed to vinyl chloride gas. Breathing high levels of vinyl chloride for a short time can cause sleepiness, dizziness, unconsciousness, and even death, if the levels are extremely high. Inhalation of vinyl chloride for long periods of time, even at low levels, can cause liver cancer, nerve damage, immune reactions, and permanent liver damage. The Occupational Safety and Health Administration (OSHA) set the maximum allowable level of vinyl chloride in workplace air during an 8-hour day in a 40-hour work week at 1 part vinyl chloride per 1 million parts of air. Vinyl chloride is also found in the water supply. Here, the EPA has stepped in and set a standard of 0.002 milligrams of vinyl chloride per liter of water (0.002 mg/L) as the maximum allowed. Wells near landfills or hazardous waste sites are the most susceptible to vinyl chloride contamination. Some experts say that water that sits in PVC (polyvinyl chloride) pipes overnight may absorb the toxin from the pipes, making the first burst of water from the faucet in the morning more likely to be toxic.

5   Radon. You can't see it, smell it, or taste it, but it may be all around you in your home. The Surgeon General's office warns that radon is the second leading cause of lung cancer in the United States and is probably responsible for up to 20,000 deaths per year. If you combine the number one cause of lung cancer—smoking—with exposure to radon, your chance of developing lung cancer is very high. Radon rises from the ground and is the byproduct of the breakdown of uranium in soil, rock, and water. This breakdown is occurring all over the United States, and it is seeping into buildings. Because people generally spend more of their time at home than at any other place, radon exposure at home poses the highest risk. The EPA recommends that everyone test their homes (below the third floor) and that all schools also test for radon. Testing kits are available at hardware stores.

6   Asbestos. Both the EPA and the International Agency for Research on Cancer of the World Health Organization have declared asbestos a proven human carcinogen. It causes lung cancer, larynx cancer, and certain gastrointestinal cancers. It also causes asbestosis, a progressive lung disease. The chances of getting any of these diseases from exposure to asbestos increase with cumulative exposure and with the length of time since the first exposure. It is estimated that by the time asbestos is eliminated from the environment, more than 200,000 people will have died because of their exposure to it. Although asbestos has been banned, it is still found in many older buildings and homes. If you have asbestos in your home and are concerned about it, contact an asbestos removal expert, as it can be very dangerous to remove the material yourself.

7   **Radiation.** Experts estimate that the average American receives about 360 millirem (millirem is the standard measurement for radiation) of radiation every year. Natural sources, including radon gas, outer space, and the earth itself, make up about 80 percent of that exposure; the remaining 20 percent comes primarily from medical x-rays. An x-ray emits about 50 millirem, while a ride in a jet from coast to coast exposes people to 5 millirem. Radiation can cause cancer as well as mental retardation or genetic defects in infants whose mothers were exposed to x-rays during pregnancy. Researchers have obtained the majority of their knowledge about radiation and cancer from studying the more than 100,000 survivors of the atomic bombs dropped on Japan. They have concluded that: 1) The more radiation a person receives, the greater the chance he or she will get cancer; 2) most cancers appear many years after the radiation exposure occurred, usually 10 to 40 years; and 3) the chance of cancer developing increases as the radiation dose increases. Scientists tend to agree that any level of radiation poses a risk.

8   **Diesel fuel.** For a real "stew" of carcinogens, look no further than diesel fuel. Diesel fuel contains hundreds of substances—some gaseous and some in the form of soot—including carbon dioxide, carbon monoxide, methane, benzene, penol, and PAHs (polycyclic aromatic hydrocarbons), all known or probable carcinogens. The California EPA calls diesel fuel a known carcinogen, while the National Toxicology Program labels it "reasonably anticipated to be a human carcinogen." The National Institute for Occupational Safety and Health (NIOSH) estimates that about 1.35 million workers are exposed to diesel fuel exhaust, including truck drivers, farm workers, vehicle maintenance workers, and mine, bridge, railroad, and tunnel workers.

9   **Tamoxifen** is a prescription drug (Novadex) that burst onto the scene as an anti-breast-cancer drug, and it appears to be quite effective for many women. However, tamoxifen also has a dark side: It has been rated a carcinogen by the National Toxicology Program because it promotes aggressive uterine and liver cancers, and it causes deadly blood clots and interferes with the functioning of the heart. Obviously, tamoxifen isn't for every woman. Women who are contemplating using tamoxifen need to weigh their risk of uterine cancer against the benefits of a lower recurrence of breast cancer or a lower risk of breast cancer if they are already at high risk for the disease.

10 **Arsenic** is a known carcinogen linked not only with cancer of the bladder, prostate, lungs, kidney, skin, and liver, but also with cardiovascular disorders and diabetes. Exposure to arsenic may be hard to avoid in some areas, because it is present in drinking water. In January 2001, the EPA revised the acceptable standards for arsenic in drinking water from 50 ppb (parts per billion) to 10 ppb, with the hope that it would help prevent cancer. Arsenic, also found in many household pesticides, is used extensively as a wood preservative. Unfortunately, President George W. Bush subsequently repealed the EPA revision.

Probable Carcinogens in Your Home

These items are listed as probable or likely carcinogens, and they appear in items commonly found in many homes. Are they in yours?

- **Formaldehyde.** Have you ever felt ill or have your eyes felt irritated after walking around for a while in a furniture or carpet store? It may not be the high prices that are making you feel ill; it may be the formaldehyde. Formaldehyde from particleboard, adhesives used in the manufacture of inexpensive wood-based furniture and other products, cushions, and carpeting can evaporate into gas.
- **Methylene chloride.** In addition to probably causing cancer, this substance is a central nervous system depressant. Methylene chloride is found in paint remover.
- **Polychlorinated biphenyls (PCBs).** The most likely sources of these probable carcinogens are paper and plastic products and electrical components.
- **Toluene diisocyanate.** This probable cancer-causing substance is found in polyurethane foam aerosols.
- **Trichloroethylene.** Has anyone ever told you that your clothes can kill you? That may be true if you get your clothes dry cleaned, as trichlomethylene is a probable carcinogen used in the dry cleaning business.

For practical ideas on reducing risk, consult the following books: *Living Healthy in a Toxic World* by David Steinman and R. Michael Wisner (Berkley, 1996); *Toxins A-Z: A Guide to Everyday Pollution Hazards* by John Harte, Cheryl Holdren, Richard Schneider, and Christine Shirley (University of California, 1991); *Home Safe Home: Protecting Yourself and Your Family from Everyday Toxics and Harmful Household Products* by Debra L. Dadd (Putnam, 1997).

chapter fifty-four

16 Reasons You Don't Want to Smoke

They make your breath stale, your fingernails yellow, your teeth stained, and your clothes stinky. And you could probably take a very nice cruise for the amount of money they cost you per year. If you still feel like lighting up a cigarette (or cigar), here are some more facts. Cigarettes and cigars contain more than 4,000 chemicals and at least 400 toxic substances, all of them delivered to a smoker's lungs and body with every puff—and every puff brings a smoker much closer to that final puff. Research shows that each cigarette reduces a smoker's life by 7 to 11 minutes, which on average translates into a life shortened by 7 to 8 years.

Smoking cigarettes affects every system in the body. When people smoke, the heat breaks down the tobacco, which results in the release of dozens of toxins. Those poisons are responsible for or play a significant role in many diseases and conditions, including those described here.

1 Lung cancer is the primary disease associated with smoking. Eighty-five percent of lung cancer cases are associated with smoking, and smokers are 12 times more likely to develop lung cancer than nonsmokers. Smokers are also more likely to get throat or mouth cancer, which rarely affect nonsmokers.

2 Atherosclerosis is the main cardiovascular disease associated with smoking. Atherosclerosis involves clogging of the arteries with fatty substances, which makes it difficult or impossible for blood to flow through them.

3 **Coronary thrombosis** is a blood clot in the arteries that supply blood to the heart. Approximately 30 percent of people with coronary thrombosis are smokers, and 90 percent of people who undergo heart bypass surgery either smoke or are ex-smokers.

4 **Stroke** occurs when the blood vessels going to the brain become blocked. Smoking damages blood vessels and causes them to constrict (narrow), which can lead to stroke.

5 **Emphysema** affects nearly 95 percent of all smokers who smoke at least one pack a day, even though they may not display symptoms of the disease. Among nonsmokers, more than 90 percent have little or no signs of the disease.

6 **Chronic obstructive pulmonary disease (COPD)**, or smoker's lung, is a decline in lung function, which causes coughing and breathlessness that get progressively worse over time.

7 **Infertility** is more common among couples who smoke. Male smokers have lower sperm counts (13 to 17% lower than nonsmokers); stopping smoking can increase sperm count by up to 800 percent.

8 **Diabetes** is aggravated by smoking, and people with diabetes are three times more likely to die of cardiovascular disease than are people without diabetes. Smokers with diabetes are also more likely to suffer nerve damage (neuropathy) and kidney disease.

9 **Colds and respiratory infections** are more common among people who smoke, because smoking increases people's susceptibility.

10 **Cervical cancer** has been linked with smoking. Carcinogens found in tobacco are found on the cervixes of women who smoke, apparently transported there by the bloodstream.

11 **High blood pressure** and smoking are a deadly combination and are related to a high incidence of heart attacks and stroke.

12 **Asthma and asthmatic bronchitis** are twice as likely to develop among children who are exposed to passive smoking every day when one or both parents smoke.

13 **Premature and low-birth-weight infants** are twice as likely to be born to mothers who smoke. These children are at high risk of respiratory disorders, jaundice, low blood sugar, and other health problems.

14 **Sudden infant death syndrome (SIDS)** occurs twice as often among infants whose parents smoke.

15 **Inflammation of the middle ear** occurs more frequently in early childhood among children whose mothers smoke.

16 **Addiction to nicotine** from a mother's smoking habit may occur among infants before they are born.

Part V

Health Statistics and Trivia You Might Need to Know

Are you a trivia enthusiast? Are you fascinated by quirky or unusual health-related facts and statistics? Some people collect baseball cards or stamps; others hoard off-the-wall knowledge.

For example, do you know how much money the U.S. government spends on medical research, or how many people died during the Black Plague? Both of these facts, and many more about medical research monies and epidemics through the ages, are available in this section.

Some trivia really isn't so trivial. For example, are some of the plants in your house poisonous? Which animals are the most dangerous? Is your pet dog safe to be around? The answers may surprise you.

Do you know someone—or are you that someone—who is expecting a baby? Then chapters on multiple births and the average height and weight by sex and age of children should be entertaining and informative. What if you're seated next to your Great-Aunt Harriet at a family gathering and you've run out of things to say? You might ask her if she's vying for a spot on the list of longest-living people in the world, an impressive list provided in this section.

chapter fifty-five

Medical Research Dollars: Where the Money Goes

Every year, Americans donate a huge amount of money to health-related charitable and research organizations. We don't know the precise amount of money that private and corporate donors make to these causes, but we can tell you where your tax dollars go. Even if you don't want to contribute to a specific research cause, the government does it for you when it takes your tax dollars. The job of distributing those tax dollars for medical research is in the hands of the National Institutes of Health (NIH).

How much does the NIH distribute to different medical research causes? Here are the figures for fiscal year 2001. You will notice that monies are now delegated to the National Center for Complementary and Alternative Medicine and the new National Human Genome Research Institute. More information about the budget can be seen at the NIH Web site: www.nih.gov/news/budget01/nih2001budget.pdf.

Fiscal Year 2001 Appropriation

Recipient	$ (in thousands)
National Cancer Institute	3,754,456
National Heart, Lung and Blood Institute	2,298,512
National Institute of Dental and Craniofacial Research	306,211
National Institute of Diabetes and Digestive and Kidney Diseases	1,302,684
National Institute of Neurological Disorders and Stroke	1,175,854

Recipient	$ (in thousands)
National Institute of Allergy and Infectious Diseases	2,041,698
National Institute of General Medical Sciences	1,535,378
National Institute of Child Health and Human Development	975,766
National Eye Institute	510,352
National Institute of Environmental Health Sciences	501,949
National Institute on Aging	785,590
National Institute of Arthritis and Musculoskeletal and Skin Diseases	396,460
National Institute of Deafness and Other Communication Disorders	300,418
National Institute of Mental Health	1,106,305
National Institute on Drug Abuse	780,833
National Institute on Alcohol Abuse and Alcoholism	340,453
National Institute of Nursing Research	104,328
National Human Genome Research Institute	382,112
National Center for Complementary and Alternative Medicine	89,138
National Center on Minority Health and Health Disparities	130,096
National Library of Medicine	246,351

Note: An additional $97 million is allocated for type I diabetes.

chapter fifty-six

24 Notorious Epidemics: Cause and Mortality

For as long as people and animals have tread on this earth, there have been diseases. Many of them merely cause annoying or uncomfortable symptoms and then go away; some linger for years, reducing the quality of life. Others strike hard and kill, often the weak, the very young, or the very old. Perhaps more terrifying, however, are diseases that sweep through an entire geographical area, affecting great numbers of people—young and old, weak and strong— seemingly without discrimination.

When a disease spreads through but is limited to a specific region, it is called an *epidemic*. When it travels through a large geographical area such as a continent or even the whole world and affects an exceptionally large number of people, it is called a *pandemic*.

Before the age of modern medicine, when researchers could use microscopes to see the tiny organisms that cause disease, people did not understand that unseen organisms were behind the widespread death and suffering. Their lack of knowledge led them to place blame on people of other religions or beliefs. In Italy during the Black Death (Black Plague), for example, frightened Christians claimed that the Muslims and the Jews were responsible for the epidemic. The situation led to some terrible atrocities.

Today, scientists understand a great deal more about the spread of disease; yet even with the great advances in medicine, epidemics and pandemics still hold many mysteries. Take AIDS, for example. Researchers have yet to definitely identify its origin, and there still is no cure or completely effective treatment.

Diseases Defined

Here's a list of eight of the best-known epidemic diseases ever to have ravaged humankind.

Bacterial Meningitis: Caused by the bacterium *Neisseria meningitidis*. Meningitis can also be caused by other bacteria, as well as by viruses.

Cholera: A severe disease spread by food and water that has been contaminated by feces. It causes severe diarrhea, which leads to extreme dehydration that results in shock, renal failure, and death.

Dysentery: A term that describes several intestinal disorders characterized by inflamed mucous membranes.

Influenza: A viral infection of the respiratory tract that causes headache, backache, fever, and weakness.

Malaria: An infectious tropical disease caused by protozoa (*Plasmodium*) that are transmitted to people through the bite of the Anopheles mosquito. Symptoms include high fever, chills, anemia, and sweating.

Plague: A term used to describe an epidemic; also, a term used to describe bubonic plague, or the Black Death, which is caused by the bacterium *Yersinia pestis*.

Smallpox: A highly infectious, potentially fatal viral disease characterized by vomiting, chills, fever, lower back pain, and skin eruptions that leave permanent scars (pocks). The last naturally occurring case was recorded in 1977 in Somalia.

Typhus: An infectious disease caused by *Rickettsia* and transmitted by mites, fleas, lice, and ticks that have fed off infected rats. Symptoms include fever, chills, severe headache, delirium, and a dark red rash.

There have been hundreds of epidemics throughout human history. The 24 most notorious ones are listed here. Will we be adding others to the list? Some experts believe we are at extreme risk for future epidemics. In *The Coming Plague* (Penguin, 1994), author Laurie Garrett says that as humans continue to fight among themselves and use up the earth's resources, "The advantage moves to the microbes' court. They are our predators and they will be victorious if we . . . do not learn how to live in a rational global village that affords the microbes few opportunities."

Here is a list of infamous plagues from history, creating some of the worst catastrophes humans have ever seen.

1 542–43 CE. The Plague (bubonic) of Justinian, named after the Emperor Justinian, lasted for about two years in Constantinople. It then spread to Italy, France, Denmark, the Rhine area, Spain, and Britain. *Death toll:* The historian Procopius reported that at the height of the epidemic, 5,000 to 10,000 people died per day in Constantinople, for a total of 70,000 over two years. The death toll in Europe is not known.

2 1347–52. The Black Death first struck Europe in 1347. The Black Death was caused by a bacterium that inhabited rats. Fleas fed off the rats, contracted the disease, and then bit humans. *Death toll:* Some estimate that 25 million people died in Europe, about one-third of Europe's population.

3 1520–21. Mexican Smallpox. *Death toll:* Experts disagree about the totals; they range from 2 million to 15 million.

4 1525–27. Smallpox epidemic in South America. *Death toll:* Approximately 200,000 Incas.

5 1542. Typhus epidemic in Hungary. *Death toll:* Approximately 30,000 Germans died while they prepared to attack the Turks in Hungary.

6 1576–81. A measles or typhus epidemic in Yucatan, Mexico. *Death toll:* Estimated 2 million.

7 1619. Smallpox epidemic in Chile. *Death toll:* 50,000.

8 1665. The Great Plague of London was the bubonic plague. Although we now know that the plague was spread by rats (specifically, the fleas on the rats), rumors that dogs and cats were responsible led to destruction of these animals, which only served to remove the rats' predators. The 1666 Fire of London helped end the Plague. *Death toll:* Officially 68,596, but experts believe the number was closer to 110,000.

9 1772–73. Persian Plague. *Death toll:* This was one of the most severe recorded epidemics of bubonic plague, with approximately 2 million deaths.

10 1779–80. A combination measles and smallpox epidemic in Mexico City. *Death toll:* 18,000.

11 1813–14. German typhus epidemics affected northern and central Germany. *Death toll:* 219,000 to 300,000.

12 1829–33. Oregon malaria epidemic. *Death toll:* Estimated to be 150,000 among the American Indian population.

13 1832–33. French cholera epidemic. *Death toll:* Estimated to be 100,000.

14 1837–40. British smallpox epidemics. *Death toll:* Approximately 42,000.

15 1846–50. Irish typhus and dysentery. *Death toll:* 800,000 to 1,100,000.

16 1848–49 and 1953–54. British cholera epidemics. *Death toll:* 54,000 to 62,000 during the first; 31,000 during the second.

17 1853. Yellow fever epidemic in New Orleans. *Death toll:* 12,000.

18 1870–75. European smallpox pandemic triggered by the Franco–Prussian War. *Death toll:* Estimated 500,000.

19 1889–90. European influenza pandemic. *Death toll:* Estimated to be 270,000 to 360,000.

20 1900–08. Indian cholera epidemic. *Death toll:* In 1900, the death toll was 805,698; thereafter, it was estimated to be 600,000 per year.

21 1901–04. Sleeping sickness epidemic in Uganda. *Death toll:* More than 250,000.

22 1918–19. Influenza pandemic. The influenza began in the United States, but as American soldiers shipped out for Europe to fight during World War I, they carried the virus with them. *Death toll:* Worldwide, an estimated 30 million people died. Nearly 20 million died in India and 500,000 in the United States; the remaining deaths occurred in various other countries.

23 1980–2000 (and it's not over yet). AIDS pandemic. *Death toll:* As of 2000, 18.8 million worldwide.

24 1996. Bacterial meningitis in Africa. *Death toll:* 17,000.

The actual number of deaths associated with any epidemic is difficult to know for certain, especially for outbreaks that occurred hundreds or thousands of years ago. Other sources may quote different figures. It's been noted in historical records that many deaths were never recorded. During the Great Plague of London, for example, thousands of slum dwellers died unnoticed; and Jews, Quakers, and other small religious groups did not report deaths to the parish church, as did larger congregations. Also, death sometimes came so quickly to so many that there was no time to count the bodies.

chapter fifty-seven

Medical Trivia:
When Conversation Drags
at Your Next Party

We've all experience awkward moments when we don't know what to say. It can happen at a party where you really don't have much in common with other guests. You've exhausted small talk about the weather and sports and don't want to get into the three taboos: religion, politics, and sex. Or maybe you're on a blind date set up by your well-meaning Aunt Millie and you're having such a dull time that you don't think you're going to make it until the main entrée is served.

These are occasions when it may be time to say, "Hey, did you know that . . . ?" For example, suppose the conversation between you and your blind date is near rock bottom and your date sneezes. You could say, "Hey, did you know that that a sneeze can exceed a speed of one hundred miles per hour? Don't ask me why I know this, but I read it somewhere and for some reason it stuck with me. Do you like trivia?"

Okay, maybe the following medical and health tidbits are not great pickup lines (unless you're at a medical convention). But they are interesting facts about the always fascinating world of health and medicine. Read them for fun. You never know when they might come in handy.

Health and Medical Trivia

- Everyone is born colorblind. That's because the cones cells, which are responsible for color detection, don't develop until an infant is about 6 to 8 months old.

- Every hair on the body has a tiny muscle that can make it stand upright.

- Humans are not the only animals known to have sex for pleasure; so do dolphins. Is that why Flipper always looked so happy?

- If the appendix doesn't do anything, why does it become inflamed in some people? This little tube that hangs about three inches from the lowest part of the large intestine sometimes collects food particles. If the particles get caught, bacteria can grow and irritate the appendix, causing it to swell.

- We acquire fingerprints even before we enter the world: They develop at three months gestation, while we're in the womb.

- A cough releases a burst of air that moves at speeds up to 60 miles per hour.

- A fingernail or toenail takes about six months to grow from base to tip. However, fingernails grow slightly faster than toenails.

- You can die of sleep deprivation before you'll die of starvation. Go without sleep for about 10 days and you'll die, but you can stop eating for weeks before death takes over.

- Humans lose about 40 to 100 strands of hair each day.

- The average human scalp has 100,000 hairs, so we can afford to lose a few each day.

- The fastest-growing hairs on the human body are those in a beard. It's been estimated that if the average man never trimmed his beard, it would grow to nearly 30 feet long during his lifetime.

- The average human drinks about 16,000 gallons of water during his or her lifetime.

- According to the Kinsey Institute (the infamous sex research group), the biggest erect penis on record measured 13 inches, while the smallest was 1¾ inches.

- The average human uses the bathroom six times per day.

- By the age of 60, most adults have lost about 50 percent of their taste buds.
- Every person has a unique tongue print as well as one-of-a-kind fingerprints.
- Every square inch of the human body has an average of 32 million bacteria living on it. That's high-density real estate.
- Every square inch of human skin has 20 feet of blood vessels.
- If you're still using stamps that you need to lick, you're consuming one-tenth of a calorie for each stamp licked. That makes self-sticking stamps a no-calorie alternative.
- Fingerprints aren't just for identification purposes: They actually provide traction for the fingers when you pick things up.
- The average American eats more than 50 tons of food during his or her lifetime. This could explain why we have an obesity problem in the United States.
- Dandruff is nothing compared with the number of dead skin cells the average person sheds: about 600,000 particles of skin every hour, which equals about 1.5 pounds per year.
- We shed and regrow outer skin cells about every 27 days, which equals about 1,000 new outer skin layers in a lifetime.
- Smiling takes less effort than frowning: 17 muscles are involved when you smile, 43 when you frown.
- Adults laugh between 15 and 100 times a day, while the average 6-year-old laughs about 300 times a day.
- The average human body contains enough fat to make seven bars of soap, enough water to fill a ten-gallon tank, and enough iron to make a three-inch nail.
- The average person releases nearly a pint of intestinal gas every day. The majority of flatulence is the result of swallowed air, and the rest is due to fermentation of undigested food. (This is not a fact to bring up during dinner.)
- The average person has enough phosphorus in his or her body to make 2,200 match heads.
- The human brain consists of about 85 percent water.
- The left and right lungs are not the same size: The left one is smaller to allow room for the heart.

- The largest cell in the human body is the ovum, the female reproductive cell, which is about 1/180 inch in diameter; the smallest is the male sperm. If you put one ovum on one side of a scale, you would need about 175,000 sperm cells on the other side to balance the scale.

- The most common blood type in the world is Type O. Less than a dozen people have been found to have Type A-H, the rarest blood type.

- The ashes of the average cremated person weigh nine pounds.

- Neanderthal people had bigger brains than we do.

- About 300 million cells die in the human body every minute.

- Reading in bad light does not damage your eyes. It can cause eye fatigue, headache, and muscular tension, but bad vision is usually the result of a defect in the eyes.

- Getting your feet wet or sitting in a cold draft do not cause a cold. Although more people get colds during the winter, experts believe that may be because cold weather forces people to stay indoors more, giving the virus a better chance to spread, and that cold weather may increase the virus's survival rate.

- Experts find that few colds are transmitted through the air and that most are passed along on the hands. Thus covering your mouth when you sneeze—if you do so with your hand—is probably much worse than not covering it at all (unless you use a tissue to cover your sneeze, of course, and discard it).

chapter fifty-eight

The *17*

Most Poisonous Plants

About 10 percent of the more than 40,000 different kinds of plants growing in the United States are poisonous to humans. This list includes botanicals that people in North America are most likely to encounter in their daily lives, especially houseplants and those found in home gardens.

Children, of course, are more likely than adults to ingest poisonous plants, especially those that have berries or attractive seeds. If a child or other individual eats a poisonous plant, do the following:

- Remove any plant parts from the person's mouth.
- Get immediate medical help. Call a Poison Control Center or 911. It is a good idea to keep your local Poison Control Center telephone number next to the phone, along with your other emergency numbers, especially if you have young children at home.
- Take the plant with you to the hospital or Poison Control Center for identification purposes.

Deadly Botanicals

Most poisonous plants fall into one of five categories: nerve poisons, internal organ poisons, mineral poisons, allergy producers, and irritants. Most of the deadliest plants are in the first two categories, and the majority of plants in this list are in those groups. They are listed alphabetically, not in order of their ability to harm or kill.

1 Caladium. This attractive plant is sometimes mistakenly called elephant's ear. It has large, heart- or arrow-shaped leaves that are bicolored: bluish-green, purplish-green, or black-violet, depending on the variety. The plant grows to heights of 2 to 5 feet and is found in tropical areas of the United States, such as Florida. It is a popular house and garden plant. Its leaves are highly toxic, as they contain the poison oxalic acid.

2 Castor bean. The beans of the castor oil plant (*Ricinus communis*) contain ricine, a potent poison. Children are attracted to the shiny, gray-brown seeds of this plant. Eating the seeds can cause violent convulsions and death from an inability to breathe. Two seeds can kill an adult. The castor oil plant grows in the southern U.S. and California as a small tree, and as a taller tree (5 to 6 feet) in the northern U.S. Its leaves are large, with five to eleven notches.

3 Dieffenbachia (dumb cane). The dieffenbachia is a popular houseplant and grows best in tropical areas of the United States. It reaches a height of about 4 feet and sports erect, unbranched, oblong leaves with white splotches. Chewing the leaves causes the mouth to swell and eventual death by asphyxiation.

4 Foxglove *(Digitalis purpurea).* This plant is cultivated throughout the United States and grows wild along the west coast. Foxglove contains digitalis, which can be helpful or dangerous depending on the amount taken. Eating too much of the plant can accelerate the heart, cause it to skip beats, or make it stop. Foxglove grows to about 6 feet in height and has clusters of leaves at the base of the stalk, along with groups of white or purple bell-shaped flowers at the tip.

5 Hyacinth *(Hyacinthus orientalis).* Pink, white, red, blue, or yellow funnel-shaped, fragrant flowers and long, narrow leaves are the trademarks of this plant, which grows from a bulb. Hyacinth is a popular house and garden plant and can be found throughout the United States. Eating any part of the plant, which contains several toxins including lycorine, causes diarrhea, nausea, and vomiting.

6 **Jasmine, Yellow jasmine** *(Gelsemium sempervirens).* Jasmine is a woody trailing or climbing vine with yellow flowers that have five rounded lobes. It is commonly seen in the southeastern United States in woodlands, thickets, and along roadways. Eating the plant causes convulsions, muscle weakness, difficulty breathing, and paralysis of the motor nerves.

7 **Larkspur** *(Delphinium nelsonii).* Larkspur is a low-growing plant (about 18 inches high) with hairy stems and upper leaves, and blue-purple flowers with spurs, thus the name. It grows throughout the United States in open woodlands and meadows. It contains the toxins methyllycaconitine and nudicauline, which affect the nervous system, causing muscle and respiratory paralysis and death.

8 **Manchineel.** The coastal lands and the Everglades of Florida are home to the manchineel, a small tree with oval leaves and red or yellow flowers. It also sports a warty bark that gives up a milky sap, and yellow or light green fruit. Both the fruit and sap contain two forms of the deadly toxin hippomane A & B. This poison causes bloody diarrhea and extremely painful gastritis, and may lead to hypovolemic (low blood level) shock.

9 **Mistletoe** *(Phoradendon serotineum).* This parasitic plant lives in many types of hardwood trees, primarily in the southern United States: from New Jersey south to Florida and west to Texas and Arizona. It has many branches and two- to three-inch long pale yellow-green leaves. The fruit (berries) are white or red and poisonous when eaten in large amounts. The toxin in the berries, called phoratoxin, causes abdominal pain and diarrhea.

10 **Oleander** *(Nerium oleander).* The oleander is an evergreen shrub with large pink or white flowers and narrow, tough leaves. It grows in the southern United States, California, and Hawaii. Eating the leaves or branches causes stomach pain, vomiting, and heart irregularities, which can lead to death. The plant contains the potent toxins oleandrin and neriine.

11 **Pokeweed** *(Phytolacca americana).* This low-growing plant has stout, purplish leaf stalks, which grow about one foot high, and green-white to purple flowers. Its dark purple to black berries are attached to its stalk. Pokeweed grows in damp woods and fields from Maine to Minnesota, south to the Gulf of Mexico. Its leaves, berries, and roots contain the toxin spanonin, which causes nausea, vomiting, and blurred vision. Death can occur if these plant parts are eaten in great quantities.

12 **Privet** *(Ligustrum vulgare).* Both the United States and Canada are home to the privet, a shrub that is popular as a hedge plant. The privet has elliptical leaves, small white flowers that grow in clusters, and black or blue wax-coated berries. The entire plant is poisonous and contains the toxin ligustrin. Eating the plant causes colic and diarrhea and can be fatal in children.

13 **Rhododendron.** Plants in the rhododendron species, which include laurels and azaleas, usually grow to a height of about 5 feet. The leaves are oblong and the flowers are funnel-shaped and come in various colors. Rhododendrons contain the toxin grayanotoxins, which causes numbness, tingling, slowed heart rate, diarrhea, confusion, muscle weakness, convulsions, coma, and death.

14 **Rhubarb** *(Rheum rhaponticum or rhabarbum).* Rhubarb is a food plant whose stalks are safe to eat but whose leaves are poisonous. The large, ovate leaves appear to be wrinkled and contain the toxins oxalic acid and anthraquinone glycosides. When eaten, the leaves cause stomach pain, vomiting, internal bleeding, convulsions, and death. Rhubarb is widely cultivated in the United States.

15 **Water hemlock** *(Cicuta species).* The water hemlock is a member of the parsley family, which also contains the wild carrot and parsnip. In fact, its leaves resemble those of carrots. The water hemlock can reach a height of 10 feet and has hollow stems covered with purple spots. It can be found throughout the United States in wetlands and along the banks of streams. The spotted water hemlock, *C. maculata,* is considered to be the most violently toxic plant in North America. Death can occur 15 minutes to 3 hours after eating the plant.

16 **Woody nightshade.** The woody nightshade—*Solanum dulcamara,* which has red berries; and *Solanum nigrum,* which has purple or black berries—grows in wooded areas throughout North America, although *S. nigrum* is native to the eastern U.S. The woody nightshade climbs like a vine and can grow up to 6 feet. Its leaves are pointed and the flowers are white, purple-white, or dark blue. Symptoms of poisoning include loss of memory, madness, kidney failure, muscle tremors, and weakness. Steroidal alkaloids such as solanine are responsible for these symptoms. Death may be the final outcome of poisoning.

17 **Yew** (*Taxus* species). There are various types of yews in this species, including Japanese, English, Western, and Canadian yews. These evergreens grow throughout the United States. All parts of the yew contain the poisonous alkaloid taxine, but the red or pink berries that are particularly attractive to children are the least toxic part of the evergreen. Yews have pointed, flat, needle-like leaves, which have the highest amount of toxin. Eating the plant can cause convulsions, difficulty breathing, and death.

chapter fifty-nine

20 Life-Threatening Animals

Lions and tigers and bears—oh my! Some of the world's most life-threatening animals, you say? Wrong! They may be big and look mean at times, and they certainly can be deadly. But lions and tigers and bears are not among the *most* life-threatening animals in the world.

We share this planet with a host of nonhuman creatures—mammals, fish, birds, amphibians, reptiles, insects, and a vast number of tiny organisms. Sometimes we get in each others' way, either intentionally or unintentionally, and occasionally such an encounter places a creature or a human in danger.

The list here consists of creatures that can be deadly to humans. They represent a very small percentage of the animals on earth, but given the amount of traveling many people do today, the chance that you may encounter one or several of the more exotic life-threatening animals in this list is certainly greater than it was decades ago. Not, of course, that we wish such an experience on you, but a heads-up now can make the difference between life and death later. If you are considering world travel, remember that Australia is the home to nine of the ten most venomous snakes in the world, and has the most deadly spiders on earth.

Then again, danger can be as close as your own backyard.

1 Anaconda. This huge snake can grow to 37-plus feet in length and weigh about 400 pounds. Its bite is not poisonous, but it can suffocate its prey in seconds. Giant anaconda are found only in South America.

2 **Black widow spider.** Drop for drop, the venom from this spider is more potent than that of a rattlesnake. The widow's bite is nearly painless, but it is followed by intense pain and rigid abdominal and other muscles, and may be accompanied by nausea, headache, and difficulty breathing. About 4 percent of those bitten die. The black widow spider is found in all 48 contiguous states and in much of the rest of the world.

3 **Blue-ringed octopus.** Although this creature is only 8 inches long, its sting can cause dizziness and shortness of breath within 5 minutes and death within 2 to 3 hours. It is found offshore of Australia, Indonesia, and the Philippines.

4 **Box jellyfish.** The box jellyfish, also known as the sea wasp, is considered the most venomous marine creature on earth. It kills more people than stonefish, sharks, and crocodiles combined. Box jellyfish live in the shallow waters off the coast of northern Australia and in the Indo-Pacific region. They can weigh up to nearly a pound and have approximately 5,000 stinging cells. Most people get stung when they bump into the jellyfish while wading or swimming. The sting causes excruciating pain and heart and respiratory failure unless antivenin is given.

5 **Brown recluse spider.** This spider has a potent venom that can easily kill a child, but adults usually survive. It can be found throughout the United States, especially in the West and Midwest.

6 **Bull shark.** This shark is one of the most dangerous in the world, and may be the most dangerous in the tropics. It is found in rivers and lakes, including the lower Mississippi River and the Amazon and Congo rivers, and along the coasts of southeast Asia, Africa, California, and New England. It would be hard to mistake this creature for a catfish or minnow in the river: It grows to about 11 feet and 400-plus pounds.

7 **Cobra.** The venom of the cobra kills by paralyzing the central nervous system of its victim. The spitting cobra first spits venom into the eyes of its victim, then bites. The king cobra bites only. Death occurs within about 20 minutes of the bite. Cobras live in Africa and Asia.

8 Cone snail. There are more than 500 species of cone snails, which can be found in the coral reefs of the Indian Ocean, Australia, the Red Sea, East Africa, and around California and New Zealand. The snail's sting releases toxins that affect the nervous system, causing pain, numbness, dizziness, vomiting, and temporary paralysis of the arms, legs, and lungs. Total paralysis of the diaphragm and death comes within several hours. Not all species of the snail are deadly. The more beautiful ones, however, are.

9 Deer. Although the Insurance Institute for Highway Safety admits that "good national statistics don't exist on how many collisions occur between deer and motor vehicles each year," the estimate is hundreds of thousands. Some states do keep records of such accidents, and Michigan is one of them. In 1999, there were 67,669 deer–motor vehicle collisions, which left 6 people dead and 2,300 injured.

10 Dogs. Tell me it's not true! Is our best friend also our enemy? Based on data from the National Center for Health Statistics and the Centers for Disease Control and Prevention, dog bites are responsible for nearly 4.5 million injuries every year. In that figure are included 20 deaths, nearly 334,000 visits to hospital emergency departments, and more than 670 hospitalizations. Every day, another 914 people seek medical care at an emergency department because of a dog bite. Between the years 1989 and 1994, there were 109 reported deaths, 57 percent of which involved children younger than 10 years old. The dogs most responsible for these statistics are pit bulls, rottweilers, and German shepherds.

11 Fire ants. Although many ant species sting, the most aggressive in the United States are imported fire ants. They attack viciously, relentlessly, and in large numbers, inflicting thousands of stings on their victims. Sometimes the victim is a person, especially anyone who happens to disturb their mounds. They also have been known to attack people while they sleep and have caused the deaths of infants and elderly people who have been unable to escape the stings. The *Annals of Internal Medicine* reports that more than 80 people have died of stings from fire ants. In 1989, there were 32 deaths from the tiny creatures in Texas, Florida, Louisiana, and Georgia.

12 Great white shark (*Carcharodon charcharias*). The great white is responsible for the most deadly shark attacks. It is found in most oceans, especially tropical and subtropical waters. It has been known to travel as far north as the New England coast.

13 Killer bees. Also known as Africanized bees, killer bees are a hybrid of Tanzanian and Brazilian bees. They were accidentally released in Brazil in 1956 and have been making their way northward. Killer bees can be found in Arizona, California, and Texas, and have killed about 1,000 people in the Americas in the last half-century.

14 Mosquito. How can something so small be life-threatening? Mosquitoes are carriers of several deadly diseases, including yellow fever, malaria, dengue fever, encephalitis, and filariasis. Mosquitoes have killed more people throughout history than all wars combined. Each year, about 1 million people around the world die of mosquito-transmitted disease, and another 250 million contract mosquito-transmitted diseases.

15 Piranha. Only 5 of the 20 known species of this Amazon native are carnivorous. Piranhas are attracted to blood and splashing, and these meat-eaters can pick all the flesh from the body of a large animal or human in minutes. Piranhas can grow to about 2 feet in length and travel in schools. They avoid being directly behind one another when they swim because they do attack and eat their own kind.

16 Poison dart frog. The tiny (about 3/4 inch long) poison dart frog lives in the South American jungles, where some of the tribal people use the frog's poison in their hunting darts. A single poison dart frog can have enough poison in the glands in its skin to kill 100 people.

17 Puffer. This fish is known as a blowfish in the U.S. and as fugu in Japan, where it is considered a gourmet delicacy. Eating a puffer can be deadly. The toxins in its intestines, liver, and ovaries are 275 times more toxic than cyanide. This toxin, called tetrodotoxin, can cause death within 6 to 24 hours after ingesting any part of the fish that contains the poison. If the chef does not properly remove the poisonous parts from the puffer before serving it up, it could be the last thing the diner eats.

18 Scorpion. The 1,300 to 1,500 species of scorpions in the world are all poisonous, but only 25 species are deadly to humans. These tiny creatures can be found everywhere: in deserts, forests, grasslands, and mountains. The venom in the scorpion's stinging tail acts on the central nervous system and paralyzes its prey. Death results because of heart or respiratory failure several hours after the sting. The largest scorpions live in southern Africa, where they grow to be up to 8 inches long. The largest in the United States are 5 inches.

19 **Stonefish.** The reefs off northeastern Australia are the main home of the deadly stonefish. The venom from just one of its spines can cause screaming, convulsions, and paralysis within minutes. The poison from several spines can be fatal if the victim is not treated immediately, and even sometimes in spite of treatment.

20 **Sydney funnel-web spider.** The female of this species is about the size of an adult human hand, and the male is slightly smaller. The Sydney funnel-web spider is so named because it is found only in Sydney, Australia, and because of the funnel-like shape of its web and nest. This deadly spider has long fangs like a snake, and the bite of the male is more toxic than that of the female. The toxin, called atraxtoxin, attacks the nerves in the spider's victim and causes muscle twitching and a profuse flow of saliva, tears, and perspiration. This leads to shock, coma, and death unless an antivenin is given.

chapter sixty

Making Babies: Counting Your Blessings by Twos and Threes and Fours

"Congratulations! It's a boy!"

"Congratulations on your new baby girl!"

Sound familiar? It should. Every year in the United States, we welcome 3,800,000 new children into the world. For parents, that means lots of dirty diapers, sleepless nights, spitting up, and bottles—work, work, work. But the work is nothing compared to the joy a child can bring.

Congratulations . . . You Have a Crowd

Now imagine a slight turn of phrase: "Congratulations. You've just had *twins!*" Or triplets, or quadruplets, or even quintuplets. That's a lot of joy to handle all at once.

The number of multiple births has been rising in the United States. Between 1980 and 1995, the number of live births of triplets tripled, and since 1971 it has quadrupled. The National Center of Health Statistics attributes this increase to two things: the use of fertility drugs, and the greater number of women older than 30 who are having children. These women are more likely to have multiple births.

MULTIPLE BIRTHS

How do multiple births occur? We'll look at the simplest of multiples: twins. There are two types of twins, and possibly a third. Identical twins are the result of one fertilized egg that has split into two after conception. Thus each individual shares all the same genes—they are essentially genetic clones of each other and so must be the same sex. Although each twin in a set will have the same hair and eye color, their fingerprints will be different, and environmental factors in the womb and after birth can have an impact on individual traits.

Fraternal twins are much more common than identical twins. They are the result of two eggs becoming fertilized, and so the result may be two boys, two girls, or one of each. (This is how higher-order multiple births occur, with multiple eggs being released and fertilized.) Some experts believe the tendency to bear fraternal twins may be inherited. Age of the mother, race, heredity, and the number of children previously borne by the mother all influence the incidence of fraternal twins.

Some researchers have suggested that there is a third type, called polar body twinning. This could be the result of an egg that splits before it is fertilized, then each half is fertilized by different sperm. The children would share the same genes from the mother and have different genes from the father. Scientists have not yet proven that polar body twinning occurs, but it could explain why some fraternal twins look as much alike as identical twins.

If you're thinking about starting a family or adding to the one you already have, or you just like to think about other people having babies, here are some facts about those multiple little bundles of joy.

THREE'S COMPANY, FOUR AND MORE'S A CROWD

- The chances of having triplets (spontaneously; without fertility drugs) is one in 7,000; for quadruplets, one in 571,000; and for quintuplets, one in 47,000,000

- Women who carry more than one child are immediately considered to be at high risk for having complications.

- According to the National Vital Statistics Report for 1980–1997:

  ➢ The number of twin births rose 52 percent (from 68,339 to 104,137).

  ➢ The number of births of triplets rose 404 percent (from 1,337 to 6,737).

➤ The rates of low birth weight, very low birth weight, and infant deaths were 4 to 33 percent higher for twins and triplets-plus, compared with single births.

➤ Twin rates in Massachusetts and Connecticut are at least 25 percent higher than in the rest of the United States.

- Babies born in triplet and higher multiple births are born smaller and earlier than are single births, and are at greater risk of infant death and life-long health problems. Infant death rates are 12 times higher for triplets than for singles.

- In 1995 alone, the 4,973 triplet and higher multiple births included 4,551 triplets, 365 quadruplets, and 57 quintuplets and greater births.

- A report in *Obstetrics and Gynecology* estimates that it is about 28 times more expensive to give birth to a baby at 25 to 27 weeks gestation than it is at 39 to 42 weeks.

- The average birth weight of a newborn triplet is 50 percent less than that of a single-birth infant. In 1995, 92 percent of triplets were born pre-term, compared with slightly more than 10 percent of single birth infants.

- The gestation period for triplets is an average of seven weeks shorter than that for single births.

- The largest rise in triplet births is among married, college-educated women older than 30.

WELL-KNOWN MULTIPLE BIRTHS

Twins

- Mario and Aldo Andretti: race car drivers
- Montgomery Clift: actor
- John Elway: pro football player
- Robin and Maurice Gibb: the BeeGees
- David and Randolph Hearst: CEO of the Hearst Corporation
- Mark and Scott Kelly: twin astronauts
- Liberace: pianist (his twin died at birth)
- John Lindsay: former mayor of New York City

- Elvis Presley: singer (his twin died at birth)
- Isabella Rosselini: actress and model
- Ed Sullivan: TV variety show host
- Kiefer Sutherland: actor (son of Donald Sutherland)
- Paul Tsongas: senator who ran for the presidency
- Abigail Van Buren and Ann Landers: advice columnists

Triplets, and So On

- Faith, Hope, and Charity Cardwell. Oldest triplets. Born May 18, 1899; Faith died in 1994, Charity in 1995, and Hope in 1997.
- Alison, Brooke, Claire, and Darcy Hansen. First set of identical girl quadruplets.
- Elisabeth Kubler-Ross, doctor and author. A triplet.
- Daniel, Michael, and Joseph Todd. They played the triplet grandsons on *My Three Sons* from 1970 to 1972.
- Amal Abdel-Fattah, in Egypt. Mother of the second known set of all-female sextuplets, which were born in November 1997.
- Hasna Mohammed Humair gave birth to septuplets in November 1997.
- Nkem Chukwu of Houston, Texas gave birth to septuplets, 5 girls and 2 boys, in December 1998. They were the world's first septuplets all to be born alive. One child died later.
- Dionne quintuplets: Annette, Cecile, Emilie, Marie, and Yvonne. Born in Canada in 1934, they were the first quintuplets known to survive infancy.
- In 1983, the first all-female sextuplets were born in England: Ruth, Jenny, Sarah, Hannah, Lucy, and Kate Walton.
- Eric, Taylor, Parker, Mason, and Hunter Guttensohn, born in 1996, believed to be the first set of all-male quintuplets born in the U.S., and the third recorded in history.
- In 1985, Alan, Brett, Connor, Douglas, and Edward Jacobssen were the first test-tube quintuplets born in the world.
- The McCaughey septuplets were born in 1997: Kenneth, Brandon, Nathan, Joel, Kelsey, Alexis, and Natalie.

TWINS: TWICE AS NICE

Here are some other interesting facts about twins:

- One-third of all twins are identical, with a nearly equal split between male/male and female/female pairs.
- One-third of twins are same-sex fraternal twins.
- One-third of twins are male/female fraternal twins.
- Slightly more than 50 percent of all twins born are male.
- More fraternal twins are conceived in July and the fewest in January.
- The rate of fraternal twins is higher in northern than in southern areas of the globe.
- Your chances of having another set of fraternal twins after giving birth to the first set is three to four times that of the general population.
- Your chances of having more than one set of identical twins are at least one in 70,000.
- When it comes to IQ, those of identical twins are usually within 5 points of each other, while those of fraternal twins can vary as much as any single-born children in the same family.

chapter sixty-one

"My, How They've Grown": Kids' Average Height and Weight by Age and Gender

Two main factors influence how children grow in height and weight: genetics and environment.

The instructions locked away in our DNA determine, to a great extent, the ultimate weight and height each person achieves in life. You can see this most obviously in the difference between the sexes. Boys and girls grow at about the same rate until the age of 10; then puberty begins for girls and stimulates a growth spurt. Boys tend to enter puberty a bit later, around age 12, when their growth surge begins. Although girls' rapid growth starts earlier, boys' lasts longer.

Environmental factors include nutrition, exercise, illness, and even the weather. Children need a well-balanced diet, augmented with supplements if necessary, to achieve their full potential for normal physical growth. Exercise has an impact because physical activity promotes stronger, denser bones. Long-term or chronic illnesses, such as diseases that affect the thyroid or pituitary glands, which regulate growth, certainly have an effect. As to the weather: Generally, children grow twice as fast in the spring as they do in the fall, but they tend to gain more weight in the fall.

Compare the Averages

How is your child growing? The following tables reflect the average height and weight for children ages 2 to 18. The figures are based on the 50th percentile, which means that for any given weight or height, 50 percent of children are heavier or taller, and 50 percent are lighter or shorter. If you have any questions about the growth rate of your child, consult your physician.

Girls		
Age	**Weight (pounds)**	**Height (feet/inches)**
2 years	24	2' 9"
3	30	3' 1"
4	35	3' 4"
5	40	3' 7"
6	45	3' 9"
7	50	3' 11"
8	55	4' 2"
9	62	4' 4"
10	70	4' 6"
11	80	4' 9"
12	90	5'
13	100	5' 1"
14	110	5' 3"
15	117	5' 4"
16	122	5' 4"
17	125	5' 4"
18	125	5' 4"

Boys

Age	Weight (pounds)	Height (feet/inches)
2 years	30	2' 10"
3	35	3' 2"
4	40	3' 5"
5	44	3' 8"
6	48	3' 10"
7	53	4'
8	60	4' 2"
9	65	4' 4"
10	73	4' 6"
11	80	4' 9"
12	90	4' 11"
13	100	5' 2"
14	110	5' 4"
15	125	5' 7"
16	135	5' 8"
17	148	5' 10"
18	155	5' 10"

chapter sixty-two

The *103*

Longest-Living People

Scientists tell us that soon people can expect to live well past the age of 100. That's a long way from where we started. Neanderthal humans lived to an average age of 18 years. The ancient Romans in 600 CE didn't fare much better: Most people didn't survive much past 30 years. Things didn't really improve until around 1900, when the average life span in England reached 46 years.

Today, according to the U.S. Census Bureau (1999) International Database, Japan leads the world in life expectancy. The average life expectancy for Japanese women is 83.35 years; for men, 77.02. Specifically, Japanese living in Okinawa live the longest: It's reported that this segment of Japan has 5.5 times more centenarians than the rest of the nation.

Australia comes in a very close second to Japan: 83.23 years for women, 77.22 for men. The United States is 24th on the list, with 79.67 years for women and 72.95 for men.

For whatever reason—good genes, healthy food, hard work, good attitude, or a daily glass of wine—a few men and women have defied the odds. They lived, or continue to live, well past the 100-year mark.

The list here contains information on people for whom there is reliable information or birth records. Other individuals are not included because their birth dates could not be verified. Maria Jeronimo, for example, was a slave who reportedly was born on March 5, 1871 in Carmo de Minas, Brazil. She died on June 14, 2000, which means she would have been 129 years old. Unfortunately, because she was a slave, no accurate record of her birth exists. Another questionable entry would have been Elizabeth Israel, reportedly born on January 2, 1875, in Dominica, a Caribbean island. Elizabeth was still alive as of March 7, 2000.

Several U.S. residents also fall into the unsubstantiated category. In July 2000, Juan Ramos, of Tampa, Florida, claimed to have been born in June 1880; and John Joe Begay, a Native American living in Navaho, Utah, said he was 114 years old. Herbert Young of Harlem, New York, who died on April 22, 1999, reportedly was born in May 1887.

Longest-Living People Trivia

In the Bible: Unsubstantiated: Aaron, Abraham, Adam, Cainan, Enoch, Enos, Isaac, Ishmael, Jacob, Jared, Jehoiada, Joseph, Joshua, Lamech, Mahalaleel, Methuselah, Moses, Noah, Sarah, Seth, Terah.

Oldest Actress in a Film: Jeanne Louise Clement, in *Vincent & Me*, at age 114.

Oldest Living Twins: Dale and Glen Mayer, born June 20, 1895, achieved that honor on January 23, 2000. They live in Alvorton and Greenville, Ohio, respectively.

Oldest Lesbian: Ruth Ellis, born July 23, 1899, died October 5, 2000 in Detroit, Michigan.

	Name	Age	Born	Died
1	Thomas Peters	111	April 6, 1745	March 26, 1857
2	Louisa K. Thiers	111	October 2, 1814	February 17, 1926
3	Delina (Ecker) Filkins	113	May 4, 1815	December 4, 1928
4	Katherine Plunket	111	November 22, 1820	October 14, 1932
5	Martha Graham	114	December 1844	June 25, 1959
6	John B. Salling	113	March 15, 1846	March 16, 1959

	Name	Age	Born	Died
7	James Henry Brett Jr.	111	July 25, 1849	February 10, 1961
8	John Mosely Turner	111	June 15, 1856	March 21, 1968
9	Johanna Booyson	111	January 17, 1857	June 16, 1968
10	Ada (Giddings) Rowe	111	February 6, 1858	January 11, 1970
11	Josefa Salas Mateo	112	July 14, 1860	February 27, 1973
12	Alice Stevenson	112	July 10, 1861	August 18, 1973
13	Mito Umeta	112	March 27, 1863	May 31, 1975
14	Rose Adelaide Heeley	111	August 26, 1864	December 24, 1975
15	Shigechiyo Izumi	120	June 29, 1865	February 21, 1986
16	Marie-Virginie (Mollet) Duhem	111	August 2, 1866	April 25, 1978
17	Sarah Ellen (Parkinson) Morgan	111	January 23, 1867	February 12, 1978
18	Fannie Thomas	113	April 24, 1867	January 22, 1981
19	Rozwlia Mielzcarak	112	1868	January 7, 1981
20	Florence Ada (Neate) Pannell	111	December 26, 1868	October 20, 1980
21	Augustine Teissier (Sister Julia)	112	January 2, 1869	March 9, 1981
22	Jane Piercy	111	September 2, 1869	May 3, 1981
23	Jeanetta Thomas	112	December 2, 1869	January 5, 1982
24	Alice Caroline Stracey Brewster	111	September 16, 1871	October 9, 1982
26	Mamie Eva (Walter) Keith	113	March 22, 1873	September 20, 1986
26	Mary Elizabeth (Wallace) McKinney	113	May 30, 1873	February 2, 1987

	Name	Age	Born	Died
27	Anna Eliza (Davies) Williams	114	June 2, 1873	December 27, 1987
28	Florence Knapp	114	October 10, 1873	January 11, 1988
29	Eugenie (Clegnac) Roux	112	January 24, 1873	June 20, 1986
30	Wilhelmine Sande	111	October 24, 1874	January 21, 1986
31	Carrie C. (Joyner) White	116	November 18, 1874	February 14, 1991
32	Caroline Maud Mockridge	112	December 11, 1874	November 6, 1987
33	Jeanne Louise Calment	122	February 21, 1875	August 4, 1997
34	Lydie Vellard	114	March 18, 1875	September 17, 1989
35	Orpha Nusbaum	112	August 13, 1875	March 30, 1988
36	Aphaeus Philemon	112	July 12, 1876	November 25, 1988
37	Birdie May (Musser) Vogt	112	August 3, 1876	July 23, 1989
38	Christina (Hoogakker) Van Druten	111	November 20, 1876	December 8, 1987
39	Maren Bolette Torp	112	December 21, 1876	February 20, 1989
40	Kate Begbie	111	January 9, 1877	September 5, 1988
41	Charlotte Marion (Milburn) Hughes	115	August 1, 1877	March 17, 1993
42	John Evans	112	August 19, 1877	June 10, 1990
43	Ettie Mae (Thomas) Greene	114	September 8, 1877	February 26, 1992
44	Mary Ann (Alder) Fewster	111	February 6, 1878	December 26, 1989
45	Rose Ellen (Sturgess) Hart	111	March 29, 1878	January 5, 1990
46	Waka Shirahama	114	March 23, 1878	June 16, 1992

	Name	Age	Born	Died
47	Jan Machiel Reyskens	111	May 11, 1878	January 7, 1990
48	Margaret (Seward) Skeete	115	October 27, 1878	May 7, 1994
49	Tane Ikai	116	January 18, 1879	July 12, 1995
50	Rosa Ann (Dossett) Comfort	113	January 21, 1879	November 6, 1992
51	Wilhelmina (Geringer) Kott	115	March 7, 1879	September 6, 1994
52	Eva (Aubert) Jourdan	112	March 25, 1880	May 6, 1992
53	Domenico Minervino	111	May 10, 1880	May 21, 1991
54	Daisy Irene (Woodward) Adams	113	June 28, 1880	December 8, 1993
55	Marie Louise Febronie Meilleur	117	August 29, 1880	April 16, 1998
56	Sarah DeRemer (Clark) Knauss	119	September 24, 1880	December 30, 1999
57	Ella Miller	119	December 6, 1880	November 22, 2000
58	Mary Electa Bidwell	114	May 9, 1881	April 25, 1996
59	Nellie (Hardman) Eby	111	May 17, 1881	January 13, 1993
60	Pauline Eugenie Chabanny	112	August 20, 1881	August 13, 1994
61	Rebecca (Ramsdale) Hewison	112	October 19, 1881	September 22, 1994
62	Estella Jones	117	November 10, 1881	June 27, 1999
63	Sister Alberta	111	January 30, 1882	April 22, 1993
64	Marie Bibeault	111	January 31, 1882	July 29, 1993
65	Annie Bannell	111	February 12, 1882	September 10, 1993
66	Florence Mary (Lennox) Deuchar	111	February 18, 1882	August 16, 1993

	Name	Age	Born	Died
67	Hulda Beata Johansson	112	February 24, 1882	June 9, 1994
68	Anicuta Batariu	115	June 17, 1882	November 21, 1997
69	Christian Montensen	115	August 16, 1882	April 25, 1998
70	Johanna Francina Zandstra	111	September 7, 1882	September 16, 1993
71	Annie Scott	113	March 15, 1883	April 21, 1996
72	Annie Emily (White) Townsend	111	May 20, 1883	September 11, 1994
73	Marguerite (Pooinsot) Petit	112	July 2, 1883	December 21, 1995
74	Lucy Jane Askew	114	September 8, 1883	December 9, 1997
75	Sue Utagawa	113	January 19, 1884	May 4, 1997
76	Suekiku Miyanaga	114	April 4, 1884	June 20, 1998
77	Asa Takii	114	April 28, 1884	July 31, 1998
78	Tase Matsunaga	114	May 11, 1884	November 18, 1998
79	Emile Fourcade	111	July 29, 1884	December 29, 1995
80	Annie (Thomas) Jennings	115	November 12, 1884	November 20, 1999
81	Helen Gertrude Haward	111	November 24, 1884	October 23, 1996
82	Anne Kathrine Matthiesen	111	November 26, 1884	March 19, 1996
83	Yasu Akino	113	March 1, 1885	February 12, 1999
84	Ruby Gilliam	113	September 21, 1885	October 22, 1998
85	Eva Morris	114	November 18, 1885	November 2, 2000
86	Minnie Ward	114	November 19, 1885	December 2, 1999

	Name	Age	Born	Died
87	Matsu Kiyo	112	January 9, 1886	November 18, 1998
88	Annie Blanche (Poole) Price	111	January 12, 1886	December 26, 1997
89	Jeanne Marie (Lagleize) Dumaine	112	March 19, 1886	January 3, 1999
90	Jeanne (Charlier) Colas	112	June 9, 1886	October 15, 1998
91	Denzo Ishisaki	112	October 20, 1886	April 29, 1999
92	Laura Hansine Svehaug	111	November 19, 1886	March 6, 1998
93	Marie-Louise "Rosea" Meunier	111	March 15, 1887	October 24, 1998
94	Ezequiel Guzman Gallardo	113	April 11, 1887	February 2000
95	Jesse Champion	112	August 15, 1887	January 12, 2000
96	Geneva (O'Kelley) McDaniel	111	August 26, 1887	April 6, 1999
97	Lempi Maria "Maija" Rothovius	112	October 2, 1887	June 17, 2000
98	Berthe (Gauthier) Sadron	111	February 18, 1888	February 27, 1999
99	Kayo Fujii	111	March 12, 1888	August 6, 1999
100	Sadayoshi Tanabe	111	October 20, 1888	January 2000
101	Karen Marie Jespersen	111	May 5, 1889	August 4, 2000
102	Edward Bernard	111	July 22, 1889	August 11, 2000
103	Anne-Marie Hemery	110	July 25, 1889	March 6, 2000

chapter sixty-three

33 Medical Breakthroughs: When They Happened

Health is our most precious possession. To attain and maintain it, we have countless remedies at our disposal. Do you have a headache? Just take a pill. Are you feeling run-down? Your doctor can draw some blood and have a lab check out its components under a microscope. Did your son fall off his bike? A trip to the emergency room for some x-rays will tell you if he'll be wearing a cast on his arm for a while. Did your dad suffer a heart attack? Sure, you're concerned, but you're also confident that the cardiac surgeons are well equipped to do his bypass operation.

We take the wealth of medical technology at our disposal for granted. As little as 100 years ago, there were no vaccines for diseases such as whooping cough, diphtheria, polio, measles, and mumps—diseases that killed people by the hundreds of thousands. Today, however, we see these diseases only occasionally in the United States. (Vaccines for these diseases were introduced in 1906, 1921–28, 1954, 1963, and 1968, respectively.) It's been only little more than 100 years since aspirin became available, yet many people today, especially those who take a pill daily to maintain heart health, can't imagine life without it.

In this chapter, we take a look at some of the most significant medical accomplishments and advancements during the past 2,000 years that in some way help us attain and maintain our health today.

Narrowing down the most significant medical breakthroughs from the thousands available to a few dozen is no easy task. Some people will likely disagree with some of the selections in this list. Omission of any event or finding is in no way a comment upon its importance. Every breakthrough, discovery, or enhancement holds some significance for someone. If you have children, you may say that each development of a vaccine that has significantly reduced the number of childhood diseases is a breakthrough. If you or someone in your family has cancer, you may want to see all the advances in cancer research on the list. As with any list on any topic, we make it personal; we put a piece of ourselves into how we see and judge it.

You will notice that the items in the list are related to conventional medicine: You will not see the introduction of acupuncture or Ayurvedic medicine in the list; nor will you see a date proclaiming the use and effectiveness of herbal medicine, aromatherapy, massage, prayer, tai chi, or yoga. That's for good reason: These are timeless medical approaches, not recent breakthroughs. True, many people in Western cultures are just discovering them and using them; but alternative approaches have been around for thousands of years in one form or another. They are a significant part of our quest for health, as you can see in many chapters in this book.

Each medical discovery—whether it's the development of a new way to view the interior of the human body or the rediscovery of an ancient healing method—is one more brick in the foundation of human health, another solid pillar upon which other medical advancements can be built and expanded.

1 400 BCE: Hippocrates, the Father of Medicine, based the practice of medicine on objective observations, with an emphasis on the doctor–patient relationship. Hippocrates refused to explain disease and illness simply as capricious acts of the gods. Thus, medicine became a science rather than a religion because of his work. He also stressed the importance of good diet and exercise, concepts that still hold true today.

2 170 CE: Galen, a Turkish doctor, proved that veins and arteries carry blood, not air. Galen had to do his research on animals, as human dissection was illegal at the time. He knew anatomy was critically important, because without it progress in medicine would be slow.

3 1543: Andreas Vesalius, an anatomist, ushered in the modern age of medicine with his anatomical studies. He corrected many of the mistakes Galen had made; yet without Galen's work, Vesalius probably wouldn't have been able to make the discoveries he did. Modern medicine is said to have begun with the publication of his book, *De Humanis Corporis Fabrica*, the first complete text-book of the human anatomy.

4 **1600 (circa):** The microscope was invented by Zacharias Janssen and Hans Lippershey, but Galileo was the first to insist it had value in medicine. The first microscope could only magnify objects 20 to 30 times, but it laid the groundwork for enhancements, which followed within the same century.

5 **1683:** Antony van Leeuwenhoek discovered and observed bacteria, using microscopes he enhanced to magnify objects 200 times or more. Leeuwenhoek's work revealed what was until then the unseen world of microorganisms and led the way for future scientists to discover the causes of disease. Although his work is considered some of the most important in the world of biology, Leeuwenhoek had no higher education or university degree behind him—just a very curious mind, which apparently was enough.

6 **1753:** James Lind discovered a cure for scurvy. This was significant at the time because scurvy was believed to be responsible for 50 percent of all shipwrecks, due to the high number of sick and dying sailors. Lind's work was important for medicine in that the type of research he conducted laid the foundation for all future studies in the area of nutrition.

7 **1798:** A smallpox vaccine was developed by Edward Jenner. This was the first "modern" vaccine and paved the way for those that followed. Today we have dozens of vaccines, and hundreds more are in the pipeline.

8 **1816:** Rene Laennec, a French physician, invented the stethoscope. The invention came about when Dr. Laennec was visited by a well-endowed young woman who had heart problems. Because the standard way to listen to the heart was to lay one's ear against the chest, and it was improper for Dr. Laennec to do this to a young lady, he rolled up a piece of paper and placed one end on her chest and the other against his ear. Surprised that he could clearly hear her heart, he soon refined his invention by making the first stethoscope out of wood.

9 **1829:** The first successful human-to-human blood transfusion was performed by James Blundell. Although blood transfusions in animals were done as early as 1665 and animal-to-human transfusions were done two years later, the death of one of the five patients who underwent the animal-to-human transfusion ended the practice until 1818. That's when Blundell discovered that blood from one type of animal could not be successfully transfused into another type of animal and that it was important to withdraw the air from the syringe when transfusing blood. Dr. Blundell performed the first successful human-to-human blood transfusion for severe postpartum hemorrhaging in 1829.

10 **1847:** Ignaz Semmelweis announced that washing hands stops the spread of disease. This seemingly simple yet critical finding has likely saved millions of lives, especially when practiced before surgery.

11 **1853:** Pravaz and Wood invented the hypodermic syringe, making it possible to safely inject substances into the body. These two scientists cashed in on the development of the hollow needle in 1844 by Francis Rynd, an Irish physician.

12 **1857:** Louis Pasteur discovered that bacteria cause disease. Note that this discovery came only 10 years after Semmelweis found that hand washing halted the spread of disease, which in many cases is caused by bacteria.

13 **1866:** Gregor Mendel discovered genes and said that these "elements" transmit heritable traits. Mendel's work is the cornerstone of modern genetics.

14 **1882:** Metchnikoff discovered white blood cells and the process known as phagocytosis and how white blood cells kill germs. His discovery led to a new understanding of how the body fights infection.

15 **1895:** X-rays were discovered by Wilhelm Röntgen. Röntgen won the Nobel Prize for Physics in 1901 for his discovery. It was the first time physicians could see structures inside the body without having to cut the body open.

16 **1899:** Felix Hoffman and Heinrich Dreser introduced aspirin. The name for this inexpensive painkiller came about by combining the letters from the ingredients: the "A" was from acetyl chloride and the "SPIR" was from the plant the researchers extracted the salicylic acid from, *Spirae ulmaria.* The "IN" was added because it was a common ending for drugs made at that time. Bayer introduced a tablet form to the market in 1915. It has been one of the top-selling drugs of all time.

17 **1902:** Hormones were discovered by William Bayliss and Ernest Starling. The first hormone discovered by Bayliss and Starling was secretin, which is produced by the small intestine. The term "hormone" wasn't used until 1905, however, and was assigned by Starling. The work of Bayliss and Starling is said to be the beginning of the field of endocrinology, which involves the work of hormones such as insulin (important in diabetes), estrogen, progesterone, thyroid hormone, and many others.

18 **1902:** The electrocardiogram was invented by Willem Einthoven, who was awarded the Nobel Prize in Physiology for Medicine in 1924. The electrocardiogram made it possible to measure precisely the electrical activity of the heart. Today's machines are based on his work and allow doctors to monitor heart function and detect damage.

19 **1906:** Sir Frederick Gowland Hopkins discovered vitamins. Hopkins was awarded the Nobel Prize in 1929 for his discovery of what were called "growth-stimulating vitamins." His work in the field of nutrition contributed greatly to our knowledge of the importance of diet today.

20 **1921:** Insulin was used for the first time to treat diabetes. Two Canadian researchers, Frederick Banting and Charles Best, were the first to experiment on a dying diabetic patient by injecting the insulin. It saved his life—fortunately for the two men. Their work made it possible for countless numbers of diabetics since that time to live a full life.

21 **1928:** Sir Alexander Fleming discovered penicillin, but it wasn't what he had in mind at the time. The discovery came when Fleming observed that the mold contaminating one of his culture plates had killed the bacteria in it. His discovery eventually made it possible for doctors to treat many otherwise fatal diseases.

22 **1928:** George Papanicolaou, M.D., presented his discovery of the Pap smear, which is used to screen for cervical cancer, herpes, human papillomavirus, and cervical dysplasia in women. Although his method was scorned for more than a decade, the test was finally put through clinical trials and the results were published in 1941. The Pap smear test is now a standard screening test for women and is recommended by the American Cancer Society. It reduced the death rate from cervical cancer by 74 percent between the 1950s, before the screening was routine, and 1992.

23 **1931:** Ernst Ruska, a German electrical engineer, invented the first electron microscope. For the first time, scientists were able to clearly view viruses and other tiny organisms and structures, magnified up to one million times more than was possible with light microscopes.

24 **1938:** Robert E. Gross completed the first successful operation for congenital (inherited) heart disease. His work is said to have initiated the modern era of cardiac surgery for people with congenital heart lesions, which affect up to 3 percent of infants born today.

25 **1953:** The DNA structure was discovered by James Watson, Francis Crick, and Rosalind Franklin. The stage was set for the surge of research into human genetics and into the genetic bases for many different diseases.

26 **1954:** The polio vaccine was created by American physician Jonas Salk. The vaccine works against all three strains of polio. Natural polio was eradicated in the Western hemisphere by 1991.

27 **1967:** The CAT scan (computerized axial tomography) was developed by Sir Godfrey N. Hounsfield, a British electrical engineer. The scan produces a detailed, three-dimensional display of the body's internal organs by combining multiple, cross-sectional x-rays taken at different angles. The original design has been improved upon, but CAT scans are still used widely today for diagnostic purposes.

28 **1967:** The first successful human heart transplant was performed by Christiaan Barnard, a senior cardiothoracic surgeon at the Groote Schuur Hospital in Cape Town, South Africa. The patient, Louis Washkansky, lived for 18 days. Dr. Barnard was a pioneer in a procedure that eventually became rather routine.

29 **1973:** Genetic engineering was born, due to the collaboration of Herbert Boyer and Stanley Cohen, who invented a technique for cloning DNA. Just a few of the medical items that developed from their achievement are a growth hormone for underdeveloped children, synthetic insulin for diabetics, and a clot-dissolving agent for people who suffer heart attacks.

30   **1982:** The first artificial heart was developed by Robert Jarvik, M.D. The first recipient was Barney Clark, age 61, who lived for 112 days with the device. After about 90 people were given the Jarvik heart, artificial hearts were banned in the United States because of complications.

31   **1995:** Artificial blood was developed by researchers at the University of Texas Health Science Center at San Antonio. The team of scientists, led by Thomas Runge, M.D., were the first to use the blood substitute, which increases the level of oxygen in the brain during cardiac surgery. Artificial blood eventually replaced the conventional saline solution, which tended to cause oxygen deficiency and excess fluid buildup.

32   **1996:** At Roslin Institute in Edinburgh, Scotland, Ian Wilmut and his colleagues successfully cloned a sheep, which they named Dolly. The ethical implications of such an event are complex, confusing, and volatile. Wilmut says he plans to use the patented cloning method to produce animals that will secrete medically valuable drugs in their milk. However, many in the medical and ethical arenas fear that this cloning will eventually lead to human cloning, which is already being promised by other researchers for the near future.

33   **1999-2000:** Human Genome Project (HGP) successfully sequenced a human chromosome. According to the Department of Energy and National Institutes of Health Human Genome Programs, which make up the project, the "information obtained as part of the HGP will dramatically change almost all biological and medical research and dwarf the catalog of current genetic knowledge."

Part VI

Alternative Views of Healing

When 46-year-old Charlene feels a headache coming on, she reaches for her feet instead of the medicine cabinet. "All I need is five minutes with my feet, and I'm pain-free and drug-free," she says.

Even though he has osteoarthritis, Bob continues to play tennis and golf every week since his retirement five years ago. "I eat a healthy diet and take vitamins," he says, "but the real secret is my acupuncturist." After an initial series of intense treatments, Bob needs only one follow-up treatment every six to eight weeks to stay medication-free and nearly pain-free.

Martha calls upon a Higher Power for her good health and that of her family. "It's not about religion, but about spirit," she says. "Prayer allows me to release stress and anxiety and brings me inner peace, which translates into better physical and emotional well-being," she explains.

The human body has a natural tendency to maintain its inner balance and harmony, but the stresses of everyday life, including poor diet, insufficient sleep, emotional and physical tensions, environmental toxins, and other abuses send the body toward disease. In this section we look at four different ways to achieve natural balance and inner peace: acupuncture and acupressure, the Eastern concept of chakras, reflexology, and prayer. Each of these approaches uses the powers within to heal the mind, body, and spirit.

The first two methods involve the idea of *chi*, which in Chinese medicine and Japanese tradition is the universal life force that flows throughout the body and is the basis of all life. Acupuncture and acupressure can influence the flow of chi at specific points on the body to achieve specific healing goals, while the seven chakras are the energy centers in the body where chi is stored and released.

Reflexology is similar to acupressure in that pressure is applied to certain sites; however, all or most of those sites tend to be on the soles of the feet, and refer to specific organs or other body parts. Prayer has been called the universal healer, and the source of this healing power can be different for every person who calls upon it for help.

A better understanding of these alternative views of healing may introduce you to paths you haven't considered before or reinforce those you already follow.

chapter sixty-four

7 Chakras: Spinning Wheels of Energy

The earth spins on its axis. Protons and electrons spin around the nucleus of an atom. Spiral galaxies spin in the heavens. And according to Hindu tradition, every human being is home to seven spinning wheels of energy called chakras. Each of these chakras has its own crystal, color, fragrance, and energy frequency or power, which determines its characteristics. Together they link our physical, mental, emotional, and spiritual selves into one life form of energy.

The concept of chakras comes to us from a 2,000-year-old Hindu tradition in India. The original meaning of the word *chakra* was "wheel" and it referred to the chariot wheels of the Aryans, the people who invaded India. Chakra was also used to refer to the cycle or wheel of time called the "kalacakra." An explanation of chakras was brought to Western societies by Arthur Avalon, an Englishman who translated some of the works of the ancient Indians on yoga and meditation.

Modern science has looked at the Hindu description of chakras and found that their locations correspond to the seven main nerve fiber bundles that radiate from the spinal column, and approximately with the positions of the endocrine glands as well. Each of the chakras acts like a valve that channels the Universal Life Force, or Universal Energy, into the body. The ideal state is to have all the chakras open to allow the flow of the Life Force through the body. The Hindus believe that emotional traumas, usually from childhood, can cause one or more of the chakras to become blocked or too open, which disrupts the flow of energy.

Because each chakra works in harmony with the others, it is necessary to restore any dysfunctional chakras to their proper frequency.

Balancing one's chakras is done to dissolve any blockages before they manifest as physical symptoms. Chakra balancing can be done in several ways. Because crystals also vibrate on their own special natural frequency, a specific crystal that correlates with an affected chakra can be placed on that chakra to help bring it into balance. Guided visualization and meditation are also used to balance the chakras. The use of color or fragrances that correlate to the chakras and physical exercises for each chakra are yet other ways to regain balance.

Here are the seven chakras and their corresponding colors, location, and powers. To understand more about the concept of chakras and their powers, read *Chakras for Beginners: A Guide to Balancing Your Chakra Energies*, by David Pond; and *Your Aura and Your Chakras: The Owner's Manual*, by Karla McLaren.

1 Root chakra. Located at the base of the spine, it supposedly contains the eight primary cells that hold all the knowledge of creation. These cells never change in a person's lifetime. This chakra grounds you to the physical world and connects your essence or soul with your body. Its color is red, its element is earth, and two of its crystals are tiger's eye and smoky quartz. When it becomes unbalanced or blocked, you may feel afraid of life or like a victim. This chakra is associated with security, health, and prosperity.

2 Spleen. Located just beneath the navel, this chakra is associated with reproductive and sexual abilities. Its color is orange, its element is water, and two of its crystals are ruby and red garnet. It is associated with emotional identity, sexual fulfillment, fluidity and grace, depth of feeling, and the ability to accept change. A blockage here shows itself as sexual guilt, reproductive disorders, or emotional problems.

3 Solar plexis. This chakra is called the seat of emotions or the power chakra. When it is blocked, the emotions expressed are anger or a sense of victimization; when healthy, it brings us self-confidence, energy, and spontaneity. Its color is yellow, its element is fire, and two of its crystals are malachite and tiger's eye. It controls our personal power, will, and metabolism.

4 Heart. This is the middle chakra and is associated with social identity and love. It integrates opposites in your universe: male/female, mind/body, ego/unity. A blockage here can show up as heart or immune system problems, or as a lack of caring. When healthy it manifests as deep love, compassion, centeredness, and tranquillity. Its color is green, its element is air, and three of its crystals are emerald, rose quartz, and green tourmaline.

5 **Throat.** This is the center of communication, self-expression, and creativity, and when it is blocked you do not communicate your emotions effectively. Gum and tooth disorders and respiratory conditions are associated with this chakra. Its color is blue, its element is sound, and two of its crystals are aquamarine and turquoise.

6 **Third eye.** This chakra correlates with the pineal gland, which is deep in the brain. The third eye has the ability to look upward and is associated with self-reflection and intuition. When it is healthy it allows us to understand things clearly. Physical symptoms of a blockage include headache, insomnia, and anxiety. Its color is indigo, its element is light, and two of its crystals are amethyst and lapis.

7 **Crown.** This chakra relates to consciousness and connects us with the universe beyond ourselves. It is related to pure awareness and all-knowing. When this chakra is developed, it brings us wisdom, knowledge, spiritual fulfillment, and bliss. Its color is purple, its element is thought, and its crystals are clear quartz and clear calcite.

chapter sixty-five

Let Us Pray:
Maximize Your Prayer Power

The word *prayer* is derived from the Latin *precari*, which means "to ask earnestly," and *precarius*, which means "obtained by begging." Prayer is associated with religious circles: churches, synagogues, mosques, temples, shrines, and other places of worship. There are designated days of the week set aside for worship, depending on your faith, as well as specific holy days when special prayers are offered.

Today we're beginning to understand that prayer can bring us more than spiritual benefits. It can affect our health in a positive way as well.

Modern Prayer

Prayer has gained the attention of the medical community. One of the most vocal advocates of the power of healing prayer and the author of several books on the topic, including *Healing Words*, Larry Dossey, M.D. has studied its power extensively. He has found convincing evidence that prayer not only works to heal people physically, emotionally, and spiritually, but does the same for nonhuman life as well. In controlled experiments, people saw their prayers answered when they prayed for grass to grow taller and for bacteria in test tubes to grow faster. "It's the best evidence of all that prayer can change the world," says Dr. Dossey.

What the Studies Show

Hundreds of studies have been done on the power of prayer in connection with health. Here are synopses of just a few of them.

- A study that Dr. Dossey credits with his initial interest in the power of prayer was conducted at San Francisco General Hospital in 1982 and 1983. For 10 months, half of a group of 393 cardiac patients received intercessory prayers while the other half did not. The group that did not receive prayers needed more antibiotics and assistance in breathing than those who received prayers.

- At St. Luke's Hospital in Kansas City, Missouri, nearly 1,000 heart patients who had serious cardiac conditions were divided into two groups: Half received daily prayers from volunteers who believed in the healing power of prayer, and the other half did not receive prayers. None of the patients knew they were part of the study. After four weeks, the researchers determined that the patients who had received prayers fared 11 percent better (in factors such as pain, pneumonia, infection, and death) than the group who did not receive prayers.

- At Barnes-Jewish Hospital in St. Louis, Missouri, 51 women attending an HIV care center were questioned about the importance of prayer in making decisions about their therapy. Ninety-two percent said prayer was an important source in their decision-making process, and 59 percent said it was more important than the doctor.

- At Duke University Medical Center in Durham, North Carolina, researchers studied the relationship between survival and older people's religious activities, such as prayer and meditation, over six years. They found that older individuals who participate in private religious activities before they become unable to perform normal daily tasks (e.g., bathing, getting dressed, personal care) appear to live longer than those who do not.

Maximize the Power

If you are interested in using prayer to heal yourself, other people, the planet, or even your pets; if you want to pray for world peace or internal tranquillity, the exact words you use or how you deliver them are not important. You may want to join in the high-tech world of prayer and maximize your prayer power, for example, or find peace in the words of prayers from other times and places. Both of these options are offered here. The first option is a list of Internet prayer sites that in some way promote healing prayers. The second is a sampling of simple healing prayers, taken from various cultures, traditions, and time periods.

Internet Prayer Sites

- Prayer Network (www.prayernetwork.com). The purpose of this site is to "empower Christians worldwide to reach the lost and hurting through personal prayer, encouragement, and praise." The site handles multilingual prayer requests 24 hours a day.

- The Healing Circle (www.thehealingcircle.org) is a free service for individuals to get healing energy and prayers. The volunteers who manage the site distribute the names of people, places, and things that need healing energy. They have healers in more than 20 countries and within the United States.

- The World Peace Prayer Society (www.worldpeace.org) is a nonprofit, nonsectarian, member-supported group that spreads the message of world peace through various programs, including the Peace Pole Project, the Peace Pals for young people, and World Peace Prayer Ceremonies. It was founded in Japan in 1955.

- The Ananda Healing Prayer Ministry (www.ananda.org). The site has a Healing Prayer Council, which offers healing prayers daily for individual and world needs. The Ministry also offers instruction in Paramhansa Yogananada's Divine Will Healing. There are opportunities to join the Healing Prayer Council and to attend retreats to learn more about healing prayer.

- Circle of Healing Purrs (www.catanna.com/healing.htm). This site is a bit different in that the operator focuses on the use of Reiki, the universal life energy, which is channeled to promote spiritual, physical, and mental well-being. That healing force is sent to cats. Anyone can send a request for healing of a cat to this site.

- Rosemary Altea Healing (www.rosemaryaltea.com). Rosemary Altea and her team of healers send their prayers out daily to individuals who submit their requests to the site. The healing team asks that recipients of healing prayers let the team know how they are progressing. Rosemary is an internationally known spiritual medium who lives in England. She is the founder of the Rosemary Altea Association of Healers, a charitable organization, and she has five healing centers in Britain.

- World Prayer Network (www.worldprayer.org). This network is associated with the Free and Unlimited Ministries in California. It is the belief of those who run the Network that the gift of conscious prayer is one of the greatest gifts people can give to themselves and to the earth.

- Healing Psalms (www.HealingPsalm.com). This site offers resources for prayer and spiritual support for people of all faiths in times of illness. Visitors are invited to share stories about their experiences with prayer and illness and to submit the names of individuals in need of healing prayers.

- The International Order of St. Luke the Physician (www.orderofstluke.org). This unique organization is a Christian healing ministry of professionals in the medical arena, clergy of the Roman, Orthodox, Anglican, and Protestant churches, and lay individuals from all walks of life. Its purpose is to promote the practice of healing as taught by Jesus Christ through various avenues, including prayer groups, workshops, healing missions, and healing services.

- The Prayer Site (www.theprayersite.com). This site is dedicated to helping anyone in the world receive healing prayer. Individuals are invited to ask for healing prayers and to offer healing prayers for others. There are forums on specific topics for prayers, such as emotional healing, trauma, heart cancer, and other illnesses.

Healing Prayers

A Navajo Prayer

O you who dwell in the house made of the dawn,

In the house made of the evening twilight . . .

Where the dark mist curtains the doorway,

The path to which is on the rainbow . . .

I have made your sacrifice.

I have prepared a smoke for you.

My feet restore for me.

My limbs restore for me.

My body restore for me.

My mind restore for me.

My voice restore for me.

Today, take away your spell from me.

Away from me you have taken it.

Far off from me you have taken it.

Happily I recover.

Happily my interior becomes cool.

Happily my eyes regain their power.

Happily my head becomes cool.

Happily my limbs regain their power.

Happily I hear again.

Happily for me the spell is taken off.

Happily I walk.

Impervious to pain, I walk.

Feeling light within, I walk.

In beauty I walk.

With beauty before me, I walk.

With beauty behind me, I walk.

With beauty below me, I walk.

With beauty all around me, I walk.

It is finished in beauty.

It is finished in beauty.

It is finished in beauty.

She Who Heals: An American Indian Healing Prayer

Mother, sing me a song
That will ease my pain,
Mend broken bones,
Bring wholeness again.
Catch my babies
When they are born,
Sing my death song,
Teach me how to mourn.
Show me the Medicine
Of the healing herbs,
The value of spirit,

The way I can serve.
Mother, heal my heart
So that I can see
The gifts of yours
That can live through me.

Prayer for Healing

(Attributed to Timothy Dailey)

Help my unbelief.
When I'm in pain, I forget that you care about me.
I forget that you have helped me through my trials.
I forget that you hold me in your arms to keep me safe.
I forget that you are feeling my pain with me.
I forget that you love me,
I forget that I am important to you.
Show me your presence—let me feel your enveloping love.
Heal my hurting soul.
Thank you for staying with me even in my unbelief.
Amen

A Physician's Prayer: Sir Thomas Browne, 1605

I have resolved to pray more and pray always,
to pray in all places where quietness inviteth: in the house, on the highway and on the street;
and to know no street or passage in this city that may not witness that I have not forgotten God.
I purpose to take occasion of praying upon the sight of any church which I may pass, that God may be worshipped there in spirit, and that souls may be saved there;
to pray for my sick patients and for the patients of other physicians;
at my entrance into any home to say, "May the peace of God abide here ";
after hearing a sermon, to pray for a blessing on God's truth, and upon the messenger;
upon the sight of a beautiful person to bless God for His creatures, to pray for the beauty of such one's soul, that God may enrich her with inward graces, and that the outward and inward may correspond;
upon the sight of a deformed person, to pray God to give them wholeness of soul, and by and by to give them the beauty of the resurrection.

Prayer for the Sick

Dear Jesus, Divine Physician and Healer of the Sick, we turn to You in this time of illness. O dearest Comforter of the Troubled, alleviate our worry and sorrow with Your gentle love, and grant us the grace and strength to accept this burden. Dear God, we place our worries in Your hands. We place our sick under Your care and humbly ask that You restore Your servant to health again. Above all, grant us the grace to acknowledge Your holy will and know that whatsoever You do, You do for the love of us.

Prayer for Peace: Jain

Lead me from Death to Life, from Falsehood to Truth.
Lead me from Despair to Hope, from Fear to Trust.
Lead me from Hate to Love, from War to Peace.
Let Peace fill our Heart, our World, our Universe.

Morning Prayer: Hindu

May all in this world be happy,
May they be healthy,
May they be comfortable
And never miserable.
May the rain come down in the proper time.
May the earth yield plenty of corn,
May the country be free from war,
May the Brahmans be secure.

Jewish Prayer

Blessed are you, Lord our God, king of the universe, who causes the bonds of sleep to fall on my eyes, and slumber on my eyelids.

May it be acceptable in your presence, O Lord my God, and God of my fathers, to cause me to lie down in peace, and to raise me up again in peace; and suffer me not to be troubled with evil dreams, or evil reflections; but grant me a calm and uninterrupted repose in your presence; and enlighten my eyes again, lest I sleep the sleep of death.

Blessed are you, O Lord, who gives light to the whole universe in your glory.

chapter sixty-six

Reflexology Points:
How to Use Them to Treat
35 Health Conditions

Feeling tense? Have a headache? Is your stomach upset? Menstrual cramps got you down? Reach for your feet!

Reflexology is an ancient therapy that is believed to have originated in China thousands of years ago. It is based on the concept that energy zones within the body can be stimulated through reflex points in the feet to promote healing to the area of the body to which the zones correspond. The entire foot has been carefully mapped out (see figures starting on page 497) so that with practice, anyone can easily learn which reflex points to press and stimulate to heal the body. Although the feet are the areas of the body most often used for reflexology, the hands and the ears also have reflex points. The feet are easy to work with, however, because you can use both hands, they are easy to access, and a foot massage feels great anytime.

The forefinger is used second most often. When doing reflexology, either on yourself or on someone else, envision that you are pressing on a pinhead. That's about the size of the point you are treating. Rotate your thumb or forefinger slightly on each point, or apply pressure and then release it many times over the same point before moving on to another point. Work each point for 3 to 5 minutes. Here are some other tips:

- Make sure your thumb and forefinger nails are short so they don't hurt you or your partner.

- Be comfortable. When doing the feet of a partner, have him or her place the foot on a pillow on a low stool or on your lap.
- Make sure your hands are warm. No one wants cold hands on their feet.
- Experiment with the amount of pressure that is right for you or your partner. Each foot has more than 7,000 nerve endings. That's a lot of feeling to deal with. Be sensitive to your partner's wishes.

Reflexology is a very safe therapy; however, there are a few caveats we'd like to share with you. Anyone with the following conditions should not be treated without first seeking professional advice from a physician or qualified reflexologist:

- diabetes, phlebitis, or thrombosis, or cancer that is being treated actively;
- pregnancy, during the first 14 weeks, especially if the individual has a history of miscarriage;
- acute stage of an infectious disease.

Refer to the figures on pages 497 and 498 to find the reflex points to relieve symptoms of the following health complaints.

1 Angina (to reduce stress and improve muscle function): Heart, lungs

2 Arthritis: Liver, gallbladder, stomach, pancreas, spleen, bladder, ureter, kidneys; also work the reflexes that correspond to the affected areas

3 Asthma: Diaphragm, heart, lungs, thoracic spine

4 Bronchitis: Diaphragm, heart, lungs, thoracic spine, liver, gallbladder, spleen

5 Carpal tunnel syndrome: Cervical spine, elbow

6 Conjunctivitis: Eyes, sinuses

7 Chilblains (painful, itchy, swollen skin, usually on the feet, triggered by cold): Heart, lungs, spine (work the feet or the hands, depending on which area is being affected)

8 Cystitis: Bladder, ureter, kidneys

9 Depression: Foot relaxation, spine, thyroid, neck, brain, adrenals, pancreas, ovaries or testes

10 Digestive problems, including irritable bowel syndrome, colitis, constipation, indigestion, and similar complaints: Liver, gallbladder, stomach, pancreas, spleen, intestinal area (ileocecal valve, ascending, descending, sigmoid, and transverse colon, small intestine)

11 Eating disorder: Foot relaxation, solar plexus, liver, gallbladder, stomach, pancreas, spleen

12 Grief: Foot relaxation, spine

13 Headache: Brain, cervical spine

14 Hormone imbalance: Thyroid, neck, brain, adrenals, pancreas, ovaries or testes

15 Incontinence: Bladder, ureter, lumbar spine, kidneys

16 Kidney stones (to relieve pain): Bladder, ureter, kidneys

17 Lumbago: Coccyx, hip, pelvis, spine

18 Mastitis: Breast

19 Menopause (transition to): Foot relaxation, thyroid, brain, ovaries, adrenals, spine, breast

20 Migraine: Brain, cervical spine, liver

21 Painful menstruation: Uterus, fallopian tubes, ovaries, lumbar spine, intestines (ascending, descending, sigmoid, and transverse colon, small intestine)

22 Palpitations: Heart, spine, diaphragm, solar plexus

23 Postnatal depression: Foot relaxation, breast, ovaries, fallopian tubes, thyroid, neck, brain, adrenals, pancreas

24 Premenstrual tension: Neck, thyroid, brain, ovaries, kidneys, groin

25 Prostate (enlarged): Bladder, ureter, kidneys, prostate gland

26 Raynaud's syndrome: Heart, lung

27 Sciatica: Coccyx, hip, pelvis, spine, sciatic nerve

28 Sinusitis: Sinuses, eyes, ears, face

29 Smoking addiction: Diaphragm, lungs, heart

30 Sore throat: Throat, sinuses, cervical spine, spleen

31 Stiff shoulder: Shoulder, cervical spine

32 Swollen feet or hands: Heart, lungs, spine

33 Tennis elbow: Shoulder, cervical spine, elbow

34 Tinnitus (ringing in the ears): Ear, sinuses, neck

35 Toothache: Teeth, pituitary

Foot Relaxation Procedure

A total foot massage using reflexology can bring the entire body into a state of relaxation. Although a total foot massage is certainly good anytime, it is especially useful when coping with conditions such as depression, eating disorders, addictions, insomnia, grief, and healing from trauma. Here's the sequence:

- Start with the right foot. Work the diaphragm area. While doing this, rock the toes back and forth across your left thumb. Repeat on the left foot.
- Support the right foot between the palms of the hands and rapidly but gently rock the foot from side to side between the hands. Repeat on the left foot.
- Support the ankle bones with the pads of your thumbs and rock the foot rapidly but gently from side to side. Repeat on the left foot.
- Using your fist, press into the sole of the right foot, using your left hand on top of the foot to brace it. Knead your fist into the sole while you squeeze the top of the foot with the left hand. Repeat on the left foot.

- Support the right heel in your left hand. Hold the top of the foot with your right hand and gently rotate the foot in a clockwise circling motion. Repeat on the left foot.

- Place the right foot between your hands and support it on the outside edge. Moving your hands like the wheels of a train, gently massage the foot. Repeat on the left foot.

- Relax the ribcage by pressing into the sole of the right foot with both thumbs. Move the fingers of both hands over the top of the foot. Repeat on the left foot.

Right Sole

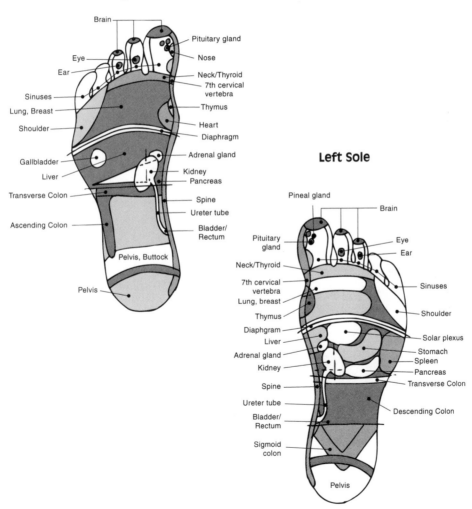

Right Foot

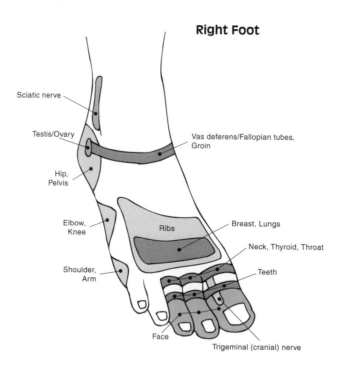

Sciatic nerve

Testis/Ovary

Hip, Pelvis

Elbow, Knee

Shoulder, Arm

Face

Vas deferens/Fallopian tubes, Groin

Ribs

Breast, Lungs

Neck, Thyroid, Throat

Teeth

Trigeminal (cranial) nerve

Left Foot

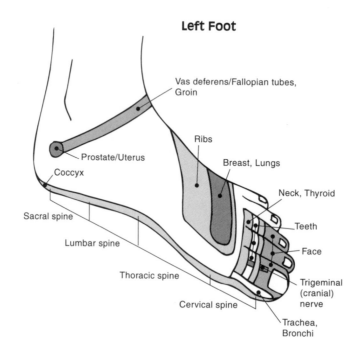

Vas deferens/Fallopian tubes, Groin

Prostate/Uterus

Coccyx

Sacral spine

Lumbar spine

Thoracic spine

Cervical spine

Ribs

Breast, Lungs

Neck, Thyroid

Teeth

Face

Trigeminal (cranial) nerve

Trachea, Bronchi

chapter sixty-seven

Getting the Point: Acupuncture and Acupressure Acupoints

When you have a headache, do you ever cradle your head in your hands, pressing your palms against your forehead? When you experience stomach pain, do you scrunch over, crossing your forearms against your abdomen? You are, in a crude way, practicing acupressure—the application of pressure to specific points on the body to restore balance—to relieve pain.

Ancient Tradition

More than 5,000 years ago, the Chinese discovered that applying pressure or needles to certain points on the body resulted in pain relief. Through trial and error (and we can only imagine how much error there was), they discovered that they could not only relieve pain, but also influence certain internal organs by stimulating certain points on the body. Thus were born the traditional Chinese medicine treatments known as acupressure and acupuncture.

The Flow of Life

Some people call acupressure "acupuncture without the needles," because both techniques are based on the same ancient Chinese concept of life energy called *chi*. Chi (or *ki* in Japanese) is the life force that flows through all life forms along invisible roadways called *meridians*. The body is in a state of balance, harmony, and health when chi flows smoothly. But when there's a bump in the road—infection, stress, poor nutrition, physical trauma, emotional upheaval—a blockage occurs, and disease, pain, depression, or other symptoms are the result.

Fortunately, thousands of years ago the Chinese developed maps of the meridians and identified about 350 sites or acupoints where energy is conducted. When you apply pressure or a needle to specific acupoints, blocked energy is released, and chi can flow freely again. Each acupoint has certain qualities, again identified by the Chinese, so an acupuncturist or acupressure practitioner knows which acupoints to stimulate, given a person's symptoms. For example, if you have a sinus headache, you will likely be treated at acupoints Large Intestine 20 and Large Intestine 4. If you want relief from menstrual cramps and bloating, the treatment acupoints are Spleen 1, 4, 6, 9, 10, and 12.

What does the large intestine have to do with headache, or the spleen with menstrual cramps, you might ask? These names and 12 others (see the list in the next section) identify the main meridians. The Chinese named them according to the organs they are believed to influence.

Western researchers, forever the skeptics, have tried to discover why acupressure and acupuncture work. Studies show that many of the acupoints are located at major crossways of the autonomic nervous system, which may partly explain how these Chinese techniques can successfully treat referred pain—pain that occurs far away from its source. Scientists have shown that stimulating acupoints with needles, pressure, or heat triggers the release of natural painkillers called endorphins. When endorphins are released, pain is relieved and blood flow is increased to the treated area. This, in turn, promotes healing.

What Acupuncture or Acupressure Can Heal

Acupuncture and acupressure do not replace conventional medicine: They cannot mend a fractured bone or cure a ruptured appendix. But they can help the body to heal itself and to return to its natural state of balance. They can promote the healing of broken bones and other physical traumas, as well as relieve stress and tension and the pain associated with countless conditions, including headache, backache, stomach cramps, menstrual pain, muscle spasms, sinusitis, and constipation. They can boost the immune system, promote blood flow, enhance energy levels, and help you sleep. Both acupuncture and acupressure are excellent complementary therapies to other treatments such as chiropractic and physical therapy, because they release the tension in the muscles and allow for faster healing. All of these benefits are available without the use of pills or injections; just a simple, relatively painless needle prick or pressure.

Acupuncture should always be done by a professional, but you can do acupressure on yourself and others (with their permission, of course). Here is a list of specific acupuncture and acupressure points (see figures on pages 506 and 507) and the health conditions you can treat when you stimulate them. Before doing acupressure on anyone, including yourself, it is recommended that you consult a qualified practitioner who can show you the technique and answer any questions you have. Then, refer to the figures and press away!

Bladder

- Bladder 2: To relieve nasal congestion, eyestrain, and headache. Press firmly for one minute on both points. Located on the inside of the eyebrows on the bony ridge.
- Bladder 10: To relieve stress. Press firmly for one minute. Located on the muscles ½ inch below the base of the skull.
- Bladder 13: To relieve stress. Press firmly with the thumbs or fingers into the muscles ½ inch outward from either side of the spine, 1 finger width below the top of the shoulder blade.
- Bladder 23: To relieve lower back pain. Press firmly for one minute using the thumbs. Located on either side of the spine, about 3 inches from the center of the back at waist level.
- Bladder 47: To relieve lower back pain. Use along with Bladder 23. Using the thumbs, press on either side of the spine, about 2 inches from the center of the back at waist level.

Conception Vessel

- Conception vessel 6: To relieve abdominal pain from constipation. Press inward as much as possible and inhale slowly. Located 3 finger widths below the navel.
- Conception vessel 12: To relieve a colicky infant. Press gently for one minute. Located about 2 finger widths above the navel.

- Conception vessel 13: To relieve middle back pain. Press firmly for one minute. Located about 3 finger widths above the navel.

- Conception vessel 14: To relieve middle back pain. Press firmly for one minute. Located about 4 finger widths above the navel.

- Conception vessel 17: To relieve croup. Gently press both points for one minute and release. Located in the center of the chest, midway between the nipples.

Gallbladder

- Gallbladder 2: To enhance hearing. Press for one minute, three to five times. Located just in front of the ears, ½ inch below the depression.

- Gallbladder 20: To relieve neck muscle stress, headache, and nasal congestion. Press both points firmly for one minute. Located about 2 inches apart on either side of the base of the skull.

- Gallbladder 21: To relieve stress. Press and hold for one minute. Located at the highest point of the shoulder muscle, midway between the spine and the outer edge of the shoulder.

- Gallbladder 34: To relieve acute pain in the thigh and groin. Press firmly for one minute. Located between the outside edge of the anklebone and the Achilles tendon.

Governing Vessel

- Governing vessel 24.5: To relieve hay fever. Press lightly for two minutes and breathe deeply. Located at the top of the bridge of the nose, between the eyebrows.

- Governing vessel 25. To relieve hiccups. First press the palms against the forehead and hold for one minute, then lightly press an index finger against the end of the nose for one minute. The point is located at the end of the nose.

Heart

- Heart 7: To promote sleep. Squeeze firmly between the thumb and index finger for one minute, then repeat on the other wrist. Located along the crease on the inside of the wrist.

Kidney

- Kidney 3: To stimulate mental activity, especially for elderly people and those with Alzheimer's, and to relieve earache pain. Press firmly for one minute using the index finger and repeat on the other foot. Located on the inside of the ankle, between the ankle bone and the Achilles tendon.

Large Intestine

- Large intestine 4: To relieve constipation, gas pains, hayfever. Use the thumb and index finger of the right hand to squeeze the web of the left hand for one minute. Located in the web between the thumb and index finger.
- Large intestine 11: To relieve constipation. Press firmly for one minute, then repeat on the other arm. Located on the outer edge of the inside elbow crease.
- Large intestine 20: To relieve congestion and swelling of sinusitis. Press both points upward and breathe deeply. Hold for one minute. Located on either side of the nose, where the nostrils flare.

Liver

- Liver 2: To relieve irritability, press steadily for one minute. Located on the top of the foot, in the web between the first and second toes.
- Liver 3: To relieve tension that may cause inflammation. Located on top of the foot.
- Liver 8: To relieve depression. Press for one minute two or three times, repeat two or three times. Located above the inside knee crease, below the knee joint.

Lung

- Lung 1: To relieve coughing spasms. Press gently for one minute on both points. Located about ½ inch below the large hollow under the collarbone on both sides.
- Lung 5: To ease coughing spasms. Bend your left elbow and make a fist. Place your right thumb on the point and press firmly for one minute and repeat on the other arm. Do three to four times.

- Lung 7: To boost the immune system and lung function. Press firmly for one minute and repeat on other arm. Located on the thumb side of the inner forearm, 2 finger widths above the wrist crease.

Pericardium

- Pericardium 3: To relax the nervous system. Press for one minute and repeat on other arm. Located in the elbow crease in direct line with the ring finger.
- Pericardium 6: To calm nerves and reduce uneasiness; to relieve general nausea. Press firmly for one minute three to five times, then repeat on the other wrist. Located in the center of the inner wrist between the two bones of the forearm, 2 finger widths from the wrist crease.

Small Intestine

- Small Intestine 3: To relieve back stiffness. Press for one minute. Located on the side of the hand below the knuckle of the little finger, between the muscle and the bone.
- Small Intestine 17: To help balance. Press lightly while breathing deeply for one minute. Repeat several times. Located just below the earlobes in the indentation at the back of the jawbone.

Spleen

- Spleen 3: To enhance memory, relief from gout. Maintain steady pressure for one minute on each foot. Located on the inside of the foot, behind the bulge associated with the big toe.
- Spleen 4: To relieve menstrual cramps and bloating. Firmly press for one to three minutes. Located on the inside arch of the foot, 1 thumb width away from the ball of the foot.
- Spleen 6: To fight blood infection; to relieve menstrual cramping and gas pains. Press with the thumb for one minute, then repeat on the other leg. Located 4 finger widths above the right inner anklebone, near the edge of the shinbone.
- Spleen 8: To improve blood flow. Press firmly for one minute and repeat on the other leg. Located 4 finger widths below the knee, on the inside of the leg.

- Spleen 9: To relieve menstrual cramps and bloating. Firmly press for one to three minutes. Located just below the knee joint on the inside of the leg, between the tibia and calf muscle.
- Spleen 10: To stimulate the immune system, relieve menstrual cramps. Press with the thumb one minute and repeat on the other leg. Located 2 thumb widths from the top of the knee, in line with the inner edge of the kneecap.
- Spleen 12: To relieve menstrual cramps and bloating. Firmly press both points for one to three minutes. Located on either side of the pubic bone.

Stomach

- Stomach 3: To relieve sinus headache. Press both points firmly for one minute and repeat three times. Located at the bottom of the cheekbones, directly under the pupils.
- Stomach 7: To relieve tension in the jaw. Press firmly for one minute. Located about 1 thumb width in front of the ears, in an indentation in the upper jawline.
- Stomach 36: To improve digestion; for constipation. Press for one minute on each leg. Located 4 finger widths below the kneecap, outside the shinbone.
- Stomach 44: To relieve foot pain. Press lightly on both feet with the index fingers for one minute, two to three times. Located in the webs between the second and third toes.

Triple Warmer

- Triple warmer 3: To relieve ear pain. Press gently and hold for one minute and repeat on the other hand. Located in the groove on the back of the hand, behind and between the fourth and fifth knuckles.
- Triple warmer 5: To relieve pain in the upper body. Press firmly for one minute, then repeat on other arm. Do two to three times. Located on the top of the forearm, 2 thumb widths from the wrist joint.
- Triple 17: To improve hearing. Press firmly for two minutes and breathe deeply. Located behind the earlobe, where the ears meet the jawbone.

Acupressure and Acupuncture Points (Front View)

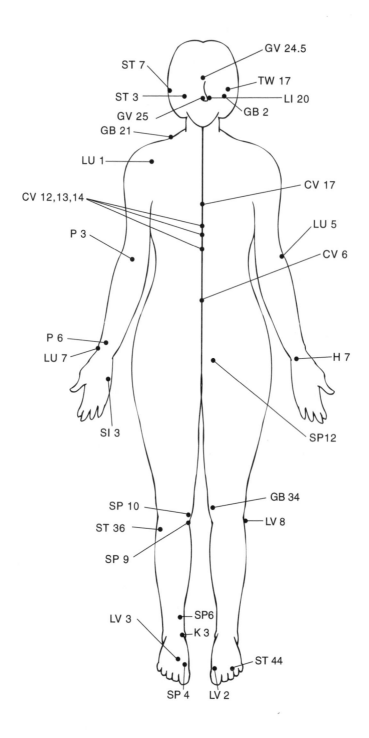

GV 24.5

ST 7

ST 3

GV 25

GB 21

LU 1

CV 12,13,14

P 3

P 6

LU 7

SI 3

TW 17

LI 20

GB 2

CV 17

LU 5

CV 6

H 7

SP12

SP 10

ST 36

SP 9

GB 34

LV 8

LV 3

SP6

K 3

ST 44

SP 4

LV 2

Acupressure and Acupuncture Points (Back View)

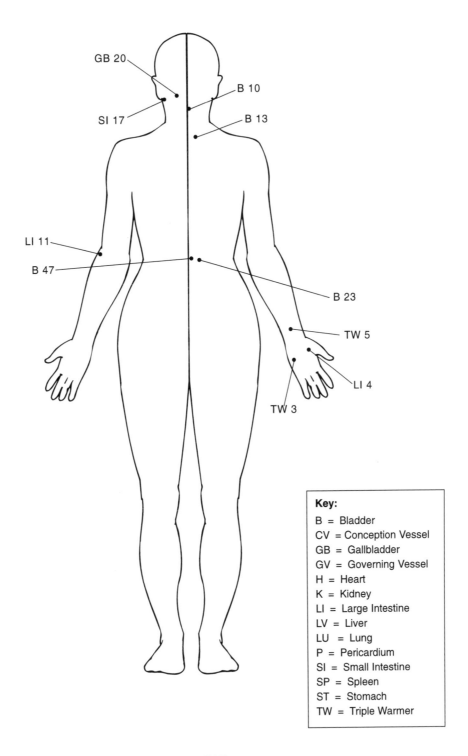

GB 20

B 10

SI 17

B 13

LI 11

B 47

B 23

TW 5

LI 4

TW 3

Key:
B = Bladder
CV = Conception Vessel
GB = Gallbladder
GV = Governing Vessel
H = Heart
K = Kidney
LI = Large Intestine
LV = Liver
LU = Lung
P = Pericardium
SI = Small Intestine
SP = Spleen
ST = Stomach
TW = Triple Warmer

Part VII

Reliable Sources

Health is one of the most popular topics for which people want information. Check out the *New York Times* best-seller list in any given week and you'll see that most of the top 10 nonfiction books are health-related. Health magazines and newsletters are doing a good business. And more and more people are buying herbs and other supplements. Demand for all these products is high, and so is the supply. The result is overload: so much information and advertising and so many products about health and related topics that we are overwhelmed.

The chapters in this section are designed to help you focus on some of the best sources for herbs and supplements, as well as reliable sources of printed materials and Web site information on health, medical, and safety issues. We suggest you consider these not only as good sources, but as launching points for further information, products, and services.

One note about Internet sites: The Internet can be an excellent source of information, with access to medical journals, articles, transcripts, press releases, newsletters, personal testimonies, discussion groups, and support groups as well as information from hospitals, clinics, health organizations, universities, charities, pharmaceutical companies, doctors, caregivers, and just plain folks who want to share their personal stories or their research findings. It's enough to make you dizzy and to wonder, how can I be sure the information I'm finding is accurate and reliable?

One nonprofit organization based in Geneva, Switzerland, helps people answer that question. The Health on the Net Foundation (HON) was developed to "build and support the international health and medical community on the Internet." To help accomplish that, it created an HON Code, which it would like health Web sites to follow. In short, these principles state:

- Any medical or health advice dispensed from the site should be given by medically qualified professionals.

- When appropriate, information should be substantiated by a source and a link to that source should be provided, if possible.

- Any information that visitors submit to the site should be kept confidential.

- Claims made about commercial products or services should be supported by unbiased evidence.
- Contact information should be clearly evident.
- All sources of contributions should be clearly identified.
- If advertising is a source of revenue, it should be clearly stated.

Web sites that meet the Health on the Net Foundation's standards have an HON Code icon on their home page. This does not mean, however, that medical or health sites without the icon contain unreliable information. In fact, there are other organizations that rate health Web sites and bestow their "seals of approval" as well, including the www.HealthAwards, a program organized by the Health Information Resource Center, a national clearinghouse and consumer health information group; and Healthlinks Select Site, which rates health links. You are urged to shop around, and to question any information that does not sound right or sounds "too good to be true." If you read information that sounds questionable, e-mail the site for backup information or references, and research your question on sites that you know are reputable. You have access to an unimaginable amount of information at your fingertips. Use it wisely.

chapter sixty-eight

Herb Sources

Herb Products

**Advanced Alternatives
for Better Health**
1344 Lansing Avenue
Lansing, MI 48915
800-945-3161
www.aabhealth.com/natural.htm

Ancient Herbs
835 Potts Avenue
Green Bay, WI 54304
888-430-4372
www.ancientherbs.com

Avena Botanicals
219 Mill Street
Rockport, ME 04856
www.avenaherbs.com

Blessed Herbs
109 Barre Plains Road
Oakham, MA 01068
800-489-4372
www.blessedherbs.com

Dances with Herbs
PO Box 1100
Idyllwild, CA 92549
www.herbanspice.com/danceswithherbs/

Dunraven House
PO Box 403
Boulder, CO 80306
303-413-9962
www.dunravenhouse.com

East Earth Trade Winds
PO Box 49315
Redding, CA 96049
800-258-6878
www.eastearthtrade.com

Gaia Herbs
108 Island Ford Road
Brevard, NC 28712
828-884-4242
www.gaiaherbs.com

The Herb Shop
247 SW G Street
Grants Pass, OR 97526
541-479-3602
www.bulkherbshoop.com

Herbal Hut
Vier Clearinghouse
2 Glenhaven Road
Glenolden, PA 19036
866-369-7404
www.herbalhut.com

The Herbalist
2106 NE 65th Street
Seattle, WA 98115
800-NW-HERBS
www.herbalconsultant.com

HerbPharm
PO Box 116,
Williams, OR 97544
541-846-6262
www.presentmoment.com/shop/
 herbpharmtable.html

High Desert Herb Company
P.O. Box 103
Hereford, AZ 85615
highdesertherbs@yahoo.com

Merz Apothecary
4716 N. Lincoln Avenue
Chicago, IL 60625
800-252-0275
www.smallflower.com

The Modern Herbalist
6900 Sesame Street
Paradise, CA 95969
530-876-1176
www.modernherbalist.com

Mountain Rose Herbs
20818 High Street
N. San Juan, CA 95960
800-879-3337
www.botanical.com/mtrose

Natural Shoppe
4114 W. Howard Avenue
Milwaukee, WI 53221
414-817-1792
www.naturalshoppe.com

Nature's Herbs
600 East Quality Drive
American Fork, UT 84003
801-763-0700
www.naturesherbs.com

Nature's Way
10 Mountain Springs Parkway
Springville, UT 84663
801-489-1500
www.naturesway.com

Raintree Nutrition
www.rain-tree.com/rtmprod.htm

Shepherd Garden Seeds
30 Irene Street
Torrington, CT 06790
860-482-3638
www.shepherdseeds.com

Solaray
1400 Kearns Blvd, 2nd Floor
Park City, UT 84060
435-655-6000
www.nutraceutical.com/about/
 solaray.cfm

Thai Herbs & Spices
PO Box 151835
Austin, TX 78715-1835
1-800-317-2715
www.thaiherb.com

Turnleaf Herb Farm
207-793-4593
www.angelfire.com/ne/turnleaf

Vitanica
PO Box 1285
Sherwood, OR 97140
www.vitanica.com

Wics & Balms
767 Purchase Street
New Bedrord, MA 02740
508-996-5669
www.wicsandbalms.com/

Wild Mountain Herbs
130 Payne Mountain Road
Tellico Plains, TN 37385
423-261-2747
rfarner@tellico.net

Yellow Emperor
PO Box 2631
Eugene, OR 97402
541-485-6664
www.yellowemperor.com

Zand Herbal Formulas
1722 14th Street, Suite 230
Boulder, CO 80302
www.zand.com

Information Sources

American Botanical Council
PO Box 144345
Austin, TX 78714-4345
512-926-4900
www.herbalgram.org

American Herbalists Guild
PO Box 70
Roosevelt, UT 84066
www.healthy.net/herbalists/

HerbNet
www.herbnet.com

Herb Society of America
www.herbsociety.org

chapter sixty-nine

Reliable Supplement Sources

All Star Vitamins
1900 Princeton Pike
Lawrenceville, NJ 08648
609-695-5570
www.allstarvitamins.com

America's Vitamin & Nutrition
778 Southwood Court
Rochester Hills, MI 48307
248-656-3782
www.americasnutrition.com

Health Quest
4761 Bayou Blvd.
Pensacola, FL 32503
850-479-7220
www.healthquestusa.com

Healthy Living by Trust Mark
44 W. Broadway #306
Eugene, OR 97401
541-736-1425
www.trustmark.org/Metagenics

Metagenics
100 Avenida la Pata
San Clemente, CA 92673
800-692-9400
www.metagenics.com

Natrol
21411 Prairie St.
Chatsworth, CA 91311
800-326-1520
www.natrol.com

Nature Wave
2201 Woodbridge Commons Way
Iselin, NJ 08830
800-816-5758
www.naturewave.com

Puritan's Pride
1233 Montauk Hwy, PO Box 9001
Oakdale, NY 11769
800-645-9584
http://puritan.com/

Swanson Health Products
PO Box 6003
Fargo, ND 58108
800-437-4148
www.swansonvitamins.com

Twin Laboratories
2120 Smithtown Ave.
Ronkonkama, NY 11779
631-630-3486
www.twinlab.com

US Health & Nutrition
1509 E City Rd 42
Burnsville, MN 55306A
612-898-6690
www.usnutrition.com

Vitacost
Boynton Beach, FL
800-793-2601
www.vitacost.com/healthshop.html

VitaNet Health Foods
12425 Market Ave N
Hartville, OH 44632
www.vitanet.net

chapter seventy

Best Web Sites for Health-Related Issues

General Health and Safety Information

- Achoo: www.achoo.com
- American Council on Exercise: www.acefitness.org
- Americas Doctor: www.americasdoctor.com/
- CNN Health Main Page: www.cnn.com/HEALTH/index.html
- Dr. Greene's House Calls: www.drgreene.com/
- Dr. Koop: www.drkoop.com
- Health-Center.com: www.health-center.com/
- Health on the Web: www.gti.net/mocolib1/health.html
- Healthfinder: www.healthfinder.gov
- Healthweb: www.healthweb.org
- Kid's Health: www.kidshealth.org
- Mayo Clinic: www.mayohealth.org
- Medical Breakthrough: www.ivanhoe.com
- Medical World Search: www.mwsearch.com
- Medscape: www.medscape.com
- MedWebPlus: www.medwebplus.com
- Mental Health Net: http://mentalhelp.net
- National Child Care Information Center: http://ericps.crc.uiuc.edu/nccic
- National Injury Information Clearinghouse: www.cpsc.gov
- National Institute for Safety and Health Information: www.cdc.gov/niosh
- National Library of Medicine: www.nlm.nih.gov

- National Women's Health Information Center: www.4women.gov
- National Women's Health Network: www.womenshealthnetwork.org
- Now You Have a Diagnosis: What's Next?: www.ahrq.gov/consumer/diaginfo.htm
- OnHealth: http://onhealth.com/home/index.asp
- Reuters Health Information Services: www.reutershealth.com
- Web MD: www.my.webmd.com
- Your Health Daily: www.yourhealthdaily.com
- Your Surgery: http://yoursurgery.com/index.cfm

Drug Information

- Consumer Drug Information: www.fda.gov/cder/consumerinfo/default.htm
- Drug InfoNet: www.druginfonet.com/index.html
- Drugstore.com: www.drugstore.com
- Internet Drug List: www.rxlist.com
- Mosby's GenRx: www1.mosby.com/Mosby/hyGenRxi
- National Institutes of Health Office of Dietary Supplements: http://odp.od.nih.gov/ods
- New Drug Database: www.virtualdrugstore.com
- Pharmaceutical Information Network: http://pharminfo.com
- Pharmacy and You: www.pharmacyandyou.org/
- United States Pharmacopoeia: www.usp.org

Diseases

- Cancer Information Services: www.cancercareinc.org
- CancerNet: http://cancernet.nci.nih.gov/
- CBS Healthwatch: www.healthwatch.medscape.com/
- Centers for Disease Control: www.cdc.gov
- Diseases, Disorders, and Related Topics: www.mic.ki.se/Diseases/index.html
- FamilyDoctor.org: http://familydoctor.org

- Health & Diseases A to Z: www.healthatoz.com
- HealthLink: Diseases and Common Conditions: www.hslib.washington.edu/conditions/
- InteliHealth: www.intelihealth.com
- Lung Cancer Online: www.lungcanceronline.org
- Mayo Health Oasis: www.mayohealth.org
- Merck Manual: www.merck.com/pubs/mmanual/sections
- National Stroke Association: www.stroke.org
- Oncolink Cancer Center: http://cancer.med.upenn.edu
- Virtual Hospital: www.vh.org
- Wellness Web: http://wellweb.com

Specific Health Organizations

- Allergy & Asthma Foundation: www.aafa.org
- Alzheimer's Disease Education & Referral: www.alzheimers.org
- American Academy of Allergy, Asthma & Immunology: www.aaaai.org
- American Academy of Dermatology: www.aad.com
- American Academy of Environmental Medicine: www.aaem.com
- American Academy of Neurology: www.aan.com
- American Academy of Ophthalmology: www.eyenet.org
- American Academy of Pediatrics: www.aap.org
- American Board of Medical Specialists: www.certifieddoctor.org
- American Cancer Society: www.cancer.org/main.html
- American College for Advancement in Medicine: www.acam.org
- American Dental Association: www.ada.org
- American Diabetes Association: www.diabetes.org
- American Heart Association: www.amhrt.org
- American Holistic Medical Association: www.holisticmedicine.org
- American Liver Foundation: www.liverfoundation.org
- American Medical Association: www.ama-assn.org
- American Osteopathic Association: www.aoa-net.org

- American Parkinson Disease Association: www.apdaparkinson.com
- Arthritis Foundation: www.arthritis.org
- Centers for Disease Control and Prevention: www.cdc.gov
- Institutes of Medicine: www.iom.edu
- National Cancer Institute: http://cancernet.nci.nih.gov/index.html
- National Eye Institute: www.nei.nih.gov/
- National Headache Foundation: www.headaches.org
- National Heart Lung & Blood Institute: www.nhibi.nih.gov/nhlbi/nhlbi.htm
- National Institute of Arthritis & Musculoskeletal & Skin Diseases: www.nih.gov.niams
- National Institute of Diabetes, Digestive, and Kidney Disorders: www.niddk.nih.gov/
- National Institute on Aging: www.nih.gov/nia/
- National Osteoporosis Foundation: www.nof.org
- National Safety Council: www.nsc.org
- Office of Alternative Medicine: http://altmed.od.nih.gov

Alternative and Complementary Medicine Sites

- Acupressure Institute: www.acupressure.com
- Alexander Technique International: www.ati-net.com
- Alternative/Complementary Medicine: www.wellweb.com/AlternativeComplementary_Medicine.htm
- Alternative Health Directory: http://dmoz.org/Health/Alternative/
- Alternative Medicine Directory: www.altmedicine.net/
- American Association of Naturopathic Physicians: www.naturopathic.org
- American Association of Oriental Medicine: www.aaom.org
- American Chiropractic Association: www.amerchiro.org
- American Lung Association: www.lungusa.org
- American Massage Therapy Association: www.amta.org
- American Polarity Therapy Association: www.polaritytherapy.org
- Association for Biofeedback: www.aapb.org
- Ayurvedic Holistic Center: www.ayurvedahc.com

- Ayurvedic Institute: www.ayurveda.com
- Feldenkrais Guild of North America: www.feldenkrais.com
- Healing People: www.healingpeople.com/ht/index.tmpl
- HealthWeb Alternative Complementary Medicine: www.medsch.wisc.edu/chslib/hw/altmed/
- Herb Research Foundation: www.herbs.org
- HerbMed: www.herbmed.org
- International Association for Reiki Professionals: www.iarp.org
- National Acupuncture and Oriental Medicine Alliance: www.acuall.org
- National Center for Complementary and Alternative Medicine: http://nccam.nih.gov/
- National Center for Homeopathy: www.homeopathic.org
- North American Society of Homeopaths: www.homeopathy.org
- Reflexology Association of America: www.reflexology-usa.org
- Wellweb: www.wellweb.com

Mental Health

- Children and Adults with Attention Deficit Disorders: www.chadd.org
- Depression and Related Affective Disorders Association: www.med.jhu.edu/drada/index.html
- Depression Clinic: http://depressionclinic.com/
- Health Center.com Mental Health: www.health-center.com/mentalhealth/defaut.htm
- Mental Health Net: http://mentalhealth.net/
- National Association of Anorexia Nervosa and Associated Disorders: www.anad.org
- National Institute of Mental Health: www.nimh.nih.gov/
- National Mental Health Association: www.nmha.org

chapter seventy-one

Best Health-Related Books

Introduction: Youth-Preserving Tips

Perls, Thomas T. *Living to 100*. New York: Basic Books, 1999.

Rowe, John W., M.D. *Successful Aging*. New York: Random House, 1998.

Part 1: Help Yourself

Adderly, Brenda D. *The Complete Guide to Nutritional Supplements*. Los Angeles: New Star, 1998.

American Medical Association. *Pocket Guide to Emergency First Aid*. New York: Random House, 1993.

Balch, James and Phyllis Balch. *Prescription for Nutritional Healing*. Garden City Park, NY: Avery, 1990.

Barlow, Wilfred, M.D. *The Alexander Technique: How to Use Your Body without Stress*. Rochester, VT: Healing Arts Press, 1990.

Boylen, Daniel J., M.D. *Sports Medicine for Parents & Coaches*. Washington, D.C.: Georgetown University Press, 1999.

Clayman, Charles B. and Raymond H. Curry, eds. *American Medical Association Guide to Your Family's Symptoms*. New York: Random House, 1992.

Columbia University College of Physicians and Surgeons Complete Home Medical Guide. New York: Crown, 1994.

Craig, Selene and editors of *Prevention*. *The Complete Book of Alternative Nutrition*. New York: Berkley Books, 1997.

Davis, Patricia. *Aromatherapy: An A-Z*. Essex, England: CW Daniel, 1992.

Duke, James A. *The Green Pharmacy*. Emmaus, PA: Rodale Press, 1997.

Feldenkrais, Moshe. *The Elusive Obvious or Basic Feldenkrais*. Cupertino, CA: Meta Publications, 1981.

Graedon, Joe and Teresa Graedon. *The People's Pharmacy Guide to Home and Herbal Remedies*. New York: St. Martin's, 1999.

Griffith, H. Winter, M.D. *Complete Guide to Sports Injuries*. New York: Berkley Publishing, 1997.

Handal, K. *The American Red Cross First Aid and Safety Handbook*. Boston: Little, Brown, 1992.

Leung, Albert Y. and Steven Foster. *Encyclopedia of Common Natural Ingredients Used in Food, Drugs, and Cosmetics*. New York: John Wiley & Sons, 1996

Levine, Suzanne M., D.P.M. *Your Feet Don't Have to Hurt*. New York: St. Martin's Press, 2000.

Lynn, Stephan G., M.D. and Pamela Weintraub. *Medical Emergency! The St. Luke's–Roosevelt Hospital Center Book of Emergency Medicine*. New York: William Morrow, 1996.

Mayell, Mark. *Natural Health First-Aid Guide*. New York: Pocket Books, 1994.

Mindell, Earl. *Earl Mindell's New Herb Bible*. New York: Simon & Schuster, 2000.

Murray, Michael. *The Healing Power of Herbs*. Rocklin, CA: Prima Publishing, 1995.

Murray, Michael T. and Joseph E. Pizzorno. *An Encyclopedia of Natural Medicine*. Rocklin, CA: Prima Publishing, 1991.

Null, Gary and Barbara Seaman. *For Women Only!* New York: Seven Stories Press, 1999.

Peirce, Andrea. *The American Pharmaceutical Association Practical Guide to Natural Medicine*. New York: William Morrow, 1999.

Rose, Stuart R., M.D. *1994 International Travel Health Guide*, 5th ed. Northampton, MA: Travel Medicine, 1994.

Smyth, Angela. *The Complete Home Healer: Your Guide to Every Treatment Available for Over 300 of the Most Common Health Problems*. San Francisco: HarperCollins, 1994.

Tierra, M. *The Way of Herbs*. New York: Pocket Books, 1990.

Turkington, Carol A. and Jeffrey S. Dover, M.D. *Skin Deep: An A-Z of Skin Disorders, Treatments and Health*. New York: Facts on File, 1998.

Valnet, Jean. *The Practice of Aromatherapy*. Rochester, VT: Healing Arts Press, 1990.

Vickery, Donald M., M.D. and James F. Fries, M.D. *Take Care of Yourself: The Complete Guide to Medical Self-Care*. Reading, MA: Addison-Wesley, 1994.

Weil, Andrew, M.D. *Health and Healing*. Boston: Houghton Mifflin, 1995.

Weil, Andrew, M.D. *Natural Health, Natural Medicine*. Boston: Houghton Mifflin, 1995.

Weil, Andrew, M.D. *Spontaneous Healing: How to Discover and Enhance Your Body's Natural Ability to Maintain and Heal Itself*. New York: Knopf, 1995.

Werbach, Melvyn R., M.D. *Healing through Nutrition*. New York: HarperCollins, 1993.

Winsor, Mari. *The Pilates Powerhouse*. New York: Perseus, 1999.

Winter, Ruth. *A Consumer's Guide to Medicines in Food*. New York: Crown Trade, 1995.

Yanker, Gary et al. *Exercise Rx*. New York: Kodansha America, 1999.

Part 2: People to See, Things to Do

Bruneton, Jean. *Pharmacognosy: Phytochemistry, Medicinal Plants*. New York: Lavoisier, 1995.

Davis, Wade. *One River*. New York: Simon & Schuster, 1996.

Goldmann, David R., M.D., ed. *American College of Physicians Complete Home Medical Guide*. New York: DK Publishing, 1999.

Graedon, Teresa and Joe Graedon. *Dangerous Drug Interactions: How to Protect Yourself from Harmful Drug/Drug, Drug/Food, and Drug/Vitamin Combinations*. New York: St. Martin's Press, 1999.

Griffith, H. Winter, M.D. *Complete Guide to Prescription and Nonprescription Drugs*. New York: Perigee, 1999.

Griffith, H. Winter, M.D. *Complete Guide to Symptoms, Illness, and Surgery*, 4th ed. New York: Body Press/Perigee Books, 2000.

Gursche, Siegfried. *Encyclopedia of Natural Healing*. Blaine, WA: Natural Life Publishing, 1997.

Hayfield, Robin. *Homeopathy for Common Ailments*. Berkeley, CA: Frog, 1993.

Joyce, Christopher. *Earthly Goods: Medicine Hunting in the Rainforest*. Boston, MA: Little, Brown & Co., 1994.

Lockie, Andrew and Nicola Geddes. *Homeopathy: The Principles & Practice of Treatment*. Great Britain and New York: Dorling Kindersley Ltd., 1995.

Margolis, Simon, M.D., ed. *Johns Hopkins Symptoms and Remedies*. New York: Rebus, 1995.

Miller, Jeanne. *The Perfectly Safe Home*. New York: Simon & Schuster, 1991.

Rose, Eric A., M.D. *Second Opinion: The Columbia Presbyterian Guide to Surgery*. New York: St. Martin's Press, 2000.

Segen, Joseph C., M.D., and Joseph Stauffer, Ph.D. *The Patient's Guide to Medical Tests*. New York: Facts on File, 1998.

Wyer, E. Bingo. *The Unofficial Guide to Cosmetic Surgery*. New York: Macmillan, 1999.

Youngson, Robert M., M.D. *The Surgery Book: An Illustrated Guide to 73 of the Most Common Operations*. New York: St. Martin's Press, 1993.

Part 3: Where to Go for Good Health

Arnot, Robert. *The Best Medicine: How to Choose the Top Doctors, the Top Hospitals, the Top Treatments*. New York: Addison-Wesley, 1993.

Beinfield, Harriet, and Efrem Korngold. *Between Heaven and Earth: A Guide to Chinese Medicine*. New York: Ballantine Books, 1991.

Burton Goldberg Group. *Alternative Medicine: The Definitive Guide*. Puyallup, WA: Future Medicine, 1993.

Korsch, Barbara M. *The Intelligent Patient's Guide to the Doctor–Patient Relationship*. New York: Oxford University Press, 1997.

Krantz, Les. *Jobs Rated Almanac*. New York: St. Martin's Press, 1999.

Lerrner, Michael. *Choices in Healing*. Cambridge, MA: MIT Press, 1994.

McCall, Timothy, M.D. *Examining Your Doctor*. Secaucus, NJ: Carol Publishing, 1996.

Part 4: Crucial Facts about the Human Body

Brand, Paul and Philip Yancey. *Pain: The Gift Nobody Wants*. New York: HarperCollins, 1993.

Diagram Group. *Man's Body: An Owner's Manual*. Chicago: Diagram Group, 1997.

Foley, Denise, et al. *Doctors' Book of Home Remedies for Children*. Emmaus, PA: Rodale Press, 1994.

Griffith, H. Winter. *Complete Guide to Pediatric Symptoms, Illness and Medications*. Los Angeles: Body Press, 1989.

Lavery, Sheila. *The Healing Power of Sleep*. New York: Simon & Schuster, 1997.

Marieb, Elaine N. *Essentials of Human Anatomy and Physiology*, 4th ed. Redwood City, CA: Benjamin/Cummings, 1994.

Mosby's Medical, Nursing, and Allied Health Dictionary, 4th ed. New York: Mosby-Year Book, 1994.

National Geographic Society. *The Incredible Machine*. Washington, D.C: National Geographic Society, 1986.

Netter, Frank H. *Atlas of Human Anatomy*. Summit, NJ: Ciba-Geigy, 1989.

Reader's Digest. *ABC's of the Human Body*. Pleasantville, NY: Reader's Digest Books, 1987.

Scialli, Anthony, M.D., ed. *The National Women's Health Resource Center Book of Women's Health*. New York: National Women's Health Resource Center, 1999.

Spock, Benjamin. *Dr. Spock's Baby and Child Care*, 6th ed. New York: Pocket Books, 1992.

Time/Life Book editors. *The Medical Advisor: The Complete Guide to Alternative & Conventional Treatments*, 2nd ed. Alexandria, VA: Time/Life, 2000.

Tortora, Gerard and Sandra Grabowski. *Introduction to the Human Body*, 5th ed. New York: John Wiley, 2001.

Woodburne, Russell and William E. Burkel. *Essentials of Human Anatomy*, 9th ed. New York: Oxford University Press, 1994.

Part 5: Health Statistics and Trivia You Might Need to Know

Altman, Linda Jacobs. *Plague & Pestilence: A History of Infectious Disease.* Springfield, NJ: Enslow Publishers, 1998.

Garrett, Laurie. *The Coming Plague: Newly Emerging Diseases in a World Out of Balance.* New York: Penguin, 1994.

Hoff, Brent and Carter Smith III. *Mapping Epidemics: A Historical Atlas of Disease.* New York: Franklin Watts, 1999.

Kohn, George. *Encyclopedia of Plague & Pestilence.* New York: Facts on File, 1995.

Traisman, Edward S., ed. *AMA Complete Guide to Your Children's Health.* New York: Random House, 1999.

Tuleja, Tad. *Fabulous Fallacies.* New York: Galahad Books, 1999.

Underwood, Lamar. *Man Eaters: True Tales of Animals Stalking, Mauling, Killing & Eating Human Prey.* New York: Lyons Press, 2000.

Part 6: Alternative Views of Healing

Bauer, Cathryn. *Acupressure for Everybody.* New York: Henry Holt, 1991.

Bruyere, Rosallyn. *Wheels of Light, Chakras, Auras, and the Healing Energy of the Body.* New York: Fireside, 1989.

Gach, Michael Reed. *Acupressure's Potent Points: A Guide to Self-Care for Common Ailments.* New York: Bantam Books, 1990.

Gillanders, Ann. *The Family Guide to Reflexology.* Boston: Little, Brown, 1998.

Goleman, Daniel. *MindBody Medicine.* Yonkers, NY: Consumer Reports, 1993.

Jarmey, Chris and John Tindall. *Acupressure for Common Ailments.* New York: Simon & Schuster, 1991.

Marcus, Paul: *Acupuncture: A Patient's Guide.* New York: Thorsons, 1985.

Norman, Laura. *Feet First: A Guide to Foot Reflexology.* New York: Simon & Schuster, 1988.

Ulett, George. *Beyond Yin and Yang: How Acupuncture Really Works.* St. Louis, MO: Warren Green, 1992.

chapter seventy-two

Best Health-Related Magazines and Newsletters

Here are some of the best consumer magazines, periodicals, and newsletters available on a variety of health-related topics. In many cases, you can get a preview of the magazine or newsletter on a Web site and subscribe from there as well.

Magazines and Periodicals

American Baby Magazine
www.americanbaby.com

American Fitness
www.afaa.com

Better Nutrition
www.betternutrition.com

FDA Consumer
www.fda.gov/fdac/fdacindex.html

Good Medicine
(Magazine of the Physicians' Committee for Responsible Medicine)
www.pcrm.org

Healthy Kids
www.healthykids.com

HerbalGram
American Botanical Council, PO Box 201660, Austin, TX 78720

Journal of Natural Hygiene
Natural Hygiene, Inc., PO Box 2132, Huntington, CT 06484
203-929-1557

Let's Live Magazine
www.letsliveonline.com

Life Extension Magazine
www.lef.org

Massage Magazine
PO Box 1500, Davis, CA 95617
916-757-6033
www.massagemag.com

Men's Health
www.menshealth.com

Natural Health
Boston Common Press Limited Partnership, 17 Station Street, Brookline, MA 02146
www.naturalhealthmag.com

New Age: The Journal for Holistic Living
www.newage.com

Twins: The Magazine for Parents of Multiples
www.twinsmagazine.com

The Vegetarian Voice
North American Vegetarian Society, PO Box 72, Dodgerville, NY 13329
518-568-7970

Vibrant Life
www.vibrantlife.com

Yoga Journal
www.yogajournal.com

Newsletters

Atlantis: The Imagery Newsletter
www.imagerynet.com/atlantis

Consumer Reports Online Health & Food
www.consumerreports.org/Categories/FoodHealth/index.html

Dr. Andrew Weil's Self-Healing Newsletter
www.drweilselfhealing.com/

Environmental Nutrition
800-829-5384
www.environmentalnutrition.com

FDA Consumer
www.fda.gov/fdac

Harvard Health Letter
www.health.harvard.edu/index.html

Harvard Women's Health Watch
www.health.harvard.edu/newsletters/backwomen.shtml

Health Style Online Monthly Newsletter
http://visitors.bestofhealth.com/newsletter/index.html

Johns Hopkins Medical Letter, Health after 50
800-829-0422
www.hopkinsafter50.com/

Julian Whitaker, M.D. Newsletter
www.drwhitaker.com/

Mayo Clinic Health Letter
www.mayoclinic.com/

McDougall Newsletter
www.drmcdougall.com/newsletter.html

Nutrition Action Health Letter
800-237-4874
www.cspinet.org/nah/

Tufts University Diet and Nutrition Letter
800-274-7581
http://healthletter.tufts.edu/

University of California at Berkeley Wellness Letter
800-829-9170
www.berkeleywellness.com

Vital Health Newsletters
www.vital-health.com/au/vitalhealth.htm

References

The resources and authorities listed here were consulted for the information contained in this book. Further information about these topics can be found on the Web sites listed for each chapter.

Introduction

Hippocrates. Mar. 2000: 14(3); Nov. 1999: 13(10).

McGill University: www.mjm.mcgill.ca/issues/v02n02/aspirin.html

MedHelpNet: www.medhelpnet.com/medhist10.html

Stabler-Leadbetter Apothecary Museum: www.apothecary.org/medical.htm

National Institutes of Health Human Genome Programs: www.nih.gov

Chapter 1

Homeopathic Educational Services: www.homeopathy.com

www.nursehealer.com/HerbsDry.htm

Jagoda, Andy, M.D. *The Good Housekeeping Family First Aid Book.* New York: Hearst Books, 2000.

Chapter 2

Medical Economics Staff. *Physician's Desk Reference for Nonprescription Drugs and Dietary Supplements.* Montvale, NJ: Medical Economics, 2000.

Merck Manual, Home Edition, section 2, chapter 13 on the Web: www.merck.com/pubs/mmanual_home/sec2/13.htm

Griffith, H. Winter, M.D. *Complete Guide to Prescription & Nonprescription Drugs,* 1999 ed. New York: Perigee, 1998.

American Academy of Family Practitioners: www.aafp.org/afp/980501ap/jacobs.html

Chapter 3

American Botanical Council: www.herbalgram.org

Adderly, Brenda D. *The Complete Guide to Nutritional Supplements.* Los Angeles: New Star Press, 1998.

Duke, James A., Ph.D. *Dr. Duke's Essential Herbs.* Emmaus, PA: Rodale Press, 1999.

Foster, Steven. *An Illustrated Guide: 101 Medicinal Herbs*. Loveland, CO: Interweave Press, 1998

Graedon, Joe and Teresa Graedon. *The People's Pharmacy Guide to Home and Herbal Remedies*. New York: St. Martin's, 1999.

Mindell, Earl. *Earl Mindell's New Herb Bible*. New York: Simon & Schuster, 2000.

Chapter 4

American Dietetic Association: www.eatright.org

Adderly, Brenda D. *The Complete Guide to Nutritional Supplements*. Los Angeles: New Star, 1998.

Murray, Michael. *Encyclopedia of Nutritional Supplements*. Rocklin, CA: Prima Publishing, 1996.

Dr. Koop Web site: www.drkoop.com

Chapter 5

American Dietetic Association: www.eatright.org

Time/Life. *The Medical Advisor*, 2nd ed. Alexandria, VA: Time/Life, 2000.

Murray, Michael. *Encyclopedia of Nutritional Supplements*. Rocklin, CA: Prima Publishing, 1996.

Chapter 6

Medical Economics Staff. *Physician's Desk Reference for Nonprescription Drugs and Dietary Supplements*. Montvale, NJ: Medical Economics, 2000.

National Institutes of Health Office of Dietary Supplements: http://odp.od.nih.gov/ods

Graedon, Joe and Teresa Graedon. *The People's Pharmacy Guide to Home and Herbal Remedies*. New York: St. Martin's, 1999.

www.supplementwatch.com

Adderly, Brenda D. *The Complete Guide to Nutritional Supplements*. Los Angeles: New Star, 1998.

Chapter 7

American Red Cross: www.redcross.org

Jagoda, Andy, M.D. *The Good Housekeeping Family First Aid Book*. New York: Hearst Books, 2000.

American Medical Association. *Complete Guide to Your Children's Health*. New York: Random House, 1999.

The Focus on the Family Physicians' Resource Council. *Complete Book of Baby &*
    Child Care. Wheaton, IL: Tyndale House, 1997.

Chapter 8

McFarlane, Rodger and Philip Bashe. *The Complete Bedside Companion: No-*
    Nonsense Advice on Caring for the Seriously Ill. New York: Simon & Schuster,
    1998.
Greif, Judith and Beth Ann Golden. *AIDS Care at Home: A Guide for Caregivers,*
    Loved Ones, and People with AIDS. New York: Wiley, 1994.

Chapter 9

American Dietetic Association: www.eatright.org
Fox, Barry. *Foods to Heal By*. New York: St. Martin's 1996.
Kradjian, Robert M., M.D. *Save Yourself from Breast Cancer*. New York: Berkley
    Publishing, 1994.
Werbach, Melvyn, M.D. *Nutritional Influences on Illness*, 2nd ed. Tarzana, CA: Third
    Line Press, 1993.

Chapter 10

The Kevala Centre: www.kevala.co.uk/
Rose, Jeanne. *The Aromatherapy Book*. Berkeley, CA: North Atlantic Books, 1992.
Worwood, Valerie Ann. *The Complete Book of Essential Oils and Aromatherapy*. San
    Rafael, CA: New World Library, 1991.

Chapter 11

American Council on Exercise: www.acefitness.org
Pilates from www.pilates.co.uk
www.gyrotonic.com
Cari Waldman, *The Detroit News*, March 28, 2000, Health section.
Mensendieck, Bess. *The Mensendieck System of Functional Exercises*. Kristianstads
    Boktryckeri, 1989.
Yanker, Gary, et al. *Exercise Rx*. New York: Kodansha America, 1999.

Chapter 12

Meuleman, E., et al. *British Journal of Urology International*. Jan. 2001; 87(1): 75–81.
    (Viagra)

HealthCentral for Viagra (March 2000)
www.plsgroup.com/dg/1e928e.htm

Chapter 13

American Heart Association: www.amhrt.org

Centers for Disease Control and Prevention: www.cdc.gov/cancer

American Institute for Cancer Research: www.aicr.org/aicr.htm

Andrew Weil, M.D.: www.drweil.com/archiveqa/0,2283,148,00.html

Willett, W.C., Colditz, G.A., and Mueller, N.E. "Strategies for minimizing cancer risk." *Scientific American*. Sept. 1996.

Talk about Sleep, Inc.: www.talkaboutsleep.com

Chapter 14

National Institute of Mental Health: www.nimh.nih.gov

Murray, Michael, N.D. *An Encyclopedia of Natural Medicine*. Rocklin, CA: Prima Publishing, 1998.

Mindell, Earl. *Earl Mindell's New Herb Bible*. New York: Simon & Schuster, 2000.

Weil, Andrew. *Natural Health, Natural Medicine*. Boston: Houghton Mifflin, 1995.

Chapter 15

Centers for Disease Control, National Center for Infectious Disease: www.cdc.gov/travel/

Chapter 16

American Podiatric Medicine Association: www.apma.org

American Association of Colleges of Podiatric Medicine, American Hospital Association, American Podiatric Medical Association, Council on Podiatric Medical Education, Podiatry Insurance Company of America, United States Bureau of the Census, and United States Department of Health and Human Services.

Graedon, Joe and Teresa Graedon. *The People's Pharmacy Guide to Home and Herbal Remedies*. New York: St. Martin's Press, 1999.

Chapter 17

Vision Council of America: www.visionsite.org

National Eye Research Foundation: www.nerf.org

Anshel, Jeffrey. *Smart Medicine for Your Eyes*. Garden City Park, NY: Avery, 1999.

Abel, Robert, M.D. *Eye Care Revolution*. New York: Kensington Publishing, 1999. Also, Abel's Web site: www.eyeadvisor.com

Chapter 18

Cleveland Clinic: www.clevelandclinic.org/dermatology/patient/faqs.htm

www.mylifepath.com

Chapter 19

American Academy of Pediatrics: www.aap.org

American Medical Association. *Complete Guide to Your Children's Health*. New York: Random House, 1999.

The Focus on the Family Physicians' Resource Council. *Complete Book of Baby & Child Care*. Wheaton, IL: Tyndale House, 1997.

Chapter 20

American Red Cross: www.redcross.org

Survival supplies: www.survivalsuppliers.com

Marine survival: www.equipped.com/marinetoc.htm

Chapter 21

American Academy of Orthopaedic Surgeons, www.aaos.org, has fact sheets on injury prevention for many popular sports. 1-800-346-2267

U.S. Consumer Product Safety Commission; 1-800-638-2772: www.cpsc.gov/

Brain Injury Association: www.biausa.org/sportsfs.htm. Provides data on brain injuries for several sports; 1-800-444-6443.

From "Knock knock: Concussions from sports injuries," RS Moser, Ph.D., *NJ Medicine*. Nov. 1998; 27–29.

Report released by National Safe Kids Campaign, Washington, D.C., on May 4, 2000. Results from the SAFE KIDS survey, entitled "Get into the Game: A National Survey of Parents' Knowledge, Attitudes, and Self-Reported Behaviors Concerning Sports Safety," released by Campaign Chairman C. Everett Koop, M.D., Sc.D.

SAFE KIDS: www.safekids.org to access facts sheets on sports and recreation injuries; 202-662-0600.

Chapter 22

National Highway Traffic Safety Association: www.nhtsa.dot.gov/hot/rollover/
2001Rollover.html

Chapter 23

Association for Safe International Road Travel: www.asirt.org

Airsafe.com: www.airsafe.com/airline.htm

www.comebackalive.com/df/dgrawait.htm

Train Safety from www.cjonline.com/stories, *Topeka-Capital Journal*. Mar. 21, 2000.

Cruise ship information: www.concierge.com

Chapter 24

National Safety Council: www.nsc.org

American Medical Association (falls): www.ama-assn.org/insight/h_focus/nemours/
safety/acciden2.htm

www.findarticles.com in the *Ladies Home Journal*

Miller, Jeanne. *The Perfectly Safe Home*. New York: Simon & Schuster, 1991.

Chapter 25

Rakel, Robert E., ed. *Conn's Current Therapy*. Philadelphia: WB Saunders, 2000.

www.mdadvice.com/library/test/medtest

www.healthanswers.com/medenc/index.asp?topic=Test

Segen, Joseph C. M.D., and Joseph Stauffer, Ph.D. *The Patient's Guide to Medical
Tests*. New York: Facts on File, 1998.

Chapter 26

Rakel, Robert E., ed. *Conn's Current Therapy*. Philadelphia: WB Saunders, 2000.

Segen, Joseph C., M.D., and Joseph Stauffer, Ph.D. *The Patient's Guide to Medical
Tests*. New York: Facts on File, 1998.

Harvard University: www.health.harvard.edu/fgh/diagnostics.shtml

www.life-line.org/health/cost.html

Everything You Need to Know about Medical Treatment. Springhouse, PA: Springhouse
Corp, 1996.

Chapter 27

American Board of Medical Specialists: www.abms.org/glossary.asp

Chapter 28

National Board for Certified Clinical Hypnotherapists: www.natboard.com

American Association of Professional Hypnotherapists: www.aaph.org

International Center for Reiki Training: www.reiki.org

American Herbalist Guild: www.naturalhealers.com

Journal of the American Geriatrics Society. December 2000.

Journal of the American Medical Association. November 1998

Journal of Clinical Oncology. 2000; 18:2505–2521.

Chapter 29

Medical Economics Staff. *Physician's Desk Reference, 2000*. Montvale, NJ: Medical Economics, 2000.

Food & Drug Administration Consumer Drug Information: www.fda.gov/cder/consumerinfo/default.htm

www.rxlist.com/top200.html

Wolfe, Sidney M., M.D. *Worst Pills, Best Pills*. New York: Pocket Books, 1999.

Griffith, H. Winter, M.D. *Complete Guide to Prescription and Nonprescription Drugs*. New York: Perigee, 1999.

Rybacki, James. *The Essential Guide to Prescription Drugs*. New York: HarperPerennial, 1999.

Chapter 30

Homeopathic Educational Services: www.homeopathic.com

Lockie, Andrew and Nicola Geddes. *Homeopathy: The Principles & Practice of Treatment*. Great Britain and New York: Dorling Kindersley Ltd., 1995.

Gursche, Siegfried. *Encyclopedia of Natural Healing*. Blaine, WA: Natural Life Publishing, 1997.

Chapter 31

Goldmann, David R., M.D., ed. *American College of Physicians Complete Home Medical Guide*. New York: DK Publishing, 1999.

Rose, Eric A., M.D. *Second Opinion: The Columbia Presbyterian Guide to Surgery*. New York: St. Martin's Press, 2000.

Youngson, Robert M., M.D. *The Surgery Book: An Illustrated Guide to 73 of the Most Common Operations*. New York: St. Martin's Press, 1993.

Wyer, E. Bingo. *The Unofficial Guide to Cosmetic Surgery*. New York: Macmillan, 1999.

Chapter 32

From an interview with Mark Plotkin.

www.accessexcellence.com/WN/NM/plotkin1.html

Encyclopedia Britannica: www.britannica.com/bcom/eb/article/4/0,5716,11724+1+11589,00.html

www.kitchendoctor.com/Chyawanprash.html

www.ahealthya.com/maca.htm/(maca)

www.delicious-online.com/D_backs/Apr_97/rainforest.cfm

www.nutrifarmacy.com/pol2.htm/(catsclaw)

www.amazon-medic.co.uk/database/data/Tayuya.html/(tayuya)

Kilham, Chris. *Tales from the Medicine Trail*. Emmaus, PA: Rodale Press, 2000.

Chapter 33

Pilgrimage: http://ebooks.whsmithonline.co.uk/encyclopedia/95/M0002495.htm

Milne, Courtney. *The Sacred Earth*. New York: Harry Abrams, 1993.

Don Pedrito shrine: www.caller.com/newsarch/news10144.html

Sacred Sites: www.sacredsites.com/index

Each site searched individually.

Chapter 34

U.S. News: www.usnews.com/usnews/nycu/health/hosptl/tophosp.htm

Dudley, R.A., et al. "Selective referral to high-volume hospitals: estimating potentially avoidable deaths." *Journal of the American Medical Association*. Mar. 1, 2000; 283(9): 1159–66.

www.100tophospitals.com

Chapter 35

American Dental Association: www.ada.org

Quackwatch: www.quackwatch.com

The Complete Book of Dental Remedies at www.healthy.net/asp/templates/article.asp?id=1793

Chapter 36

Acupuncture and Oriental Medicine Alliance: www.acuall.org

QuackWatch: www.quackwatch.com

Medical Reporter: http://medicalreporter.health.org/tmr0495/chooseapcp.html

Health Grades: www.healthgrades.com/Healthtools/HowToChoose/
    HG_choose_phys.cfm#Checklist/Questions

Chapter 37

American Medical News: www.ammednews.com

Acupuncture and Oriental Medicine Alliance: www.acuall.org/colleges.htm

Alternative Dr.com: www.alternativedr.com/naturopathy/index

American Association of Naturopathic Physicians: www.naturopathic.org

www.heall.com/links/clinics.html (integrative medicine)

Chapter 38

MSNBC site on *Self's* survey on healthiest cities.

From: www.smallmarketmeetings.com/town%20mtgs/madison.html

From: http://content.health.msn.com/content/article/1728.53282

www.channel4000.com/news/stories/news-19991208-010045.html, "Men's Fitness."

Money magazine, 1995, "Safest and most dangerous places in the U.S."

Chapter 39

www.fieldingtravel.com/df/dngrjobs.htm

Bureau of Labor Statistics: http://stats.bls.gov/special.requests/ocwc/cfar0020.txt

Occupational Safety & Health Administration: www.osha.gov/oshstats/bls/txts/cfar0015.txt

Chapter 40

National Organ Procurement and Transplantation Network: www.organdonor.gov

BusinessWeek on-line, March 20, 2000.

www.findarticles.com/m1590/8_56/59086803/p1/article.jhtml

Tortora, Gerard and Sandra Grabowski. *Introduction to the Human Body*, 5th ed. New
    York: Wiley, 2001.

Chapter 41

www.historyofhair.com/abouthair.html

National Geographic Society. *The Incredible Machine*. Washington, D.C.: National Geographic Society, 1986.

Reader's Digest. *ABC's of the Human Body*. Pleasantville, NY: Reader's Digest Books, 1987.

Tortora, Gerard and Sandra Grabowski. *Introduction to the Human Body*, 5th ed. New York: Wiley, 2001.

Chapter 42

International Association for the Study of Pain: www.halcyon.com/iasp/

Brand, Paul and Philip Yancey. *Pain: The Gift Nobody Wants*. New York: HarperCollins, 1993.

Caudill, Margaret. *Managing Pain before It Manages You*. New York: Guilford Press, 1995.

Chapter 43

American Family Physician. June 1993: 47: 8: 1759.

www.howstuffworks.com/question447.htm (drinking ice water)

Web M.D.: http://onhealth.webmd.com/fitness/briefs/item%2C76484.asp

www.foodfit.com/fitness/archive/askFitness_may04.asp

Brody, Jane. *Jane Brody's Good Food Book*. New York: Norton, 1985.

Chapter 44

Fast-Food Facts: www.kenkuhl.com/fastfood/

Chapter 45

Goldmann, David R., M.D., ed. *American College of Physicians Complete Home Medical Guide*. New York: DK Publishing, 1999.

Clayman, Charles B. and Raymond H. Curry, eds. *American Medical Association Guide to Your Family's Symptoms*. New York: Random House, 1992.

Columbia University College of Physicians and Surgeons Complete Home Medical Guide. New York: Crown, 1994.

Chapter 46

Healthgate: www.healthgate.com/sym/index.shtml

Segen, Joseph C., M.D., and Joseph Stauffer, Ph.D. *The Patient's Guide to Medical Tests*. New York: Facts on File, 1998.

Margolis, Simon, M.D., ed. *Johns Hopkins Symptoms and Remedies*. New York: Rebus, 1995.

Chapters 47 to 49

Goldmann, David R., M.D., ed. *American College of Physicians Complete Home Medical Guide*. New York: DK Publishing, 1999.

Traisman, Edward S., M.D., ed. *American Medical Association Complete Guide to Your Children's Health*. New York: Random House, 1999.

Schiff, Donald, M.D. and Steven P. Shelov, M.D. *American Academy of Pediatrics: The Official, Complete Home Reference Guide to Your Child's Symptoms*. New York: Villard, 1997.

Columbia University College: http://cpmcnet.columbia.edu/texts/guide/hmg07_0019.html

Mayo Clinic: www.mayohealth.org/mayo/9606/htm/pid.htm

http://209.52.189.2/article.cfm/women_and_depression/39791

"Phobia." *Journal of the American Academy of Child and Adolescent Psychiatry*. 2000; 39: 721–726.

Chapter 50

Editors of Time/Life. *The Medical Advisor*. Alexandria, VA: 2000.

Goldmann, David R., M.D., ed. *American College of Physicians Complete Home Medical Guide*. New York: DK Publishing, 1999.

Clayman, Charles B. and Raymond H. Curry, eds. *American Medical Association Guide to Your Family's Symptoms*. New York: Random House, 1992.

Columbia University College of Physicians and Surgeons Complete Home Medical Guide. New York: Crown, 1994.

Chapter 51

National Institute on Deafness and Other Communication Disorders: www.nidcd.nih.gov/health/kids/decible/decible.html

Occupational Safety & Health Administration

National Council on the Aging

Hearing Alliance of America: www.hearingalliance.com

H.E.A.R.

Temple University Dept. of Civil/Environmental Engineering: www.temple.edu/departments/CETP/environ10.html

Bay Area Reporter newspaper, March 30, 2000.

Chapter 52

Hauri, Peter, Ph.D. *No More Sleepless Nights*. New York: Wiley, 1996.

National Sleep Foundation: www.sleepfoundation.org

Chapter 53

National Library of Medicine: www.nlm.nih.gov/medlineplus/skincancer.html

New England Journal of Medicine. May 28, 1998; vol. 338, editorial (asbestos).

Cancer Network: www.cancernetwork.com/CanMed/Ch025/025-3.htm

www.Emagazine.com/september-october_1998/0998gl_ecohome.html

National Tribal Environmental Council: www2.ntec.org/air/factsheet3.html

Environmental Protection Agency: www.epa.gov/radiation/

Warde, John. *The Healthy Home Handbook*. New York: Times Books, 1997.

Chapter 54

Chaturvedi, S., et al. "Ischemic Stroke Prevention." *Current Treatment Options in Neurology*. May 1999; 1(2):113–26.

Ebrahim, S. "Cost-effectiveness of stroke prevention." *British Medical Bulletin*. 2000; 56(2): 557–70.

Vine, Marilyn. *Fertility Sterility Journal*. 1994; 6(1): 35–43.

American Journal of Public Health. 1993 (info on cigarettes and colds).

www.netdoctor.co.uk/health_advice/facts/smokehealth.htm

http://answermd.com/HealthAndVitality/SMOKE_CERVIX.HTML

Chapter 55

National Institutes of Health: www.nih.gov/news/budget01/nih2001budget.pdf

American Diabetes Association: www.diabetes.org/ada/drwg/drwgsummary.html

Chapter 56

Altman, Linda Jacobs. *Plague & Pestilence: A History of Infectious Disease*. Springfield, NJ: Enslow Publishers, 1998.

Garrett, Laurie. *The Coming Plague: Newly Emerging Diseases in a World Out of Balance*. New York: Penguin, 1994.

Hoff, Brent and Carter Smith III. *Mapping Epidemics: A Historical Atlas of Disease*. New York: Franklin Watts, 1999.

Kohn, George. *Encyclopedia of Plague & Pestilence*. New York: Facts on File, 1995.

UNAIDS HIV/AIDS Report on the Global HIV/AIDS Epidemic, June 2000. From: www.gmhc.org (Gay Men's Health Crisis).

Harvard University: www.uhavax.hartford.edu/~bugl/histepi.htm

Chapter 57

From: Trivia about the Human Body (through About.com portal)

Tuleja, Tad. *Fabulous Fallacies*. New York: Galahad Books, 1999.

Chapter 58

Cornell University, Poisonous Plants Page: www.ansci.cornell.edu/plants/plants.html

Food & Drug Administration, Center for Food Safety and Applied Nutrition, Poisonous Plant Database: http://vm.cfsan.fda.gov/~djw/readme.html

University of California, San Diego, Poisonous Plants: http://health.ucsd.edu/poison/plants.htm

Chapter 59

National Center for Injury Prevention & Control: www.cdc.gov

Centers for Disease Control: www.cdc.gov

Insurance Institute for Highway Safety, report of April 3, 1993 (vol. 28, no. 4).

Weiss, H., et al. "Incidence of dog-bite injuries treated in emergency departments." *Journal of the American Medical Association*. Jan. 7, 1998; 279(1): 51–53.

Humane Society of the U.S.: www.hsus.org

Detroit News. Sept. 2000: http://detnews.com/2000/metro/0009/29/d02-127181.htm

www.usroads.com/journals/rmj/9705/rm970503.htm

Chapter 60

National Organization of Mothers of Twins Clubs: www.nomotc.org/twins.htm

Luke, Barbara, et al. "The cost of prematurity: A case-control study of twins vs. single-tons." *American Journal of Public Health*. June 1996; 86(6): 809–14.

www.epregnancy.com/info/multiples/multiples.htm

www.usatoday.com/life/health/doctor/lhdoc038.htm

Chapter 61

Miller, Steve Z. and Bernard Valman. *Columbia University College of Physicians and Surgeons Children's Medical Guide*. New York: DK Publishers, 1997.

Traisman, Edward S., ed. *AMA Complete Guide to Your Children's Health*. New York: Random House, 1999.

Chapter 62

Gerontology Research Group: www.grg.org

National Centenarian Awareness Project: www.adlercentenarians.com

Chapter 63

www.sacredcenters.com

Pond, David. *Chakras for Beginners: A Guide to Balancing Your Chakra Energies*. St. Paul: Llewellyn Publications, 1999.

McLaren, Karla. *Your Aura and Your Chakras: The Owner's Manual*. York Beach, ME: Samuel Weiser, 1998.

Chapter 64

www.prayernetwork.com

www.crosssource.com/prayer.html

www.thehealingcircle.org

www.worldpeace.org

www.ananda.org

www.catanna.com/healing.htm

www.worldprayer.org

www.orderofstluke.org

www.infoholisticonline.com (prayers) (Permission received March 9, 2001.)

Harris, William, et al. *Archives of Internal Medicine*. October 25, 1999.

Crane, J.R., S. Perlman, et al. "Women with HIV: Conflicts and synergy of prayer within the realm of medical care." *AIDS Educational Preview*. Dec. 2000; 12(6): 532–43.

Stewart, D.E., et al. "Attributions of cause and recurrence in long-term breast cancer survivors." *Psychooncology*. Mar-Apr 2001; 10(2): 179–83.

Helm, H.M., et al. "Does private religious activity prolong survival? A six-year follow-up study of 3,851 older adults." *Journals of Gerontology Series A: Biological Sciences and Medical Sciences*. Jul. 2000; 55(7): M400–405.

Chapter 65

Reflexology Association of America: www.reflexology-usa.org

Gillanders, Ann. *The Family Guide to Reflexology*. Boston: Little, Brown, 1998.

Wills, Pauline. *The Reflexology Manual: An Easy-to-Use Illustrated Guide to the Healing Zones of the Hands and Feet*. Rochester, VT: Healing Arts Press, 1995.

Chapter 66

American Association of Oriental Medicine: www.aaom.org

Editors of Time/Life. *The Medical Advisor*. Alexandria, VA: 2000.

Gach, Michael Reed. *Acupressure's Potent Points: A Guide to Self-Care for Common Ailments*. New York: Bantam Books, 1990.

Chapters 68 to 72

American Federation for Aging Research

National Institute on Aging: www.nih.gov/nia/

National Association for Therapeutic Humor

Calorie Restriction: www.msnbc.com/news/180101.asp#BODY

Claflin, Edward, ed. *Age Protectors*. Emmaus, PA: Rodale Press, 1998.

Gottlieb, Bill. *Alternative Cures*. Emmaus, PA: Rodale Press, 2000.

Optometrist Marc Grossman, codirector of the Integral Health Centers in Rye and New Paltz, New York.

Julian Whitaker, M.D., founder and director of the Whitaker Wellness Center in Newport Beach, California.

Michael Janson, M.D., author of *The Vitamin Revolution* and *Dr. Janson's New Vitamin Revolution*.

Medicine and Science in Sports and Exercise. 2000; 32: 2005–2011.

Vitamin C: Reported by www.medscape.com on November 13, 2000.

Christian J. Gillin, M.D., professor of psychiatry at the University of California, San Diego.

Larry Dossey, M.D., author of *Prayer Is Good Medicine*.

Andrew Weil, M.D., author of *Natural Health, Natural Medicine*.

Index

Systemic lupus erythematosus
(SLE):
between ages 20–40, 409–410
risk for developing, 374

T
Tai chi to reduce anxiety, 96
Tamoxifen as carcinogen, 429
Tanning beds, avoiding, 118
Teething, homeopathic remedies
for, 245
Telephone numbers, emergency,
119–120
TENS, 344
Test, definition, 176
Testicular cancer:
between ages 20–40, 410
risk for developing, 374
Thallium stress test and imaging,
171–172
Therapeutic touch practitioners,
211
Thiamin, 33
Thoracentesis, 189
Thoracic surgeons, 192
Throat:
culture, 172
sore, homeopathic remedies
for, 244
Thrush in infant, 391
Thyroid panel, 172
Thyroidectomy, 259
Tincture, 83
definition, 4
of herbal remedies, 18
TMJ (temporomandibular joint
syndrome), pain of, 346
Tobacco smoke as carcinogen,
427
Toes, ten tips for, 109–111
Toluene diisocyanate as probable
carcinogen, 430
Tonsillectomy, 259
Tonsillitis:
between ages 1–12, 401
homeopathic remedies for,
245
Tooth fillings, 190

Toothache, homeopathic reme-
dies for, 246
Toxins:
detoxifying, xx–xxi
in homes, xxi
Trabeculectomy, 259
Train travel, risk factors in,
146–147
Transfusion, blood, 179–180
Travel, tips for staying healthy
and disease-free,
97–108
airplane travel, 98–99
diarrhea, 97–98
Outbreak Notices of CDC,
101
pregnant travelers, 99–100
vaccinations, 100
undeveloped regions, guidelines for, 100–108
Africa, 103–105
Asia, 107–108
Australia, 106
Caribbean, 102–103
Central America, 103
East Asia, 107
Europe, 105–106
Indian subcontinent, 108
Mexico, 103
Middle East, 108
Outbreak Notices of
CDC, 101
South America, 101–102
South Pacific, 106
Southeast Asia, 107
vaccinations, 102
Traveling, safest and riskiest ways
of, 144–149
airplane in U.S. and abroad,
145–146
bicycling in U.S., 148
boats, 147
cruise ships, 147–148
minivans in developing coun-
tries as riskiest, 144
motorcycles in United States,
145
intoxicated drivers, 149

piracy factor, 145, 147 (*see
also* Piracy)
Safety of Life at Sea
(SOLAS), 147
trains in U.S., 146–147
vehicular traffic in U.S.,
148–149
cars, 148–149
school buses, 149
trucks, large, 149
alcohol-related, 148–149
Trichloroethylene as probable
carcinogen, 430
Trivia, 435–480
animals, life-threatening,
453–457
epidemics, notorious,
439–443
health and medical trivia,
444–447
longest-living people,
466–472
medical breakthroughs,
473–479
medical research money,
where it goes, 437–438
multiple births, 458–462
poisonous plants, 448–452
weight and height averages
for children, 463–465
Trucks, large, risk factors of, 148
Tuberculin skin test, 172
Tummy tuck, 250
Tylenol, 9
Typhus, 440

U
U.S. Consumer Product Safety
Commission (CPSC),
137
U.S. Department of Health and
Human Services, 426
U.S. Public Health Service, 36
Ulcer treatment, over-the-
counter, 12–13
Ulcerative colitis, risk of develop-
ing, 374
Ulcers, pain of, 346
Ultrasound tests, 172